CURRENT THERAPY

IN NUTRITION

KHURSHEED N. JEEJEEBHOY, M.B., B.S., PhD.,
F.R.C.P.(EDIN), F.R.C.P.(C), F.R.C.P.(LOND)

Professor of Medicine
University of Toronto Faculty of Medicine
Chief
Division of Gastroenterology
Toronto General Hospital
Toronto, Ontario, Canada

1988

B.C. Decker Inc • Toronto • Philadelphia

Publisher

B.C. Decker Inc
3228 South Service Road
Burlington, Ontario   L7N 3H8

B.C. Decker Inc
320 Walnut Street
Suite 400
Philadelphia, Pennsylvania   19106

Sales and Distribution

United States
and Possessions

The C.V. Mosby Company
11830 Westline Industrial Drive
Saint Louis, Missouri   63146

Canada

The C.V. Mosby Company, Ltd.
5240 Finch Avenue East, Unit No. 1
Scarborough, Ontario   M1S 5P2

United Kingdom, Europe
and the Middle East

Blackwell Scientific Publications, Ltd.
Osney Mead, Oxford OX2 OEL, England

Australia

Harcourt Brace Jovanovich
30–52 Smidmore Street
Marrickville, N.S.W. 2204
Australia

Japan

Igaku-Shoin Ltd.
Tokyo International P.O. Box 5063
1–28–36 Hongo, Bunkyo-ku, Tokyo 113, Japan

Asia

Info-Med Ltd.
802–3 Ruttonjee House
11 Duddell Street
Central Hong Kong

South Africa

Libriger Book Distributors
Warehouse Number 8
"Die Ou Looiery"
Tannery Road
Hamilton, Bloemfontein 9300

South America
(non-stock list
representative only)

Inter-Book Marketing Services
Rua das Palmeriras, 32
Apto. 701
222–70 Rio de Janeiro
RJ, Brazil

Current Therapy in Nutrition
ISBN 0–941158–94–2

Library of Congress catalog card number: 87–72966

10 9 8 7 6 5 4 3 2 1

CONTRIBUTORS

JOAN AIRD, B.A.Sc., R.P.Dt.

Manager, Patient Food Services, McMaster University Medical Center, Chedoke-McMaster Hospitals, Hamilton, Ontario, Canada
Dietary Supplements

SHARON A. ALGER, M.D.

Fellow, Division of Clinical Nutrition, Albany Medical Center, Albany, New York
Celiac Disease

SELWYN J. BAKER, M.B., B.S., M.D.(Melb), F.R.A.C.P., F.R.C.P.C.

Professor, Department of Medicine, University of Manitoba Faculty of Medicine; Chief, Division of Gastroenterology, St. Boniface General Hospital, Winnipeg, Manitoba, Canada
Iron Deficiency Anemia
Megaloblastic Anemia

ELBRIDGE BILLS, B.Sc.

Medical Student, Emory University School of Medicine, Atlanta, Georgia
Congestive Heart Failure

GEORGE L. BLACKBURN, M.D., Ph.D.

Associate Professor of Surgery, Harvard Medical School; Chief of Nutrition, Metabolism Laboratory and Director of Nutrition Support Service, New England Deaconess Hospital, Boston, Massachusetts
The Unconscious Patient

ABBY S. BLOCH, M.S., R.D.

Director, Clinical Nutrition Support Kitchen, Memorial Sloan-Kettering Cancer Center, New York, New York
Head and Neck Cancer

MARGARET P. BOLAND, M.D., F.R.C.P.C.

Assistant Professor, Department of Pediatrics, University of Ottawa School of Medicine; Active Staff, Children's Hospital of Eastern Ontario, Ottawa, Ontario, Canada

Cystic Fibrosis

DON C. BONDY, M.D., F.R.C.P.

Professor of Medicine, University of Western Ontario Faculty of Medicine; Division Head, Division of Gastroenterology, University Hospital, London, Ontario, Canada

Gastric Surgery

GORDON P. BUZBY, M.D.

Assistant Professor of Surgery, University of Pennsylvania School of Medicine; Active Staff, Hospital of the University of Pennsylvania, Philadelphia, Pennsylvania

Preoperative Nutritional Support

KATHRYN M. CAMELON, B.A.Sc., R.P.Dt.

Registered Professional Dietitian, Toronto General Hospital, Toronto, Ontario, Canada

Common Hyperlipoproteinemias

DONALD O. CASTELL, M.D.

Professor of Medicine, Bowman Gray School of Medicine; Chief, Gastroenterology Section, North Carolina Baptist Hospitals, Winston-Salem, North Carolina

Esophageal Disease

GEORGE W. CHRISTY, M.D.

Resident in Medicine, Emory University School of Medicine, Atlanta, Georgia

Congestive Heart Failure

MERVYN DEITEL, M.D., F.R.C.S.(C), F.A.C.S., F.I.C.S.

Professor of Surgery and Professor of Nutritional Sciences, University of Toronto Faculty of Medicine; Surgeon, St. Joseph's Health Center and Staff, Hillcrest Hospital, Toronto, Ontario, Canada

Head and Neck Surgery

MARTIN EASTWOOD, M.B., M.Sc., F.R.C.P.(Edin)

Reader in Medicine, University of Edinburgh; Consultant Physician,
Gastrointestinal Unit, Western General Hospital, Edinburgh, Scotland
Colonic Disease

EBEN I. FEINSTEIN, M.D.

Clinical Associate Professor of Medicine, University of
Southern California School of Medicine; Attending Physician,
Los Angeles County-USC Medical Center,
Los Angeles, California
Chronic Renal Failure
Acute Renal Failure

ROBERT M. FILLER, M.D., F.A.C.S., F.R.C.S.(C)

Professor of Surgery, University of Toronto Faculty of Medicine;
Surgeon-in-Chief, Hospital for Sick Children, Toronto, Ontario, Canada
The Pediatric Surgical Patient

JOSEF E. FISCHER, M.D., F.A.C.S.

Christian R. Holmes Professor of Surgery and Chairman, Department of
Surgery, University of Cincinnati College of Medicine; Chief of Surgery,
University of Cincinnati Hospital–Christian R. Holmes Division,
Cincinnati, Ohio
Hepatic Encephalopathy

C. RICHARD FLEMING, M.D.

Professor of Medicine, Mayo Medical School, Rochester, Minnesota;
Consultant in Gastroenterology, Mayo Clinic, Jacksonville, Florida
Home Parenteral Nutrition

ANN T. FOLTZ, R.N., D.N.S.

Instructor, School of Nursing, Duke University Medical Center,
Durham, North Carolina
Metastatic Cancer

STEVEN M. FOWLIE, M.B., M.R.C.P.(UK)

Clinical Tutor, University of Edinburgh Faculty of Medicine; Medical Registrar, Gastrointestinal Unit, Western General Hospital, Edinburgh, Scotland
Colonic Disease

PAUL E. GARFINKEL, M.D., F.R.C.P.(C)

Professor, Department of Psychiatry, University of Toronto Faculty of Medicine; Psychiatrist-in-Chief, Toronto General Hospital, Toronto, Ontario, Canada
Anorexia Nervosa and Bulimia Nervosa

DAVID S. GOLDBLOOM, M.D., F.R.C.P.(C)

Assistant Professor, Department of Psychiatry, University of Toronto Faculty of Medicine; Staff Psychiatrist, Toronto General Hospital, Toronto, Ontario, Canada
Anorexia Nervosa and Bulimia Nervosa

RICHARD J. GRAND, M.D.

Professor of Pediatrics, Tufts University School of Medicine; Chief, Division of Pediatric Gastroenterology and Nutrition, The Floating Hospital, New England Medical Center, Boston, Massachusetts
Growth Retardation in Inflammatory Bowel Disease

MARJORIE GREEN, B.A., R.P.Dt.

Ambulatory Care Dietitian, Toronto General Hospital, Toronto, Ontario, Canada
Normal Diet and Desirable Intake

PAUL D. GREIG, M.D., F.R.C.S.(C)

Assistant Professor, Department of Surgery, University of Toronto Faculty of Medicine; Staff Surgeon, Division of General Surgery, Toronto General Hospital, Toronto, Ontario, Canada
Total Parenteral Nutrition
Hepatic Surgery

PEGGI A. GUENTER, R.N., M.S.N., C.N.S.N.

Nutrition Support Clinical Nurse Specialist, Philadelphia Veterans Administration Medical Center, Philadelphia, Pennsylvania
Home Enteral Nutrition

JOAN E. HARRISON, M.D., F.R.C.P.(C)

Professor, University of Toronto Faculty of Medicine; Director, Medical Physics Laboratory, Toronto General Hospital, Toronto, Ontario, Canada
Metabolic Bone Disease

JENNY HEATHCOTE, M.B., B.S., M.D., F.R.C.P., F.R.C.P.(C)

Associate Professor, Department of Medicine, University of Toronto Faculty of Medicine; Staff Gastroenterologist, Toronto Western Hospital, Toronto, Ontario, Canada
Acute Hepatitis

RICHARD V. HEATLEY, M.D., M.R.C.P.

Senior Lecturer in Medicine, Department of Medicine, The University of Leeds, St. James's Hospital, Leeds, England
Inflammatory Bowel Disease

STEVEN B. HEYMSFIELD, M.D.

Associate Professor of Medicine and Director of Weight Control Unit, Obesity Research Center, Columbia University College of Physicians and Surgeons, New York, New York
Congestive Heart Failure

ROBERT I. HILLIARD, M.D., F.R.C.P.(C)

Associate Professor, Department of Pediatrics, University of Toronto Faculty of Medicine; Active Staff, Division of General Pediatrics, Hospital for Sick Children, Toronto, Ontario, Canada
Failure to Thrive

LYN J. HOWARD, M.A., B.M., B.Ch.(Oxon), F.R.C.P.(UK), F.A.C.P.(USA)

Professor of Medicine, Associate Professor of Pediatrics, and Head, Division of Clinical Nutrition and Pediatric Gastroenterology, Albany Medical College of Union University, Albany, New York
Celiac Disease

JON I. ISENBERG, M.D.

Professor of Medicine and Head, Gastroenterology Division, University of California School of Medicine, San Diego, California
Peptic Ulcer Disease

ELIZABETH JACOB, M.B., B.S.(Madras), F.R.C.Path., F.R.C.P.C.

Associate Professor, Department of Medicine, University of Manitoba Faculty of Medicine, Winnipeg, Manitoba, Canada
Iron Deficiency Anemia
Megaloblastic Anemia

TOM JAKSIC, M.D., Ph.D.

Clinical Fellow in Surgery, Harvard Medical School; Nutritional Support Service, New England Deaconess Hospital, Boston, Massachusetts
The Unconscious Patient

MARK T. JAROCH, M.D.

Staff Surgeon, Akron Clinic, Akron, Ohio
Gastrointestinal Fistula

KHURSHEED N. JEEJEEBHOY, M.B., B.S., Ph.D., F.R.C.P.(Edin), F.R.C.P.(C)., F.R.C.P.(Lond)

Professor of Medicine, University of Toronto Faculty of Medicine; Chief, Division of Gastroenterology, Toronto General Hospital, Toronto, Ontario, Canada
Short Bowel Syndrome
Intestinal Pseudo-Obstruction
Jaundice
Diet Therapy Complications

ALEXANDRA L. JENKINS, B.Sc., R.P.Dt.

Research Associate, Department of Nutritional Sciences, University of Toronto Faculty of Medicine; Clinical Nutritionist, St. Michael's Hospital, Toronto, Ontario, Canada
Dietary Fiber

DAVID J. A. JENKINS, D.M., B.Ch., D.Phil.

Professor, Departments of Medicine and Nutritional Sciences, University of Toronto Faculty of Medicine; Staff Physician, Division of Endocrinology, St. Michael's Hospital and Associate Physician, Division of Gastroenterology, Toronto General Hospital, Toronto, Ontario, Canada
Dietary Fiber

SUSAN JONES, R.D.

Dietitian, Nutrition Support Team, Abington Memorial Hospital, Abington, Pennsylvania
Home Enteral Nutrition

ANNE B. KENSHOLE, M.B., B.S., F.R.C.P.(C), F.A.C.P.

Associate Professor, University of Toronto Faculty of Medicine; Medical Director, Tri-Hospital Diabetes Education Center, Toronto, Ontario, Canada
Diabetes

NICHOLAS A. LEYLAND, B.A.Sc., M.D.

Chief Resident, Department of Obstetrics and Gynecology, Toronto General Hospital, Toronto, Ontario, Canada
Nutrition in Pregnancy

ARTHUR LEZNOFF, M.D., C.M., B.Sc., M.Sc., F.R.C.P.(C)

Associate Professor, Department of Medicine, University of Toronto Faculty of Medicine; Attending Staff Physician, St. Michael's Hospital, Toronto, Ontario, Canada
Allergy and Intolerance

SUSANA MOLINA, M.D.

Staff Scientist and Head, Pediatric Program, Center for Studies of Sensory Impairment, Aging and Metabolism, Research Branch of the Guatemala National Committee for the Blind and Deaf; Attending Physician, Nutritional Rehabilitation Ward, "San Juan de Dios" General Hospital, Guatemala, Guatemala
Nutritional Assessment of the Child

KATHLEEN J. MOTIL, M.D., Ph.D.

Assistant Professor of Pediatrics, Baylor College of Medicine; United States Department of Agriculture/Agricultural Research Service, Children's Nutrition Research Center; Active Staff, Section on Nutrition and Gastroenterology, Texas Children's Hospital, Houston, Texas

Growth Retardation in Inflammatory Bowel Disease

DANIEL W. MURPHY, M.D.

Clinical Instructor of Medicine, Bowman Gray School of Medicine, Winston-Salem, North Carolina

Esophageal Disease

DANIEL W. NIXON, M.D.

Professor of Medicine, Emory University School of Medicine, Atlanta, Georgia

Metastatic Cancer

JOHN PATRICK, M.B., B.S., M.D.

Associate Professor of Biochemistry and Pediatrics, University of Ottawa School of Medicine; Active Staff, Children's Hospital of Eastern Ontario, Ottawa, Ontario, Canada

Cystic Fibrosis

KAREN PAUL, B.A., R.P.Dt.

Research Dietitian, Toronto General Hospital, Toronto, Ontario, Canada

Normal Diet and Desirable Intake

YVONNE PAYNE, B.Sc., R.D.

Nutritionist, Cardiac Clinic, Grady Memorial Hospital, Atlanta, Georgia

Congestive Heart Failure

MAX PERLMAN, M.B., F.R.C.P.(Lond), F.R.C.P.(C)

Associate Professor, Department of Pediatrics, University of Toronto Faculty of Medicine; Senior Staff Neonatologist, Division of Neonatology, Hospital for Sick Children, Toronto, Ontario, Canada

Feeding the Preterm Infant

CAROL C. PODUCH, B.Sc., R.P.Dt.

Senior Dietitian, Clinical Investigation Unit, Toronto General Hospital, Toronto, Ontario, Canada
Therapeutic Dietetics
Normal Diet and Desirable Intake

JERRY RADZIUK, M.D., Ph.D., C.M.

Associate Professor, McGill University Faculty of Medicine; Research Division Head, Division of Gastroenterology, Royal Victoria Hospital, Montreal, Quebec, Canada
Gastric Surgery

ROGER G. P. REES, B.M.Sc., M.R.C.P.

Senior Research Fellow, Department of Gastroenterology and Nutrition, Central Middlesex Hospital, London, England
Chronic Neurologic Disease

ROBERT M. A. RICHARDSON, M.D., F.R.C.P.(C)

Associate Professor, Department of Medicine, University of Toronto Faculty of Medicine; Staff Nephrologist, Toronto General Hospital, Toronto, Ontario, Canada
Hypertension

JOHN L. ROMBEAU, M.D.

Associate Professor of Surgery, University of Pennsylvania School of Medicine, Philadelphia, Pennsylvania
Home Enteral Nutrition

MOSHE SHIKE, M.D.

Assistant Professor of Medicine, Cornell University Medical College; Associate Attending Physician, Memorial Sloan-Kettering Cancer Center, New York, New York
Head and Neck Cancer

JERRY SHIME, B.A., M.D., F.R.C.S.(C)

Associate Professor, Department of Obstetrics and Gynecology, University of Toronto Faculty of Medicine; Obstetrician and Gynecologist-in-Chief, Women's College Hospital, Toronto, Ontario, Canada
Nutrition in Pregnancy

ROBIN SILVERSTEIN, B.Sc., R.P.Dt.

Consulting Dietitian and Staff Dietitian, Toronto General Hospital, Toronto, Ontario, Canada
Normal Diet and Desirable Intake

DAVID B. A. SILK, M.D., F.R.C.P.

Consultant Physician and Co-Director, Department of Gastroenterology and Nutrition, Central Middlesex Hospital, London, England
Enteral Nutrition and Products
Chronic Neurologic Disease

NOEL W. SOLOMONS, M.D.

Senior Scientist and Scientific Coordinator, Center for Studies of Sensory Impairment, Aging and Metabolism, Research Branch of the Guatemala National Committee for the Blind and Deaf; Formerly: Affiliated Investigator, Divison of Nutrition and Health, Institute of Nutrition of Central America and Panama, Guatemala, Guatemala
Nutritional Assessment of the Child

EZRA STEIGER, M.D.

Head, Section of Surgical Nutrition, Department of General Surgery, Cleveland Clinic Foundation, Cleveland, Ohio
Gastrointestinal Fistula

GEORGE STEINER, B.A., M.D., F.R.C.P.(C)

Professor of Medicine and Physiology, University of Toronto Faculty of Medicine; Director, Division of Endocrinology and Metabolism, Toronto General Hospital, Toronto, Ontario, Canada
Common Hyperlipoproteinemias

NORMAN STEINHART, B.Sc., M.D.

Fellow in Clinical Nutrition, University of Toronto, Toronto General Hospital, Toronto, Ontario, Canada
Drug-Nutrient Interactions and Drug-Induced Nutrient Deficiencies

SUSAN M. TARLO, M.B., B.S., M.R.C.P.(UK), F.R.C.P.(C)

Assistant Professor, Department of Medicine, University of Toronto Faculty of Medicine; Staff Physician, Respiratory Division, Toronto General Hospital and Gage Research Institute, Toronto, Ontario, Canada
Allergy and Intolerance

THEODORE B. VAN ITALLIE, M.D.

Professor of Medicine, Columbia University College of Physicians and Surgeons; Co-Chief, Division of Metabolism and Nutrition, St. Luke's-Roosevelt Hospital Center, New York, New York
Obesity

BRAD W. WARNER, M.D.

Resident in Surgery, Department of Surgery, University of Cincinnati Medical Center, Cincinnati, Ohio
Hepatic Encephalopathy

JAMES D. WOLOSIN, M.D.

Clinical Instructor, Division of Gastroenterology, University of California School of Medicine, San Diego, California
Peptic Ulcer Disease

STANLEY H. ZLOTKIN, M.D., Ph.D., F.R.C.P.(C)

Associate Professor, Departments of Pediatrics and Nutritional Sciences, University of Toronto and Research Institute, Hospital for Sick Children; Staff Physician, Division of Clinical Nutrition, Department of Pediatrics, Hospital for Sick Children, Toronto, Ontario, Canada
Feeding the Preterm Infant
Total Parenteral Nutrition in Pediatrics

PREFACE

Nutrition as a modality of therapy has become an established way of treating or of supplementing the treatment of many conditions. Unfortunately, most texts dealing with nutrition are either theoretical or biased towards a narrow area. Thus, anyone attempting to learn the details of nutritional therapy must undertake a tedious search for information. In addition, therapy often involves important personal and practical details, which do not find their way into published texts. In recognition of these problems, we have attempted in *Current Therapy in Nutrition* to provide the reader with a text that discusses and informs, in succinct terms, the reader about the role of nutrition in the treatment of a variety of disorders. The authors selected are experts in their chosen area, and they have presented the role of nutrition in their field of expertise as is practiced currently. Brevity and practicality have been emphasized rather than theoretical details. The latter can be followed up by the interested reader from the brief list of suggested reading.

The field of nutrition has changed from being an obscure science to a conceptual one that has permeated the entire social fabric of North America. This explosion of interest has, unfortunately, raised unreal expectations of nutritional therapy and has resulted in the use of unproven and, at times, dangerous measures. This text tries to place the role of nutrition in proper and balanced perspective and also to define those areas in which it is perhaps not the primary, or best, mode of therapy.

I would like to thank Dr. Alan Bruce-Robertson for his thoughtful comments and untiring editorial efforts. Thanks are also due to Mrs. P. Dobson, J. Chrupala, and J. Whitwell for helping with the countless problems required to make this effort possible.

Khursheed N. Jeejeebhoy
Toronto, October 9th, 1987

CONTENTS

DIETARY CONSTITUENTS, TECHNIQUES AND PRODUCTS

NUTRITION AND GASTROINTESTINAL DISEASE

Nutrition and Liver Disease

Nutrition and Surgery

Nutrition and Renal Disease

NUTRITION AND METABOLIC DISORDERS

NUTRITION AND CANCER

OTHER CONSIDERATIONS

NUTRITION AND PEDIATRICS

DIETARY CONSTITUENTS, TECHNIQUES AND PRODUCTS

THERAPEUTIC DIETETICS

CAROL C. PODUCH, B.Sc., R.P.Dt.

The therapeutic dietitian in the acute care setting attempts to bridge the gap between food as nutritional support and food as an integral component of normal daily life. Diet is the common base for all three modes of nutritional support—oral, enteral, and parenteral. Meals represent more than just a means of supplying physiologic requirements; food is a focal point of many social occasions and a primary means of family interaction. With this in mind, a review of the steps in the provision of dietetic care seems warranted for all members of the nutrition support team.

THE DIET HISTORY

Just as the physician obtains a medical history on admission, so the dietitian should obtain a detailed diet history during the first patient interview. This is the basis for further intervention and development of a "clinical feel" for the patient's ability, or lack thereof, to meet their nutritional needs via oral intake. A number of methods for determining nutrient intake have been developed over the past 40 years. These include:

1. Diet history
2. Twenty-four hour recall
3. Food frequency questionnaires
4. One month purchase record
5. Food records (3 or 7 days)

Whereas it is beyond the scope of this discussion to review the pros and cons of these methods, suffice it to say that it is impossible to obtain an absolutely accurate nutrient intake history. The practitioner must accept that there will be some inconsistencies between reported and actual intake. For most clinical applications a diet history following the Burke method described in 1947 provides sufficient data. This involves obtaining a "usual" day's intake with a cross check to ensure that major food groups are not omitted. The dietitian can then expand the scope of the history to obtain a general feel for the patient's deviations from this pattern during times of acute illness or stress. Additionally, it is useful to determine weekly food patterns, taking into account weekend alterations and restaurant meals, as well as activity patterns that affect energy consumption and utilization. Upon concluding this portion of the interview, the dietitian should have an understanding of the course of the patient's illness and the role food has played throughout this period. The ultimate goal is to determine:

1. Whether or not weight loss is consistent with caloric deficit based on expected energy expenditure for the "normal" individual.
2. The patient's capacity to meet nutritional requirements via diet. For example, a patient whose estimated needs based on Harris-Benedict calculations are 2,000 calories per day but whose maximum intake by diet history has been 600 to 800 calories per day clearly is not a candidate for oral diet as the sole means of nutritional support.
3. Whether or not dietetic manipulation maximizes oral caloric intake and allows the patient to increase a marginal intake. For example, a patient whose estimated requirements are 2,000 calories per day based on the Harris-Benedict equation, whose appetite is fair, and whose estimated intake has been 1,400 to 1,600 calories per day may be able to meet his nutritional needs by increasing caloric density. Assuming the patient enjoys eating the required foods and his physical condition allows this mode of support, a trial of diet therapy is warranted prior to more costly and invasive enteral or parenteral feeding.

BEDSIDE NUTRITIONAL ASSESSMENT

Whereas the value of biochemical assessment versus clinical judgment remains somewhat controversial, there are a number of parameters that can provide a basis for a particular treatment plan. Most parameters are merely common sense; however, if they are overlooked the dietetic plan is doomed to failure. Both the patient's ability to meet his caloric needs via diet and his current nutritional status must be considered in determining a course of action.

Considerations in formulating a treatment plan are as follows:

1. Is the patient grossly underweight (i.e., less than 80 percent of ideal body weight based on Metropolitan Life Insurance tables)?
2. Has there been a dramatic recent weight loss (i.e., loss of 10 percent or more of normal body weight within 3 months without an intentional reduction of calories)?
3. Does the patient have a potential source of nutrient loss such as malabsorption syndrome, short gut, fistulas, inflammatory bowel disease, wounds with chronic protein loss, or irradiation to the abdomen?
4. Has the patient undergone several days of starvation as the result of being kept NPO for tests?
5. Does the patient have increased metabolic needs due to burns, trauma, infection, or protracted fever?

If any of these conditions are present, the need for a reliable means of nutrition support is intensified. Whereas diet is the easiest and least expensive means of support, assessment of actual intake in the hospital setting is likely to take many days without clear-cut benefit to the patient in terms of clinical improvement. In these cases, it is preferable to "feed first and ask the dietetic questions later."

In addition to the diet history and the clinical considerations previously noted, it is useful to conduct a brief physical examination during the initial visit with a patient. Although hospital dietitians are generally unable to order biochemical tests, they can, and should be, looking for the physical signs and symptoms of malnutrition. Table 1 reviews clinical findings suggestive of malnutrition.

FORMULATING THE NUTRITIONAL CARE PLAN

Regardless of the mode of nutritional support selected, a patient at nutritional risk should be followed by a professional dietitian. Often en-

TABLE 1 Signs and Symptoms of Malnutrition

General appearance	Lethargy, inattention, apathy, irritability, disorientation, pallor, growth retardation, shrunken temporal muscles
Posture	Sagging, slumped shoulders, drawn-up knees, bending of ribs
Hair	Dry, brittle, dull and lusterless, easily plucked, abnormally distributed, depigmented
Eyes	Pale conjunctiva, dry wrinkled conjunctiva, dull, Bitot's spots, poor night vision
Lips	Cracked, dry, angular stomatitis/cheilosis
Tongue	Magenta, beefy red, impaired taste, swollen, absent papillae, smooth, white/grey coating
Gums	Red, inflamed, bleed easily
Teeth	Brown patches, loose-fitting dentures, loose or missing teeth, chipped or worn teeth
Extremities	Calf tenderness, cramps in hands and feet, low or absent knee/ankle reflex, poor muscle tone, edema, bowleg, knock knee, diminished thigh muscle
Hands/Nails	Spoon-shaped nails, brittle nails, diminished muscle mass
Abdomen	Obese, distended, hard
GI function	Change in appetite, elimination habits, and/or bowel sounds
Skin	Dry, flabby, pale, flaky, sandpaper feel, easy bruising, decubitis ulcers, depigmented spots, rash on arms and legs, petechiae, pressure sores, poor wound healing
Activity	Reduced energy and activity
Neurological status	Forgetful, loss of vibratory sense

teral feeding or peripheral parenteral nutrition is utilized in conjunction with oral diet and, in that case, the dietitian should have daily contact with the patient. Although enteral or parenteral nutrition is the sole means of nutritional support, the dietitian should periodically monitor intake, weight gain, and nutritional adequacy. If the eventual goal is to resume oral diet as the sole means of support, the dietitian will assume an integral role in the transitional feeding process.

In formulating the dietetic care plan, the practitioner must keep a number of practical considerations in mind. The dietetic plan is only as good as the patient's ability to consume the food provided. Many patients who have lost significant weight will have difficulty eating because of ill-fitting dentures, and gums, lips, and tongue may be sore due to nutrient deficiency. It may be useful to offer softer foods or, better yet, for the institution to provide a soft, yet palatable menu focusing on nutrient-dense foods. Timing and volume of meals and snacks are important: some patients prefer three large meals and appreciate the opportunity to "rest" in the interim, while other patients are overwhelmed by large portions and consequently refuse to eat. Clearly, small meals and frequent snacks are preferable for these patients. Generally speaking, energy intake is best maximized in a six-small-meal pattern when calorically dense foods are the primary focus. All the better if active family support is available and favorite foods from home are on hand for the patient.

A number of defined formula diets are available for use and in fact are heavily relied on in most institutions. Their value is that they provide a "balanced diet in a can," hence assuring dietary adequacy, and are easy to prescribe and evaluate. As long as the patient is able to consume prescribed foods routinely, the diets are worth using; however, the diets are often too heavy or sweet and may be repulsive to a slightly nauseated patient. Flavor fatigue is common, so that providing various supplements in a cyclic pattern may be helpful, although consumption of a defined formula diet may cause reduced intake at the following meal or even mild anorexia. Patients may benefit by waiting an hour or so after consuming a defined formula feeding before having a meal. Similarly, patients being supported by a combination of oral diet and parenteral or enteral feedings may benefit from a cyclic regimen. Tube feedings may be given 30 to 60 minutes prior to mealtime to allow the patient to develop the capacity for upcoming meals. Total parenteral nutrition can be given in 12- to 16-hour periods during the night, again so that appetite is stimulated for daily meals.

Finally, the dietetic practitioner must consider the feasibility of achieving energy goals via diet. For example, when a number of tests are scheduled that require holding meals or keeping the patient NPO for prolonged periods it may be beneficial to recommend a peripheral parenteral system or a cyclic enteral feeding approach until such time as diet may be relied on to provide adequate energy and nitrogen. In any event, whatever the initial plan, it is effective only with careful monitoring and follow-up care.

FOLLOWING THE NUTRITION CARE PLAN

In assessing the adequacy of a dietetic care plan it is imperative that a target calorie intake (TCI) be defined. One method is the following:

TABLE 2   Harris-Benedict Formula for Caloric Intake

Men = 66 + (13.7 W*) + 5H* − (6.8 A*)
Women = 655 + (9.6 W) + (1.8 H) − (4.7 A) + stress and activity factor

*W = weight in kilograms; H = height in centimeters; A = age in years.

However, other methods have been defined and are equally useful. The target number obtained should be viewed as an estimate of requirements. Caloric intake and weight must be routinely monitored in follow-up. If the patient is unable to achieve his TCI after a reasonable trial of dietary intervention, an alternative mode of support is indicated. All too often further ground is lost as the result of indecisiveness regarding the effectiveness of the dietetic plan. If within 7 to 10 days of close monitoring and revision of the initial care plan, the patient is unable to achieve TCI, it is time to provide intensified nutritional support via the enteral and parenteral routes.

DISCHARGE PLANNING

The very nature of nutritional support implies the need for long-term follow-up. In many instances the management of patient care is greatly affected by the patient's ability to adhere to a dietary regimen. Yet past experience with weight reducing and diabetic diets indicates that most individuals are unable to make significant lifestyle changes to achieve a permanent alteration in their food intake patterns. It has been estimated that as few as 5 percent and no more than 20 percent of patients prescribed a weight reducing diet actually lose weight and maintain the loss following conventional dietetic counseling. If this holds true for therapeutic management in cases such as postsurgical trauma and short bowel syndrome, in all likelihood the patient will require more frequent hospital admissions or more frequent visits to the physician's office due to an unsatisfactory clinical course. For this reason, careful teaching by a skilled dietetic practitioner seems indispensible.

It is unrealistic to expect patients to modify lifelong habits after a 1-hour counseling session. However, all too often diet counseling is undertaken on the day of discharge when the patient is preoccupied with all the details of leaving the hospital. It is little wonder that he or she is unable to remember, let alone adhere to, a prescribed diet. A far superior approach is to have the dietetic consult early in the hospital stay, thus allowing several visits with the patient and family. Preferable even to early consultation, however, is to have the dietitian function as an integral component of the health care team. By developing a close rapport with staff physician, nurse, and pharmacist, the dietitian will be able to tailor counseling sessions to the information imparted by the rest of the team. In this way, patients develop confidence in the advice they are given and regard dietetic information as an integral part of the treatment plan. Attendance at bedside rounds is most helpful in establishing this link in the patient's mind.

DIETETIC COUNSELING

Assuming that the dietitian has obtained baseline data (weight history, diet history, food preferences, social profile) early in admission and has had intermittent follow-up, the counseling session is merely a component of the diagnosis and treatment process during admission. It is time to bridge the gap between the foreign hospital environment where decisions are made for the patient and the home setting where the patient must function autonomously.

It must be kept in clear view that the dietetic plan is only as good as the patient's ability to adhere to it. Factors to be considered include lifestyle, family support, finances, work schedule, and individual motivation. Lifestyle considerations include whether or not the patient travels, is involved in sports activities, socializes frequently, or eats in restaurants with regularity. If so, he or she must be given guidance in making appropriate selections during these occasions. Family support is most helpful if undertaken constructively; unfortunately, all too often this can be a source of conflict or stress. If the patient lives in a family environment it is useful for the dietitian to conduct the counseling session in their presence, giving guidelines for positive reinforcement. When finances are limited, advice must be altered to provide a plan that the patient can afford, particularly when a high-calorie high-protein diet is warranted. Often the patient's work schedule will affect eating habits. Finally, advice must be given with the patient's motivation in mind. Some people require detailed instructions in order to feel comfortable that they are following their diets accurately, while others are overwhelmed by too much information. For these latter patients the dietetic practitioner must select the most critical information for hospital counseling and hope to cover more information on outpatient follow-up appointments.

One of the most critical components of good counseling is making the information "real" for the patient. A diet sheet of printed information cannot answer the day to day questions and problems that are bound to arise. A useful alternative is to give the patient a copy of the diet provided in the hospital and to follow up with mealtime visits. With the food in front of the patient, pertinent questions will often arise and the dietitian will be able to clarify the dietetic plan on the spot. Along these same lines, counseling with food models will help the patient to visualize portions and meal composition required for adherence. During counseling, the dietitian should be developing a comfortable rapport with the patient and family, thus facilitating outpatient follow-up.

OUTPATIENT FOLLOW-UP

Because dietetic modification tends to be a long-term proposition, community follow-up is essential for compliance. It is ideal if the inpatient dietitian is able to follow the patient as the closest link to the health care team who devised the treatment plan. However, this is not routine in many hospitals. Resources are available in the community such as public health nutritionists and outpatient clinics staffed by professional dietitians. In any event, the dietetic plan should be reassessed after discharge until the practitioner is certain that compliance is feasible and that the patient understands the diet. Usually this can be accomplished in two or three visits with subsequent follow-up by phone. However, if the plan is particularly complicated or the patient is having difficulty following the diet, a longer follow-up period may be indicated.

SUGGESTED READING

Block G. A review of validations of dietary assessment methods. Am J Epidemiol 1982; 115:492–505.

Glasswood RG. Nutrition assessment: a critical review. Top Clin Nutr 1986; 1(4): 16–27.

Schwartz DB. Critical care patients: what is critical knowledge for dietitians? Top Clin Nutr 1986; 1:1–7.

Snetsellar LG. Nutrition counselling skills, assessment, therapy and evaluation. Baltimore, MD: Aspen Systems Corp, 1983.

American Society for Parenteral and Enteral Nutrition. Standards of practice, nutritional support dietitian, nutrition in clinical practice, A.S.P.E.N., 1986.

NORMAL DIET AND DESIRABLE INTAKE

CAROL C. PODUCH, B.Sc., R.P.Dt.
ROBIN SILVERSTEIN, B.Sc., R.P.Dt.
KAREN PAUL, B.A., R.P.Dt.
MARJORIE GREEN, B.A., R.P.Dt.

This chapter focuses on dietary guidelines relative to risk reduction for overall morbidity and mortality from various pathologic conditions. Comments in this chapter are restricted primarily to the adult population; the special needs of the elderly and of pregnant and lactating women are not addressed. Topics discussed in terms of general recommendations for preventive medicine and dietary guidelines include coronary heart disease, hypertension, weight control, osteoporosis, and cancer. Information is also included regarding fluid requirements and the emerging topic of sport nutrition.

DIETARY CONSIDERATION IN CORONARY ARTERY DISEASE

In the chapter *Common Hyperlipoproteinemias* the diagnosis and treatment of various lipid disorders are described, and dietary and ancillary drug therapy are outlined in some detail. However, further comment is warranted in this section in reference to normal or desirable intake for the general population. Recommendations for the general population are given by the National Institutes of Health in their Consensus Development Conference Statement: "Many compelling lines of evidence link blood cholesterol to coronary heart disease. There is also good evidence from epidemiologic studies that the relationship between level of cholesterol and level of risk for coronary heart disease covers virtually the entire cholesterol distribution for the U.S. population. In fact, recent epidemiologic studies suggest that the relationship holds even at the lower end of the spectrum of cholesterol levels found in our population."

The Japanese population, in comparison with the U.S. population, has a much lower average cholesterol level and a much lower frequency of coronary heart disease. Finns, on the other hand, have a much higher average cholesterol level and a much greater risk of coronary heart disease than do U.S. citizens.

Furthermore, Japanese who have migrated to Hawaii and to San Francisco have higher cholesterol levels and a higher risk of coronary heart disease than nonmigrants. Compilation of all the available data suggests that it will be beneficial to lower the blood cholesterol of the average American.

Dietary Recommendations

Dietary recommendations include the following:

1. Men, women, and children over the age of 2 should reduce the percentage of calories from fat from 40 percent to 30 percent of total intake.
2. Calories from saturated fat should be reduced to 10 percent or less of total calories.
3. Dietary cholesterol should not exceed 250 to 300 mg daily.
4. Calories from polyunsaturated fat should be increased but should not exceed 10 percent of total calories.

This diet is consistent with recommendations from the American Heart Association and the Atherosclerosis Study Group of the Inter-Society Commission on Heart Disease Resources. Of course, other cardiovascular risk factors such as obesity, smoking, high blood pressure, and physical inactivity must be addressed.

Means of implementing dietary recommendations in the general population include the following:

1. Dietary modifications should be made for all members of the family over the age of 2.
2. Educational services should be readily available in the community as should nutrient composition data for foods.
3. Specific food items consistent with the recommended diet should be available, accessible, and affordable.
4. The food industry should accelerate efforts to develop, produce, and market leaner meats and other foods including products with reduced total fat, saturated fat, and cholesterol content.
5. Restaurants, including fast-food outlets, should make foods satisfying these diet recommendations available to their customers as should government and school food programs.

To aid in achieving the SC goals, the National Heart, Lung and Blood Institute (NHLBI) of the National Institutes of Health (NIH) launched the National Cholesterol Education Program (NCEP) in November 1985. The program focuses on professional and patient education, public education, work site programs, and school-based education.

DIETARY CONSIDERATIONS FOR THE PREVENTION OF HYPERTENSION

In recent years much attention has been given to the role of diet and nutrition in the control and prevention of hypertension. It has been estimated that between 10 and 20 percent of North American adults are hypertensive. Three major nutritional factors are relevant in terms of controlling potential hypertension: (1) weight control in the obese, (2) moderation in alcohol intake, and (3) moderation in sodium intake.

Obesity

Obesity has been clearly shown to enhance potential development of hypertension. Obese patients undertaking weight loss programs have historically had little success in achieving and maintaining their ideal body weight. However, the clinician may have greater success in controlling potential obesity in the lean patient by encouraging decreased intake of fats, alcohol, and simple sugars and encouraging regular aerobic exercise. These recommendations should be routine and information should be readily available to patients during office visits.

Alcohol

Although the exact mechanism is debatable, the role of excess alcohol consumption in the development of hypertension has received recent attention. Data derived from the epidemiological survey studies in the United States indicate that both abstainers and heavy alcohol users have an increased incidence of hypertension. Additionally, blood pressure in hypertensive alcohol-dependent patients has been shown to return to normal with abstinence. Patients at risk for hypertension should restrict intake to one drink daily (10 g of alcohol), while alcohol-dependent patients are best advised to abstain.

Sodium

Much controversy revolves around the value of universal sodium-restricted diets. Among the 10 to 20 percent of North Americans who are hypertensive there appears to be sodium-sensitive and sodium-insensitive subgroups. This leaves a large percentage of the population who are not hypertensive or who cannot be managed by salt restriction alone. It is important that the practitioner have realistic goals for sodium restriction. The average sodium intake is estimated to be between 139 and 244 mmol (3 and 6 g) per day. To control hypertension sodium intake should be in the 60 to 90 mmol (1.4 to 2.1 g) per day range, but this may be extremely difficult to achieve, given today's trends toward sodium-laden fast and convenience foods. Many food manufacturers have begun to market low-sodium products, and this trend should be encouraged as lifestyle habits are unlikely to allow for the elimination of convenience foods. Although the benefit of a universal low-sodium diet remains controversial, a high-sodium diet appears to have no benefit for normal individuals. Consequently, the safest approach appears to be the achievement of a 60 to 90 mmol sodium diet. Most patients would benefit from individualized dietary counseling by a qualified dietitian in this regard.

STRATEGIES FOR WEIGHT CONTROL

Weight control is a lifelong investment in better self-image and better health. Billions of dollars are spent by individuals to lose unwanted and unhealthy excess weight. Weight reduction diets appear with great regularity, flooding book shelves with promises of weight loss, internal cleansing, and increased energy. While there are diet programs available that promote safe healthful weight loss, many are inadequate for protein, calories, vitamins, and minerals compared to the Recommended Dietary Allowances. The result of this pursuit of weight loss is often frustration, frequent weight gains above the original weight, and more importantly a loss of a positive self-image.

For these reasons an ongoing alertness on the part of the physician who is the primary care giver to include weight control as part of individual medical care is important. Weighing the patient at every office visit will provide a basis for assessment of weight changes and will inspire confidence in the patient that the physician cares about this ever-increasing problem on an individual basis. Critical times for special attention to weight control are following pregnancy and lactation, cessation of smoking, changes in lifestyle, periods of anxiety and depression, and increase in use of alcohol. Encouragement given early enough can prevent the accumulation of excess weight.

Etiologic Factors

Eating problems, which may lead to weight gain or less frequently weight loss, include (1) skipping meals, (2) excessive between-meal snacking, (3) too-large or too-small regular food portions, (4) use of food for comfort or to relieve stress or boredom, (5) food-centered activities, and (6) lack of interest in food.

Weight Reduction Strategies

Behaviour modification techniques that have been shown to be most effective are (1) keeping records of food intake, (2) substituting alternate activities, (3) preplanning meals, (4) increasing walking and other exercise, and (5) keeping food out of sight.

Strategies for reducing energy intake include the following:

- use skim or 2 percent milk
- avoid high-fat dairy products such as cream, sour cream, ice cream, high-fat cheeses, and yogurt
- decrease intake of high-energy foods such as cakes, pastries, chocolate, nuts, and candy
- increase intake of fruits and vegetables
- decrease use of fats and oils in cooking and decrease intake of fried foods and high-fat foods such as nuts and potato chips
- use cooking methods that require less fat such as broiling, roasting, barbecuing, or steaming
- reduce intake of high-fat meats such as luncheon meats and sausage; choose instead fish, poultry, or lean meats
- increase use of whole grain breads and cereals
- limit between-meal snacks

A checklist of the intake of the four food groups will provide the physician with information for assessment of problems or deficits in the current diet. The physician should encourage inclusion of all the food groups in the diet so that future deficiencies do not occur. The patient should be encouraged to exercise on a daily basis as tolerated. How these goals can be met requires a decision on the part of the patient and the physician. When more extensive counseling is required, it is appropriate that the patient be referred to a dietitian/nutritionist or to an approved weight loss program. The loss of 10 to 20 lbs provides a more immediate goal for the patient and is more likely to be successful.

DIETARY CONSIDERATIONS IN THE PREVENTION OF OSTEOPOROSIS

The purpose of this section is to assist the health care provider in defining the patient population at risk for and planning a diet to minimize life-long risk of the development of osteoporosis in the nonosteoporotic individual. Calcium intake and requirements will be the primary focus; however, it should be clearly pointed out that osteoporosis has a multifactorial etiology. Bone loss is more common in people with the following characteristics:

1. Sex—Most cases occur in women, but men occasionally are diagnosed.
2. Age—Young women sometimes have osteoporosis but the vast majority are over 50.
3. Body Type—Osteoporosis is more common in shorter and lighter women, perhaps due to smaller bone mass.
4. Race—The condition occurs most frequently in white women, particularly those who are fair.
5. Exercise—Sedentary people have less dense bone than active people.
6. Drinking/Smoking—Excessive intake of caffeine and alcohol appear to increase risk. Smoking has also been shown to contribute to the condition.

Calcium Requirements

Calcium requirements have been the subject of extensive investigation. The current recommended daily nutrient intake (RDNI) for calcium in Canada is 350 to 400 mg in the first year of life, 500 to 900 mg from 1 to 9 years, 1,000 to 1,100 mg from 10 to 12 years, 700 to 900 mg for adolescents, 700 to 800 mg for the 25 to 49 age group, and 800 mg for those over the age of 50. However, the adequacy of these levels has been questioned. Heaney et al recommend 900 to 1,000 mg for premenopausal adult women and 1,200 to 1,500 mg for postmenopausal women. While requirements are as yet ill defined, it is clear that a poor calcium intake will result in increased parathyroid hormone and increased skeletal calcium resorption.

Nutritional Factors

In clinical practice patients at risk for the development of osteoporosis should be defined and screened for nutritional factors that may contribute to bone loss. This can be done for all age groups. Factors to consider include:

TABLE 1 Calcium Content of Selected Calcium-Rich Foods

Food	Amount	Calcium (mg)
Milk		
Whole	1 cup	288
Nonfat (skim)	1 cup	296
Cheese		
Cheddar	1-inch cube	129
Cottage	4 oz	110
Swiss	1-inch cube	139
American	1-inch cube	122
Ice cream	1 cup	194
Yogurt	1 cup	272
Oysters, raw	1 cup	226
Salmon, canned	3 oz	167
Sardines	3 oz	372
Broccoli	1 stalk	158
Collards, cooked*	1 cup	289
Mustard greens*	1 cup	193
Spinach, cooked*	1 cup	200
Turnip greens*	1 cup	252
Rhubarb*	1 cup	212
Almonds	½ cup	160
Tofu	3½ cups	128

* Oxalic acid may cause calcium to be poorly absorbed.

1. Calcium Intake — (See above recommendations for levels required.) Table 1 provides calcium contents of foods commonly consumed and may be a useful benchmark for screening. Many North American adults consume less than 600 mg Ca^{++} per day according to nutritional surveys.
2. Vitamin D — The main source of vitamin D is in the skin where it is produced in response to sunlight. It occurs naturally in fish, eggs, and chicken liver. Milk is supplemented with vitamin D.
3. Protein — Excessive amounts of protein, particularly of animal origin, may increase calcium loss.
4. Caffeine — Caffeine consumption in excess of six cups of coffee daily has been associated with increased urinary losses.
5. Alcohol — Increased alcohol intake has been associated with bone loss.
6. Fluoride — Less than 3 ppm added to the water supply has been found to be beneficial for the preservation of bone mass and bone strength. Fluoride supplements are not recommended.

Adequate calcium can be obtained from a well-balanced diet following Canada's Food Guide. There is no evidence to support the use of calcium supplements, and they are contraindicated for those at risk for hypercalcemia or hypercalciuria.

DIETARY CONSIDERATIONS FOR DECREASED RISK OF CANCER

Laboratory and epidemiologic studies indicate that dietary factors are related to cancer risk and prevention. International population migration studies show that a change in diet during adulthood can affect cancer risk. Thus, researchers are trying to establish an optimal diet to minimize cancer risk. At present, no optimal diet is known that would guarantee that cancers are not developing. The solution to this dilemma seems to be to recommend a prudent diet that will reduce total energy, fat, salt, and alcohol intake and increase intake of complex carbohydrates, fruit, and vegetables. This diet is further described in the chapter summary.

Total Energy Intake. A reduction in total energy is recommended because obesity is associated with an increase in cancers of the uterus, gallbladder, kidney, stomach, colon, and breast. However, it is difficult to determine whether the state of obesity or the consumption of a diet with increased energy density affects risk. It is also not known whether weight reduction will lower risk.

Fat. A high total fat intake seems to be the most important dietary factor increasing the risk of cancer, especially of the breast, colon, and prostate. Excessive intake of both saturated and polyunsaturated fat enhances tumor growth. Fat may affect hormone levels and together they may have a symbiotic role in the development of breast, uterine, ovarian, and prostate cancer. The role of fat in colon cancer is related to its effect on both bile acid secretion and gut flora.

Salt, Nitrite, Nitrate, and Smoke. Countries such as China and Japan that have a high consumption of salt-cured or pickled foods have an increased incidence of stomach and esophageal cancers. These cancers are also higher in parts of the world where nitrate and nitrite are prevalent in food and water (e.g., Colombia). Therefore, a reduced intake of salt- and nitrite-treated foods (e.g., cured meat) is recommended. Smoked foods such as ham contain tars that are potentially carcinogenic. Barbecuing may be dangerous when fat dripped on coals results in compounds such as benzopyrene being deposited on the food. Barbecue coals should be a few inches from the food and should not be allowed to flame up.

Alcohol. Heavy drinkers, especially those who are also cigarette smokers, are at unusually high risk for cancers of the oral cavity, larynx, and esophagus. Alcohol abuse can result in cirrhosis, which sometimes leads to liver cancer. Alcohol intake may also be a risk factor for breast cancer.

Complex Carbohydrates, Fruits, and Vegetables. Increasing intake of these foods is consistent with good nutritional practice, but research into a protective role for dietary fiber, vitamin A, carotenoids, vitamin C, and brassica vegetables (broccoli, cabbage, cauliflower) is ongoing and results are not conclusive. Scientists who do not support a protective role for fiber in colon cancer suggest that a low-fiber diet tends to be high in fat, which may play a more prominent role in elevating cancer risk. Carotenoids from vegetable sources (carrots, squash), not from animal retinol, may reduce the risk of lung cancer. There is meager support for the role of vitamin A and C in prevention. Vitamin E and minerals such as selenium, zinc, iron, and copper are also being investigated. At present, studies show that selenium may have some promise for reducing the risk of some cancers, especially breast cancer. Because of the potential hazard of selenium poisoning its medically unsupervised use as a food supplement is not recommended.

WATER—A MOST IMPORTANT NUTRIENT

Of all the required nutrients, water is the most common and it is essential for life. Perspiration, although at times a nuisance, is one way that water benefits the human body. It lowers body temperature as it evaporates on the skin, allowing heat to escape. As an essential component of all body fluids, water makes up 80 percent of our blood supply. Fluids such as blood and lymph transport oxygen and other nutrients and carry waste away. Saliva and digestive juices are needed to moisten food and make it easier to swallow, and water in the bowel promotes bowel regularity thus aiding in the prevention of constipation. It also provides a cushion for intestinal organs. This function is particularly important in pregnancy when amniotic fluid surrounding the growing fetus provides insulation and protection. In many municipalities, water provides a source of fluoride for the prevention of dental caries.

Sources

Most of our water intake (about 1,000 to 1,500 ml daily) comes directly through drinking water and other beverages. About 700 to 1,000 ml of our daily intake comes from the food we eat: fruits and vegetables, for instance, are approximately 80 percent water. For most adults the total daily intake from all sources averages 2,100 to 2,500 ml.

Daily Requirements

For adults, the general requirement is considered to be approximately 2,500 ml (or 10 cups) per day. It can be calculated as 35 ml per kilogram body weight for adults, 50 to 60 ml per kilogram for children, and 150 ml per kilogram for infants. Requirements vary with the amount of water lost by the body. Factors that influence loss are body size, physical exertion, and environmental temperature and humidity. The need for water is increased when a fever is present or if there is excessive sweating, vomiting, or diarrhea. Thirst is an example of the body's wisdom, a reminder to replace lost water. Water should be used for drinking only in areas where it has been tested and treated if necessary to ensure its safety.

SPORTS NUTRITION

As more people are becoming involved in exercise-related activities, there is an increased need for sound dietary information to replace popular misconceptions held by atheletes. The information presented below is intended to provide a background to the health professional to assist in advising the recreational and competitive athlete.

Energy

Energy needs will vary from athlete to athlete depending on age and intensity, frequency, and duration of activities. A balance of energy intake with energy expenditure will serve to maintain weight. However, when a daily intake above 21,000 kJ (35,000 kcal) is required for the serious athlete, it may be difficult to train and consume all the food necessary in one day.

Carbohydrates

A diet in which more than 45 percent of total energy comes from complex carbohydrates should be encouraged for the recreational athlete. Athletes in training for prolonged endurance events should increase their carbohydrate intake to 60 percent or more of total energy.

Carbohydrate Loading. Carbohydrate loading, also known as glycogen loading, loading, and supercompensation is advantageous only for endurance athletes exercising continuously for greater than 90 minutes. The traditional method of loading involves a 7-day plan beginning with a low-carbohydrate diet combined with aggressive training followed by an increase in dietary carbohydrate toward the day of the event with a decrease in exercise. The side effects of this method of loading are depression, lethargy, hypoglycemia, nausea, fatigue, loss of muscle tissue, and electrocardiographic changes. The preferred method of carbohydrate loading consists of a basic 350-g carbohydrate diet 7 days prior to an event with an increase to approximately 600 g carbohydrate 3 days before and until the event. Training should be maximized 7 days before an event, tapering down to complete rest the day before the event. The regimen may not be appropriate for all athletes, particularly those with diabetes or heart disease or under adolescence. It should only be attempted a few times per year and is beneficial only for endurance events. In both methods of loading, 3 g of water are stored with each gram of glycogen, which may contribute to weight gain, stiffness, cramps, and fatigue.

Protein

Athletes consuming a diet based on the recommendation that 15 percent of total energy come from protein sources will easily meet their increased needs of approximately 1 g per kilogram per day. Intakes above this may exacerbate dehydration, contribute to a high fat intake, and reduce the percentage of carbohydrate consumed. Athletes concerned about increasing muscle size should be informed that only an increased workload applied to the muscle will achieve this, not an increased protein intake.

Vitamins and Minerals

The need for vitamins and minerals can be met through the consumption of a balanced diet. Athletes consuming low-energy diets and female or amenorrheic athletes may require specific counseling by a dietitian-nutritionist as they may be consuming inadequate amounts of nutrients such as iron and calcium.

Hydration

Cold water is the recommended beverage for the majority of athletes and should be consumed prior to, during, and after exercise. Since the thirst mechanism may become blunted with exercise, a rehydration plan should be established. Electrolyte requirements can be met through the daily diet. Exceptions may occur under extreme environmental conditions and with heavy exercise as undertaken in triathalons. Triathletes should begin to increase their sodium intake approximately a week before their event by salting food. While concentrated sugar solutions should be avoided, a combination of commercial sports drinks and water may be used in extreme temperature conditions.

Ergogenic Aids

There is presently a lack of evidence supporting the various claims that certain substances enhance performance. These aids may be expensive and if they replace a balanced nutrition program may have health and performance consequences. Alcohol is not recommended for athletes and caffeine may be consumed in moderation or not at all.

Recommendations for diet and preventive medicine can be summarized for this discussion as follows:

1. High-fiber, high-complex carbohydrates— Vegetarian meals, low in cholesterol and saturated fats (e.g., without cheese and eggs) should be included in weekly menus.
2. Decreased total fat and cholesterol— Meals should be prepared with a minimum of fried foods and excess fat. Polyunsaturates should be moderately increased.
3. Adequate calcium— There is no contraindication to taking the equivalent of three 8-oz. glasses of milk daily and consequently this should be advised.
4. Weight control— Total energy (calorie) intake should be limited and physical activity encouraged.
5. Fluid intake— Adequate fluid intake is advised. In most cases thirst will define intake required.
6. Sodium— Moderate sodium intake (60 to 90 mmol per day) should aid in the control of undiagnosed hypertension.
7. Alcohol— Intake should be moderate, no more than one drink daily. Abstinence is advisable for specific patients.

SUGGESTED READING

American Dietetic Association. Nutrition for physical fitness and athletic performance for adults. JADA 1987; 87(7):933–939.

Haggerty PA, Blackburn GL. A critical evaluation of popular low calorie diets in America: part 2. Top Clin Nutr 1987; 2(2):46.

Heaney RP, Gallagher JC, Johnston CC, et al. Calcium nutrition and bone health in the elderly. Am J Clin Nutr 1982; 36:986–1013.

Hudiburgh NK. A multidisciplinary approach to weight control. JADA 1987; XX:444

Matkovic V, Kostial K, Simonivoc I, et al. Bone status and fracture rates in two regions of Yugoslavia. Am J Clin Nutr 1979; 32:540–549.

Health and Welfare Canada. Recommended nutrient intakes for Canadians, 1983.

Saunders JB, Beevers DG, Paton A. Alcohol induced hypertension. Jancet 1981; 2:653–656.

Stamler R, Stamler J, Grimm R, et al. Nutritional therapy for high blood pressure, final report of a four-year randomized controlled trial in the Hypertension Control Program. JAMA 1987; 257:1484–1491.

Symposium on nutritional aspects of exercise. Clin Sports Med 1984; 3(3).

---

* For further information on the NCEP contact the National Cholesterol Education Program, National Heart Lung and Blood Institute, National Institutes of Health, C-200, Bethesda, Maryland 20892.

DIETARY SUPPLEMENTS

JOAN AIRD, B.A.Sc., R.P.Dt.

After it has been determined that a patient is unable to ingest enough food to meet energy goals, an alternate method of nourishment must be used. If food can be digested and absorbed through the gastrointestinal (GI) tract and the use of the GI tract is not contraindicated, the first alternate method that should be tried is to supplement the oral diet with an enteral nutrition product* or modular component.†

The main advantage of using oral supplementation instead of tube feeding is the reduced chance of complications such as aspiration. In addition, using the GI tract is more efficient for nutrient utilization and preservation of the small intestinal mucosa than the parenteral route.

THE ROLE OF THE PHYSICIAN

Often the physician will be assessing the patient's need for supplementation. Here is a series of questions and answers to aid in the decision-making process.

1. Is the patient consuming enough? If not, changes in the current diet to improve intake should be tried first. See the following section for ideas.
2. If this is unsuccessful after 1 to 2 weeks and supplementation is necessary, what product should be selected? First, determine the category of product needed, i.e., blenderized diet, intact nutrients with or without lactose, defined or elemental formulas, high-energy, high-protein formulas, specialized formulas, components. Second, find out what products are available locally and are priced reasonably. Third,

---

* An enteral nutrition product can serve as a source of the major nutrients needed to support life when instilled into the gastrointestinal tract.
† A modular component contains one or two of the energy substrates carbohydrate, protein, and fat. Vitamin and mineral modules are also available.

review the factors under product selection to ensure that an appropriate product is recommended. Prior to recommending a formula, taste it.
3. How much supplementation is realistic? The majority of patients cannot drink more than three cans per day (750 ml or 24 oz).
4. What parameters should be monitored for tolerance?
5. If the patient cannot afford the product, what assistance is available? Financial assistance will vary from area to area. Contact a social worker in the local public health department, local chapters of charitable organizations, local community groups, and the local hospital for assistance.

THE ROLE OF THE DIETITIAN

In the hospital environment, the dietitian has two major additional roles in the area of dietary supplements. The first is the development of an enteral formulary for the institution. The dietitian(s) in the facility may determine the formulary independently or as a member of a multidisciplinary committee (members consisting of representatives from nursing, pharmacy, dietetics, medical staff, and administration), and jointly decide what products to stock. A standardized formulary is desirable because it is not practical or cost effective to stock all of the four dozen products currently available. The number of products in a formulary generally ranges from 2 to 30, with a median of 10. The formulary should be located on all wards for easy access by doctors and nurses and updated regularly.

The second role is as a member of the health care team responsible for the individual patient. In addition to the duties outlined in the preceding article, the dietitian must determine whether a modification in the current diet will meet the energy goal. For example, a patient may simply need to have likes and dislikes catered to. A high-energy, high-protein milkshake, Carnation Instant Breakfast, between meal snacks or favorite foods from home may be sufficient to improve the patient's intake. If not, the dietitian must:

1. Determine what category of supplement is required and, if necessary, what product within the category. Factors to consider in the selection of the category include digestive and absorptive capacity,

including lactase deficiency, major organ status, medical condition or disease state past and present, surgical interventions, medication and other therapy, the patient's cultural background, and the patient's nutritional requirements.
2. Establish realistic goals for consumption of the formula. Often the patient cannot or will not drink as much of the supplement as would be ideal. The dietitian can recommend a reasonable goal.
3. Monitor the patient's intake and tolerance of the supplement.
4. Determine if the formula needs to be changed or discontinued, or if an alternate mode (i.e., tube feeding) is needed.
5. Communicate the goals of the patient's nutrition care plan and the patient's progress to the other members of the team.

If the patient is discharged with the supplement, the dietitian should:

1. Assist the patient in finding local suppliers.
2. Direct the patient to the appropriate hospital or community resource for financial assistance.
3. Provide the patient with as many suggestions as possible for enhancing the palatability of the product on a long-term basis.

THE ROLE OF THE NURSE

The support of the hospital nursing staff is essential: they spend the most time with the patient and they are usually on the ward when the supplement is received and/or consumed. The role of the nurse is to:

1. Ensure that the canned supplement without a pull tab is opened; ensure that the supplement with the pull tab can, in fact, be opened by the patient (e.g., an arthritic may still need assistance); provide the patient with straws or a glass.
2. Store the supplement for the patient if he does not want to drink it immediately. The nurse should make the ambulatory patient aware of the location of the product and should advise the bedridden patient to ring when the supplement is desired.
3. Ensure the microbiologic safety of the formula at the ward level. Once the can is opened or the package reconstituted, the formula is perishable and should be kept on ice or refrigerated. The unconsumed por-

tion should be discarded after 24 hours.

4. Support and encourage the patient to drink the product; communicate that it is part of the overall medical therapy.
5. Ensure that the patient consumes only the prescribed formula. For example, if the formula is not on the patient's meal tray or available on the ward, then the nurse should order some from Nutrition Services rather than give the patient another product, as the nutritional composition of the substitute may not be appropriate.
6. Accurately document the patient's oral intake, including the supplement, so that accurate energy intakes can be calculated by the dietetic assistant/dietitian.
7. Document the tolerance of the feeding and any complications, such as nausea, vomiting, abdominal cramps, or diarrhea.

INDICATIONS FOR USE

A list of indications for supplementation is given in Table 1.

AVAILABLE PRODUCTS

Compared with the institutionally prepared milk-based supplements of the 1960s, the formulas available today are usually commercially prepared. They are also free from bacterial contamination, conveniently packaged (e.g., can, package, bottle, or tetrapack), with known nutritional composition and an extended shelf life (unopened, usually about 1 year). One classification scheme for enteral nutrition products is presented in Table 2. Unfortunately, there is no standard terminology for these products.

The blenderized diets are a mixture of pureed meat, vegetables, fruit, cereal, and oil and require normal digestion and absorption.

The intact nutrients with or without lactose, and the high-energy, high-protein products also require normal digestion and absorption. Protein sources include egg albumin, casein, soy protein isolate, and lact albumin. Carbohydrate sources include corn syrup, sucrose, maltodextrins, glucose, fructose, soy polysaccharides, and hydrolyzed corn starch. Corn oil, soybean oil, MCT oil, and mono- and diglycerides provide the fat.

TABLE 1 Indications for Supplementation

Decreased Oral Intake	Increased Nutritional Needs	Increased Losses
Anorexia	Burns	Malabsorption syndrome
Developmental delay affecting chewing and swallowing	Cancer	Short bowel syndrome
Distorted taste	Cystic fibrosis	Diarrhea
Inflammation	Fever, sepsis, infection	Steatorrhea
Poor appetite due to cancer, depression, respiratory disease	Postoperative healing	
Stroke	Protein-calorie malnutrition	
Vomiting	Stress, trauma	
Pain		

TABLE 2 Classification of Enteral Nutrition Products

Blenderized Diets	Intact Nutrients with Lactose	Intact Nutrients without Lactose	Defined or Elemental	High-Energy High-Protein	Specialized
Compleat	Meritine Liquid	Ensure	Flexical	Ensure HN	Hepatic
Compleat Modified	Meritine Powder	Enrich[†]	Flexical HN	Ensure Plus	Hepatic Aid
Vitaneed	Sustacal	Entrition	Pepti 2000	Ensure Plus HN	Travasorb Hepatic
	Sustagen	Fortison	Vital HN	Fortical	Renal
	Sustacal Pudding	Isocal	Vivonex	Isocal HCN	Amin Aid
		Isosource	Vivonex HN	Isotein HN	Travasorb Renal
		Osmolite	Vivonex T.E.N.	Magnacal	Stress
		Renu		Osmolite HN	Trauma Aid
		Travasorb		Sustacal HC	Other
		Travasorb MCT		Travasorb HN	Portagen
				Twocal HN	Pulmocare
					Pre-Fortison
					Fortison Low
					Sodium

* There may be compositional differences between Canadian and American products.
† Contains fiber

The defined or elemental diets can be given to patients with impaired GI function. The protein comes from crystalline amino acids, hydrolyzed whey, meat and soy, or hydrolyzed casein; the fat from soy, MCT, or safflower oil; the carbohydrate from sucrose, corn syrup, tapioca starch, cornstarch, glucose oligo- and polysaccharides, and maltodextrins.

The protein source for the specialized hepatic formulas is high in branched chain amino acid concentrations. The renal formula protein source is mainly essential amino acids.

In the past 10 years, modular components have increased in availability and usage. Products currently available are listed in Table 3.

PRODUCT SELECTION

The dietitian often recommends the category of product to use to the physician, based on the information listed earlier. The factors listed below pertain to the enteral products themselves and may be given lesser or greater importance depending on the therapeutic needs of the patient.

Palatability

Palatability is a crucial factor, but it is highly subjective and highly variable. One patient may find the taste of a bland, mildly vanilla fla-

TABLE 3 Modular Components

Carbohydrate	Caloreen
	Nutrisource
	Polycose
	Sumacal
Carbohydrate and Protein	Citrotein
Carbohydrate and Fat	Controlyte
	Duocal
Protein	Nutrisource
	Promix
	Propac
Fat	MCT oil
	Microlipid
	Nutrisource

vored product pleasant and tolerable since he has a low tolerance for sweet tastes; another patient may state that the product tastes like chalk. One patient finds the taste of a defined formula refreshing, while another will refuse to drink more than one sip. Generally speaking:

1. Formulas with fiber (i.e., blenderized diets and Enrich) are less palatable than those without fiber.
2. The more intact the protein, the more palatable the product.
3. Liquid formulas are more palatable than powdered formulas.
4. Formulas consisting of intact nutrients with or without lactose and the high-energy supplements are the most palatable.
5. The palatability of defined or elemental formulas is a major drawback for oral consumption.
6. Modular products are usually added to other solids or liquids when given orally. There still may be a taste change; e.g., the food may be a bit sweeter or dryer.

To determine what product(s) the patient likes, the patient should be allowed to participate in the selection. The dietitian should let the patient sample and choose from among the various products in the appropriate feeding category.

In some instances, the dietitian may have to organize the purchase of a product not in the formulary for a patient. If the patient has consumed a particular product for months at home or in another facility and enjoys it and refuses to drink anything else, it is appropriate to give that formula to the patient.

Aftertaste is important. Patients often refuse products because of a chalky, oily, or artificial aftertaste.

Taste fatigue can occur. Some very sweet or highly flavored formulas are palatable initially or when taken in small amounts, but if the product must be taken for a long time, a bland-tasting product may be better. When taste fatigue occurs, the dietitian should again let the patient sample alternatives. The dietitian may decide it is more advantageous to give the patient a 3-day break with no supplements at all than have to deal with a patient who refuses to drink any form of supplement.

Tips to Improve Palatability. For most patients, the key to palatability is to drink the supplement cold, i.e., directly from the refrigerator. The formula should be kept cold by putting the can or glass in an ice bath at the bedside. However, there still may be a few patients who like the feeding at room temperature. The other key is to sip the supplement, like a liqueur, which helps avoid some of the intolerance symptoms such as abdominal cramps and diarrhea.

Another major way to enhance palatability is to add flavorings. Ideas that have been successful include:

- grape juice, lemon juice, orange-pineapple flavoring added to defined or elemental formulas
- blending defined or elemental formulas with ice
- rum or rum flavoring added to an eggnog flavored supplement
- syrups such as banana or butterscotch for bland-tasting supplements
- maintaining a variety of flavors of the commonly used supplements in the formulary
- purchasing the flavor packets that are available for some products
- adding commonly available foods, such as peanut butter, jam, jelly crystals, instant coffee, fresh fruit, ice cream, or sherbet
- using the enteral nutrition products in recipes, such as in soups, puddings, muffins, and frozen pudding pops
- putting the supplement in a vacuum bottle to keep it cold

Dietitians and physicians should use the resources of the sales representatives of the enteral nutrition product companies. They have tear sheets and recipe books that other facilities have successfully used for additives.

Nutritional Composition

The physician and dietitian must be cognizant of the energy substrate sources and their quality for each supplement. This is because the substrate source will directly affect the choice of product. For example, a patient with a casein allergy would require a supplement with an egg albumin or soy protein source. A patient with impaired digestive and absorptive capacity may benefit more from a peptide protein source than from an intact protein or crystalline amino acids. Modular products allow supplementation of one nutrient in the diet and provide the freedom to alter the nutrient source. The dietitian should also know the percentage of calories or energy contributed by the substrates, as this will also affect the category selection. Knowledge of special features of each supplement is also mandatory (e.g., presence or absence of trace elements in the product).

Osmolality

Osmolality is defined as the number of osmoles of particles (solute) in a kilogram of solvent. Carbohydrate, protein, and electrolytes effect the osmolality of an enteral nutrition product. Osmolality is of lesser importance for orally supplemented patients than for tube-fed patients. However, it should remain a factor in product selection, especially for severely debilitated patients, patients with gastrointestinal problems, and patients whose guts have not been used for a while. Most of the ideas listed earlier to improve palatability also increase the osmolality of a formula.

Cost

Although cost is not a major factor for inpatients, when a patient uses a supplement at home for an extended period of time, cost can become the primary concern, as many of the supplements are very expensive. If a patient cannot afford the commercial product and if the product is not covered by a medical plan and other sources of financial assistance are unavailable, the dietitian may have to provide recipes and ideas that the patient can use at home, instead of buying the commercially available formula.

Ease of Opening the Container

If the patient cannot open the container and if the nurse is not available to perform the task, the supplement obviously cannot be consumed. Pull tabs have been a major step forward; however, there are still many patients who are not strong enough or lack the manual dexterity to use them. The tetrapack supplements with attached straw are an innovative approach. Again, some patients may not be able to use this method. One advantage of the pull tab and tetrapack is that they are convenient for children who need long-term supplementation to take to school.

Ease of Preparation

The easier the formula is to prepare, the better, as there will be less chance of error. There are still a number of powdered products on the market with ambiguous mixing instructions. To promote accuracy, the dietitian should develop recipes for commonly used volumes of the product.

Viscosity

This is another subjective factor. The high-energy, high-protein supplements are thicker and more viscous. These are preferred by some patients and strongly disliked by others. If the hospital formulary or local pharmacy stocks only these products, diluting the supplement will reduce the viscosity.

Odor

Although this is another subjective factor, the distinctive odor of the crystalline amino acids in the defined or elemental formulas may cause the patient to refuse the product. One way to overcome this is to serve these formulas in a covered styrofoam cup with a straw.

PATIENT MONITORING

The patient must be monitored to ascertain that:

1. The energy goal is being met.
2. The patient is tolerating the feeding.
3. The metabolic and nutritional parameters (e.g., electrolytes, intake/output, serum albumin) are within the acceptable clinical range for the patient.

It is imperative that the dietitian carry out a 3 to 7 day energy intake assessment. Regularly reviewing, interpreting, and acting on the available clinical information is also essential. The dietitian should discuss tolerance of the formula with the patient frequently. If the patient is not achieving his energy goal by the end of 1 week, further intervention should be discussed with the physician and patient such as supplemental or total tube feeding.

COMPLICATIONS

These are uncommon since most patients can tolerate enteral nutrition products orally, as long as they are consumed slowly and adequate fluids are ingested. The main complications include nausea, vomiting, diarrhea, and psychologic distress. Gulping a formula may cause increased gastric emptying resulting in nausea and/or vomiting. This can be averted by drinking the formula slowly. Diarrhea, often stated to be caused by a high osmotic load from the supplement, may in fact be a result of other causative factors, including enteric infection, such as *Clostridium difficile* infection, bacterial contamination of the formula, decreased serum albumin, medications, and lactose intolerance, and should be investigated. If the osmotic load is causing problems, it should first be verified that the patient is drinking the formula slowly. After that, changing to a lower osmolality supplement may help. Psychologic manifestations may include confusion and depression. If a dietitian has not visited with the patient, he/she can be confused when the meal tray arrives with an additional item on it. The key is to involve the patient from the start, explaining everything to him/her. If the patient sees no progress, depression may result. One solution is to show the patient his/her weight and/or energy intake progress.

SPECIFIC DISEASE STATES

A discussion of some specific conditions and special circumstances follows.

Burns

Nutritional supplementation in the burn patient requires a high degree of individualization. The need for supplementation is based on the following considerations:

Preburn Considerations
- the patient's usual eating habits and nutritional status
- cause of injury

Postburn Considerations
- severity and location of burn(s)

- inhalation injury
- implications of surgery
- patient positioning post grafting
- gastrointestinal complications
- pain management
- psychological status

These factors can affect the patient's ability to eat, chew, or swallow, frequency of eating, appetite, food preferences, digestion, and gastric motility. If the patient is unable to meet the energy goal because of these or related problems, nutritional supplementation is indicated. The most satisfactory approach is one that combines hospital-prepared supplements (e.g., high-energy, high-protein milkshakes or desserts) and commercial products.

Cancer

The nutritional status of the cancer patient is affected by the type of cancer treatment—surgery, radiation and/or chemotherapy, and the area of the body affected. The consequent problems, such as nausea, vomiting, stomatitis, dry mouth, taste abnormalities, diarrhea, lactose intolerance, and pain, must be considered when recommending liquid supplements. The degree of weight loss, proposed treatment, and prognosis determine how supplements are to be used. Two ways of using supplements in the nutrition care plan are:

1. Oral food intake is considered the primary source of nutrients, and supplements are used as a snack to ensure adequate nutritional intake. They may be used daily or when the patient assesses his usual intake as inadequate.
2. Supplements are considered the primary source of nutrients, supplying 1,500 to 2,000 kcal with oral food as a secondary source.

Patients with nausea, severe stomatitis, or excess saliva may prefer a high-protein clear supplement or glucose polymer added to cool, clear liquids.

Diabetes

The choice of dietary supplement for the diabetic who is catabolic or unable to tolerate his/her usual diet will depend on several factors, such as palatability, residue content, and nutrient source. Carbohydrate constitutes the largest percentage of energy (45 to 92 percent) in most formulas, and the source varies from sucrose to glucose oligosaccharides. A large proportion of simple sugars will increase the likelihood of osmotic-induced diarrhea and poor glycemic control. Fat will help to delay gastric emptying and lower glucose fluctuations. Many patients will continue to be managed on subcutaneous injections of insulin. The dietitian's role will involve designing a feeding schedule to approximate the patient's usual diet. The amount of carbohydrate should be kept as consistent as possible.

Gastrointestinal Problems

The choice of supplements for GI patients is determined by the presence or absence of lactose intolerance, the need for increased specific macro- or micronutrient intake, the protein source, and ultimately, the acceptance and tolerance of the commercial products available. In liver disease, the use of modular supplements appears attractive when, in the presence of precarious nutritional status, the protein and sodium content of the diet has to be controlled while maximum energy should be provided to the patient. However, practical experience has shown that these supplements are often poorly accepted due to their unpalatability. Furthermore, these supplements do not contribute a significant amount of extra energy, as these patients frequently exhibit poor appetite, which impairs their ability to ingest an adequate amount of food, including supplements.

Acute Renal Failure

If minimal protein of high biologic value and high energy is desired, a specialized formula such as Amin-Aid should be considered. If a high-protein product and a limited volume of food are desired, a high-energy, high-protein formula, such as Isotein HN, Magnacal, or Ensure Plus should be considered. Examples of lower-protein products that may be appropriate are Isocal, Osmolite, or Ensure. These products contain variable amounts of minerals but not excessive amounts of sodium, potassium, and phosphate. Additional energy can be supplied by fat or carbohydrate in modular components.

Chronic Renal Failure

Predialysis. Individuals in this category are generally on protein-controlled, high-energy regimens. Control of sodium and phosphorus, variable control of potassium, and freedom in fluid intake is the usual therapeutic nutritional procedure. If minimal protein of high biologic value and high energy is desired, a product such as Amin-Aid is appropriate as a supplement. Examples of other appropriate supplements are Ensure and Citrotein.

Hemodialysis. Individuals on this therapy generally require less rigid control of protein but greater control of all electrolytes, particularly sodium, potassium, and phosphorus, and fluid restriction. Appropriate supplements include Ensure or Ensure Plus, Isotein HN, or Magnacal.

Intermittent or Cyclic Peritoneal Dialysis. This therapy requires adequate protein to replenish losses through the peritoneum but strict control of sodium, potassium, phosphorus, and usually fluids. The degree of control will depend upon residual renal function and the frequency of dialysis. Examples of appropriate supplements are Ensure Plus, Isotein HN, or Magnacal.

Continuous Ambulatory Peritoneal Dialysis (CAPD). Individuals on this therapy require adequate protein to replenish daily losses through the peritoneum. At the same time, peritoneal absorption of dextrose from the dialysate provides significant energy from simple carbohydrates. Daily dialysis permits a more liberal intake of sodium, potassium, phosphorus, and fluids. Meritine, Ensure Plus, Isotein HN, and Magnacal are appropriate supplements. Additional protein supplements to consider are the protein modules such as Propac and Promix. Energy supplementation can also be provided by the fat or carbohydrate modular components.

Respiratory Disease

Individuals with respiratory disease often suffer from weight loss. This can, in whole or in part, be attributed to the lack of available oxygen necessary for the metabolism of food and/or fatigue resulting from the increased work of breathing, which leaves the patient too tired and too disinterested to eat. Such an individual who is physically able to eat but unable to eat enough can benefit from oral supplementation. Careful dietary management should concentrate on weight maintenance or restoration and the reduction of nutritional risk to which these patients are exposed. In a situation where the patient is volume restricted either by decreased capacity or by necessity (i.e., fluid restriction), more energy-dense supplements such as Ensure Plus or Magnacal would be appropriate.

Fluid-restricted patients can also be supplemented by a semisolid product, such as Sustacal Pudding. Respiratory-distressed patients sometimes report that milkshake type formulas, such as Ensure, Meritine, and Sustacal, cause increased production of mucus. While this is a subjective conclusion, it must be taken into account when providing a product that will be consumed. Citrotein or products with a thinner consistency should also be offered. The investigations concerning the provision of low-carbohydrate, high-fat enteral nutrition products to respiratory patients presently are concerned only with mechanically ventilated patients on total tube feeds. The recommendations have not yet been extended to the orally supplemented respiratory patient.

Children

Oral nutritional supplements are not normally used for infants under 1 year of age due to the increased osmotic and renal solute loads. With children, the nutritional goal is to provide adequate energy and protein for catch-up growth. The physician or dietitian should appeal to the child's desire to grow. Supplements that look, taste, and feel similar to something they are currently familiar with are often more readily acceptable. For example, the tetrapack is very popular as children are familiar with fruit drinks in this form.

SUGGESTED READING

Gordon AM. Enteral nutritional support. Postgrad Med 1982; 72:72–82.

Nutrition Support Services Survey, 1986. Clinical product, procedures, and practices. Nutr Supp Serv 1986; 10:9–11.

Weinmann-Winkler S, Dudrick S. Enteral nutrition history—past, present, future. Nut Supp Serv 1986; 6:7–8.

DIETARY FIBER

DAVID J. A. JENKINS, D.M., B.Ch., D. Phil.
ALEXANDRA L. JENKINS, B.Sc., R.P.Dt.

The dietary fiber hypothesis as we know it today was developed over the last 20 years by Denis Burkitt and Hugh Trowell after a lifetime of medical work in Uganda. They noticed very different patterns of non-infectious disease and related them to the dietary habits of the Ugandans. The most visible effect of this dietary difference was the large fecal output produced. Thus the recorded differences in disease patterns became linked to the nondigestible part of the diet, evidenced by larger fecal outputs. In this way, emphasis was placed on the nonabsorbable fraction of the diet and its relation to gut function and disease. The hypothesis of Burkitt and Trowell owed much to Surgeon Captain Cleave of the British Navy and Alec Walker and D. G. Campbell in South Africa, all of whom considered that the refining of carbohydrate foods diminished their nutritive value. The original hypothesis suggested a role for fiber in the maintenance of good health and the prevention or treatment of a wide range of disorders and diseases including constipation, diverticular disease, colon cancer, gallstones, obesity, coronary heart disease, and diabetes. Since that time, research has been undertaken and considerable confirmatory evidence has been adduced to support a role for fiber in maintaining health and ameliorating the effects of many diseases. As a result, official bodies such as Health and Welfare Canada have endorsed the advice to increase consumption of fiber-rich foods, both by the general public and by those suffering from constipation, diverticular disease, and diabetes. A role for fiber is also seen in the treatment of hyperlipidemia.

Definition

Dietary fiber can be defined as plant polysaccharides and lignin, which are resistant to hydrolysis by human digestive juices. A variable proportion of this material is fermentable by the colonic bacteria, and as with herbivorous animals, the resulting short-chain fatty acids may be absorbed for use by the tissues of the body.

All unprocessed plant materials (and to some extent most processed materials) contain dietary fiber, which comprises the cell wall materials, the nonstarch storage polysaccharides, and the gums and mucilages that coat the outside of plants for repair purposes or as a further protective coat in the case of aquatic plants.

Classification. Originally, the only fiber estimation used was "crude fiber," which is still the figure given in the majority of food tables. It refers largely to cellulose and lignin and was developed to describe forage for ruminant animals. Dietary fiber is a much more inclusive term that is applied to human nutrition. The figure for crude fiber does not bear a constant relationship to dietary fiber: the dietary fiber figure may be three- to tenfold more than the crude fiber figure depending on the food source.

The first extensive dietary fiber figures were found in the tables of McCance and Lawrence under the heading Unavailable Carbohydrate. The current tables of McCance and Widdowson (revised by Paul and Southgate) remain the most extensive.

Perhaps the most useful classification of dietary fiber is as soluble and insoluble fractions. Most foods contain both in varying proportions, but purified (e.g., pectin or guar) or partially purified (e.g., wheat bran) preparations are produced to serve specific functions (e.g., as bulk additives to cereal products, as thickeners in jams, ice cream, and salad dressings, or as therapeutic agents).

Soluble Fibers. The water soluble forms of dietary fiber (Table 1) include the gums, mucilages, and pectic substances that increase the viscosity of solutions and are found in fruit (pectin), legumes, and beta glucan-containing cereals such as barley and oats. These forms of fiber may exert metabolic effects, including reducing postprandial blood glucose and insulin, reducing serum lipids, notably low-density lipoprotein (LDL) cholesterol, and in general, being readily fermented in the colon with the generation of short-chain fatty acids (SCFA), which are themselves absorbed. In the process of absorption, the SCFA may enhance colonic divalent cation absorption (e.g., Ca^{++}, Mg^{++}, Zn^{++} and vitamin K uptake). At the same time, the reduction in pH may regulate the growth of colonic microflora (especially *Salmonella*), reduce the solubility of bile acids, and especially in the case of butyrate, provide a source of metabolizable energy for the enterocytes lining the colon. Because of the completeness of fermentation of most soluble fibers, they have little or no effect on fecal weight. Indeed in the case of pectin, this soluble fiber has been used as an antidiarrheal agent.

TABLE 1 Purified Soluble Fibers and Foods High in Soluble Fiber

Soluble Fiber	
Foods	*Purified Supplements*
Oats	Pectin
Barley	Guar
Dried beans	Locust bean gum
Dried peas	Konjac mannan
Dried lentils	Xanthan gum
Okra	Tragacanth
Persimmons	

Insoluble Fibers.   These fibers (Table 2) include those in which cellulose is a major component and in which various fiber types are combined with lignin. Important sources in the human diet include whole grain or whole meal wheat, rye, and rice products. In the milled form (as in whole meal bread) they enhance motility in the upper gastrointestinal tract, increasing the rate of gastric emptying and small intestinal transit. Their effect on macronutrient absorption is small in comparison with the soluble fibers, although they tend to hold water in the lumen of the bowel. Possibly due to the phytic acid often associated with these fibers, their effect in reducing divalent cation (mineral and trace element) absorption is of greater importance. In the colon they continue to retain water and salts in the lumen of the bowel, and because they are relatively resistant to colonic fermentation, carry their water and minerals with them and so increase stool bulk. Use of large amounts of insoluble fiber, as in the Iranian diet (rich in unleavened high-phytate whole meal flat breads), has been associated with Zn^{++} deficiency. Negative Ca^{++} and Fe^{++} balances are well documented on high-cereal fiber diets. It must be emphasized that the levels of fiber intake have been high and the diets restricted. In addition, had soluble sources of fiber been used at the same time, the interaction might have made more minerals available for colonic absorption. Nevertheless, this does sound a cautionary note for the use of insoluble fibers in those (such as the elderly) whose mineral status may already be precarious.

TABLE 2 Semi Purified (and Purified) Insoluble Fibers and Foods High in Insoluble Fiber

Insoluble Fiber	
Foods	*Supplements*
Whole meal or whole grain:	Bran:
Wheat bread	Wheat
Rye bread	Rye
Pumpernickel bread	Rice
Brown rice	(Cellulose)
Brown pasta	(Lignin)
Wheat breakfast cereals	

SPECIFIC FIBER USES

The original hypothesis suggested that the disorders noted in Table 3 were associated with a deficiency of dietary fiber. This hypothesis has had a major impact on the advice given to the general public and on the treatment of constipation, diverticular disease, and diabetes. In addition, the advice was aimed at the prevention of cardiovascular disease and diet-related cancers. It has been suggested that fiber has a role in the treatment of irritable bowel syndrome and Crohn's disease and that patients with dumping syndrome and renal and hepatic disease may benefit from fiber supplements or high-fiber diets. Conditions in which fiber may have a role in dietary management are listed in Table 4.

TABLE 3 Some Disorders Originally Believed To Be Related to Fiber Deficiency

Constipation	Coronary artery disease	Hiatus hernia
Appendicitis	Diabetes mellitus	Varicose veins
Hemorrhoids	Obesity	Deep vein thrombosis
Colon cancer	Diverticular disease	Gallstones

TABLE 4 Disorders in Which Fiber May Have a Role in Dietary Management or Prevention

Constipation	Diabetes	(Peptic ulcer disease)
Irritable bowel syndrome	Hyperlipidemia	(Gallstones)
Diverticular disease	(Obesity)	(Dumping syndrome)
(Crohn's disease)*	(Azotemia)	(Hepatic encephalopathy)
(Colon cancer)		

* The relation between dietary fiber and the disorders in parentheses is hypothetical and requires confirmation.

Healthy Individuals

There are two reasons why the healthy individual may benefit from increased dietary fiber. First, there is a recommendation that the general population should take at least half their dietary calories from carbohydrate sources, and the higher fiber starchy foods are nutritionally sound foods. Second, specific fibers may have physiologically useful attributes in the maintenance of health and the prevention or treatment of certain diseases as already outlined.

To increase fiber intake, the general population is advised to consume at least half its caloric intake as carbohydrate, preferably as starchy foods with associated fiber. Fat should make up less than 30 percent of calories with a polyunsaturated/saturated ratio of 1:0 with protein intake held at approximately 15 percent. An attempt should be made to select carbohydrate foods from among the legumes, unrefined cereals (including wheat, barley, oats, rye, and corn), and root vegetables whenever possible and to include substantial amounts of low-calorie vegetables (e.g., broccoli, cauliflower, zucchini) and leafy green vegetables. These general guidelines can be modified to suit individual tastes and needs.

Constipation

When organic causes have been eliminated, an increase in fiber in the diet often ameliorates this condition. The most effective fiber appears to be wheat bran due to its high pentosan content. Particle size appears to be important, with the coarser wheat brans being most effective (diameter greater than 0.5 mm). This particle size is found in most whole meal breads and many breakfast cereals containing wheat bran. Of these cereals, All-Bran has one of the highest wheat fiber contents. In general a 1 g increase in wheat fiber intake results in a 3 to 4 g increase in fecal output. Thus for every 1 g of All-Bran eaten (over 30 percent fiber), there is an increase of 1 g in fecal weight. Some individuals do not tolerate wheat fiber well. Among the problems noted is pruritus ani, presumably due to the abrasive nature of the bran particles. Use of fiber of the type found in leafy vegetables such as cabbage or dried legumes may be beneficial for these patients since the increase in fecal bulk it induces may in part be due to the accompanying increased bacterial mass of the feces. For still others, a high-fiber diet may be insufficient of itself, and a bulk laxative such as Metamucil (psyllium husk) may be most effective or best tolerated.

Rather than adding only the most effective fiber sources to the diet, the ideal way to increase fecal bulk is to improve the diet in general. As is true for the general population, fat calories should be reduced and carbohydrate calories increased. In general, use should be made of whole grain cereals—not only wheat, but also oats and barley, which contain soluble fiber. Also, what may be new starchy foods, such as legumes, should be introduced into the diet and a substantial intake of green leafy vegetables should be consumed daily. Perhaps the key benefit of this prescription, aside from a general dietary improvement is that the risk of negative mineral balance, which can occur with wheat fiber as the single fiber source, is less likely. As mentioned, this is of importance to elderly patients.

Irritable Bowel Syndrome

There is little consistent evidence that high-fiber diets play an important role in the management of irritable bowel syndrome. Nevertheless, many experienced clinicians support its use. In the absence of other clear indications for therapeutic intervention, high-fiber diets of the sort suggested for the treatment of constipation may prove useful. Due to the discomfort sustained while the gut adapts to a higher fiber intake and the fluctuating nature of the syndrome, it is advised that a long-term trial of 3 months or more be undertaken before discarding this approach.

Diverticular Disease

There is now considerable support for the use of high-fiber diets in the treatment of diverticulosis, where previously low-fiber diets were recommended. It has been claimed that bran reduces the motility indices and intestinal pressures generated within the colon and the recurrence of diverticulosis after sigmoid myotomy, but there have been few double-blind randomized crossover studies. Notably, one study fulfilling relatively strict criteria of control failed to detect any symptomatic improvement in patients with diverticular disease taking fiber. However, the patients in the study had very mild symptoms, and even the increased flatulence on taking fiber may have confused interpretation of the symptom score. In addition, the increase in fiber intake was very small. For the present, therefore, there seems to be no good reason for eliminating fiber from the diets of patients with diverticulosis. On the other hand, the volume of positive reports suggests again that the opportunity should be taken to place the patient on the nutritionally sound, mixed-fiber diet recommended for the treatment of constipation.

Crohn's Disease

Although it is not disputed that in the acute phase bowel rest appears to be the treatment of choice, the long-term dietary management options are less clear. Prompted by studies suggesting that the preillness diet in Crohn's disease was low in fiber, a trial of a high-fiber, low-sucrose diet was undertaken with apparently beneficial effects. Over a 5-year period the disease was under better control and the need for surgical intervention was reduced to one-quarter of the historical controls. Perhaps of greatest interest, increased fiber was given regardless of strictures and no episodes of obstruction were reported. These studies, although not confirmed, suggest that the use of cereal fiber in the diets of patients with Crohn's disease is not contraindicated. Nevertheless, care should be taken with leafy vegetables such as cabbage, which appear to pose more of a problem in causing obstruction in the gut.

Colonic Polyps and Cancer

Studies are under way to determine the influence of high-fiber diets on polyp recurrence in individuals who have undergone polypectomy, although fiber is only one contender for a protective effect. The epidemiologic association of colon cancer with fat and meat consumption is far stronger, and hence reduction of intake would be predicted to have a more marked effect. Other hypotheses include a protective effect for calcium. At present, however, all recommendations offered are subject to further testing.

Gallstones

It has been claimed that the use of wheat bran may decrease the lithogenecity of the bile by increasing the chenodeoxycholic acid content of the bile acid pool and reducing the proportion of lithocholic acid. This observation has not been tested in an intervention trial.

Diabetes

This is an area in which there has been considerable research activity with both purified fiber supplements and high-fiber diets. The use of high-fiber diets has had the support of the major diabetes associations and has ushered in an era of high-carbohydrate diets. The current recommended macronutrient profile is shown in Table 5. The emphasis has been on saturated fat reduction with the caution that protein intake should be held at or near the minimum daily requirement. This is the background diet against which the fiber level should be measured. The soluble types of fiber have been recommended.

Soluble fiber supplements such as guar and pectin have been used with success, but commercial preparations are not universally available and it is likely that formulations will have to be modified to achieve the same level of efficacy demonstrated in the early trials. In addition, it is unlikely that maximum effectiveness will ever be achieved with viscous supplements unless they are in a form in which they can be properly mixed with the food to allow a delay in luminal diffusion from the bulk phase to the enterocyte.

High-fiber diets composed of regular foods have been strongly endorsed and are being generally prescribed. The simple view is that soluble fiber in commonly used foods will produce the same spectrum

TABLE 5 Macronutrient Profile of the Diabetic Diet

Recommended Daily Intakes (ADA 1986)	
Carbohydrate	55–60% calories
Protein	0.8 g/kg body weight
Fat	<30% calories
Polyunsaturated	6–8% calories
Saturated	<10% calories
Cholesterol	<300 mg/day
Sodium (elemental)	<3 g/day

of activity seen with the purified fiber supplements when incorporated into foods. While this does not appear to be entirely correct, certain types of high-fiber foods do nevertheless appear to have beneficial effects on diabetic control. However, it appears that many other fiber-associated factors (Table 6), in addition to fiber itself, confer these characteristics on the foods. Thus, foods with high amylose content, large particle size, or high phytate or lectin content, irrespective of fiber content, may lower postprandial blood glucose levels. An attempt has therefore been made to classify foods according to their postprandial glycemic effect. The glycemic index for each food is expressed as a percentage of the glycemic response to an equal amount of carbohydrate given as white bread (Table 7). Also included in Table 7 are the foods high in soluble fiber. For obvious reasons the diet for diabetics, as for any other patient group must be individualized and thus foods can be selected from Table 7 according to the patient's own tastes. The diet should conform to the overall nutrient profile outlined in Table 5. A good starting point is the high-fiber diet as recommended for healthy individuals in the general population. As potentially useful foods are introduced into the diet, these can be monitored by the patient using home glucose monitoring. The physician should also be aware that patients taking insulin may need to adjust insulin dosage as blood glucose control improves.

Hyperlipidemia

Purified Supplements. Viscous fibers (guar, pectin, locust bean gum, and konjac mannan) have all been used successfully to reduce low-density lipoprotein (LDL) cholesterol. When this has been used in a starchy food formulation (crisp bread/melba toast or spaghetti), the LDL

TABLE 6 Food Factors Associated with Modifying the Glycemic Response of Starchy Foods

Cooking	Antinutrients:
Particle size	Phytates
Degree of hydration	Lectins
Amylase content	Saponins
Amylopectin content	Tannins
Dietary fiber	Amylase inhibitors

TABLE 7   Glycemic Index (GI) Ranking of Some Common Starchy Foods as Higher (Class I), Intermediate (Class II), and Lower (Class III) Groups

Class I (GI > 90)	Class II (GI 70–89)	Class III (GI < 69)
Most breads	All-Bran	Pumpernickel bread
Plain crackers	Oatmeal	Most pasta
Most breakfast	Most cookies	Parboiled rice
cereals	(biscuits)	Most legumes (dried)
Most potatoes	Rice	Nuts
Millet	Buckwheat	Barley
Corn chips	Sweet corn	Bulgur (cracked wheat)
	Boiled new	
	potatoes	
	Yams	
	Sweet potatoes	

cholesterol reduction was also associated with falls in very low-density lipoprotein (VLDL) triglyceride. The nonfood formulations are commercial agglomerates of these fibers in the form of coarse grain powders, which do not hydrate as rapidly as the native materials in powder form. The native materials are not palatable but may be incorporated into fruit juices to form jellies, added to soups or dairy products (milk or yogurt) or baked into breads. A total intake of 15 to 20 g daily is usually required for an effect on serum lipids; the effect, if present, is usually readily discernible within 1 to 2 weeks. The success of this approach is both individual and formulation specific. It is necessary to maintain strict caloric control, since if the formulation contains calories, there is a temptation to take the supplement in addition to the regular diet. When taken with fat, the formulation negates the lipid-lowering effect, possibly by preventing hydration of the fiber. Use-limiting side effects such as flatulence and abdominal distension tend to subside with time.

High-Fiber Diets.   As with the diabetic diet, the diet for the hyperlipidemic patient should conform to guidelines laid down for the treatment of individual hyperlipidemias. High-fiber diets have shown promise in the control of both LDL cholesterol and VLDL triglyceride. The triglyceride-lowering effect of these diets is a much more constant finding than that seen with purified supplements. The dietary additions and modifications again include the high-fiber dietary changes advocated for the general population. Certain foods such as dried legumes (beans, peas, and lentils) and concentrated sources of viscous fiber such as oat bran seem to be particularly useful in reducing serum cholesterol. Thus a cup of oat bran for breakfast and 1 to 2 cups of dried legumes during the rest of the day may reduce serum cholesterol by 10 to 20 percent or more. Serum triglyceride may be reduced by such a maneuver. The same fiber prescription advocated for diabetics is useful in the management of hypertriglyceridemia.

Dumping Syndrome

Although relatively uncommon nowadays with the extensive use of H_2 receptor blockade and the reduced dependency on gastric surgery for peptic ulcer disease, there are still a number of intractable cases of dumping syndrome. For these, a viscous fiber source such as pectin may prove useful at a dose of 5 g once or twice daily (with major meals). This can be taken with water at the start of the meal. It tends to reduce the hypovolemic phase by impeding the effect of osmotically active small intestinal contents, and in so doing, results in a more sustained rate of absorption. In addition, pectin results in less gastrointestinal hurry, a lower insulin response, and less of a lag phase to the blood glucose response. For the maximum effect, the patient should take more frequent small meals with the major fluid intake between meals.

Peptic Ulcer Disease

Epidemiologic evidence from India suggested that peptic ulcer disease was less common in individuals who ate a high cereal fiber diet than in those who ate white rice. Later clinical trials carried out in Norway demonstrated that duodenal ulcer recurrence was significantly lower in patients on a high-fiber diet. The prescription included a high wheat fiber bread eaten in exchange for other breads and a breakfast cereal of either a high wheat fiber porridge or one made of wheat barley, rye, and oats, all containing unprocessed fiber. Studies have also shown that such diets may have a role together with drug therapy in the initial treatment of peptic ulcers, but the results have not been as clear cut.

Renal Disease

Studies have indicated that blood urea levels could be reduced in uremic patients by 15 to 20 percent when given 20 g arabinogalactan or 7 g ispaghula daily. Decreased urinary urea is also observed in healthy volunteers consuming high-fiber diets. This presumably relates to the break in the enterohepatic nitrogen cycle in which urea diffuses into the colon, is split to NH_3 and is reabsorbed to be used by the liver either for reamination of the carbon skeleton of amino acids or for urea synthesis once more. The presence of carbohydrate as an energy substitute in the colon allows the bacteria to fix the NH_3 nitrogen for bacterial proteins, which are then eliminated in the stool, providing an alternative route for the loss of urea N_2. This appears the likely explanation for the lower urea levels, since there is no comparable percentage increase in protein loss as seen from the small intestine of ileostomates on higher-fiber diets.

Studies in the area of fiber and renal disease are only beginning, and no clear guidelines can be given at present. Caution must be taken to monitor electrolytes since many fiber sources may also be rich in K^+ and patients may run the risk of developing hyperkalemia.

Liver Disease

Increasing fiber intake seems appropriate for patients with liver disease for two reasons: First, the studies showing the beneficial effects of vegetable protein in the treatment of patients prone to hepatic encephalopathy focused attention on fiber as a possible beneficial attribute of foods containing vegetable protein. It was reasoned that, as in renal disease, the trapping and elimination of NH_3 results from increased carbohydrate entering the colon and providing a substitute for bacterial fermentation and cell synthesis. Use of the synthetic liquid "fiber" lactulose is already standard clinical practice. Second, carbohydrate intolerance is common in patients with cirrhosis, including frank diabetes. For this reason diets recommended for diabetic patients seem appropriate in hepatic disease. Actual fiber trials in this area remain to be reported.

Blood Pressure

There is evidence that high-fiber diets of the sort advocated for the general public may lower blood pressure. The mechanism is at present unclear and the effect is small. Further studies are required before such dietary manipulation becomes routine therapy.

To conclude this discussion, the move to increase dietary fiber in both health and disease is linked to the recommendation that carbohydrate intake in general be increased. Many potentially useful and often neglected high-fiber foods can be used to increase carbohydrate intake. In terms of dietary modification, the basic fiber prescription therefore is similar in each situation. There are, however, specific situations where certain types of foods appear more appropriate; for example, insoluble cereal fiber for constipation-related problems and soluble legume and cereal fiber for metabolic disorders such as diabetes and hyperlipidemia. In addition, the indications for pharmacologic use of purified fiber types and components are just emerging.

SUGGESTED READING

American Diabetes Association. Nutritional recommendations and principles for individuals with diabetes mellitus: 1986. Diabetes Care 1987; 10:126–132.

Rampton DS, Cohen SL, Crammond V de B, et al. Treatment of chronic renal failure with dietary fiber. Clin Nephrol 1984; 21:159–163.

Report of the expert advisory committee on dietary fibre. Ottawa: Health and Welfare Canada, 1985.

Shaw S, Womer TM, Lieber CS. Comparison of animal and vegetable protein sources in the dietary management of hepatic encephalopathy. Am J Clin Nutr 1983; 38:59–63.

Vahouny GV, Kritchevsky D. Dietary fiber: basic and clinical aspects. New York: Plenum Press, 1986.

ENTERAL NUTRITION AND PRODUCTS

DAVID B. A. SILK, M.D., F.R.C.P.

It has been 10 years since Bristian and colleagues published their papers showing that up to 50 percent of hospitalized medical and surgical patients had some evidence of nutritional deficiencies. One interpretation of their findings was that up to 50 percent of their patients were "malnourished" and therefore in need of nutritional support. Subsequently, it has become clear that it is difficult to agree on what actually represents clinically significant malnutrition. Moreover, even if agreement is reached, it may not be clear that outcome will be affected by providing nutritional support. This is so because in the hospitalized patient, malnutrition often arises as a consequence of the underlying disease process, which may often not be amenable to correction. It is not surprising that it is frequently not possible to clearly define the indications for instituting nutritional support.

Once the decision has been made to provide nutritional support, it can be given by the enteral or parenteral route. Clinical experience during the last decade has confirmed that enteral nutrition is an efficient way of providing nutritional care to patients with normal or near normal gastrointestinal function, and experience in our own unit has shown that over three-fourths of all patients receiving nutritional support have been fed enterally. Table 1 presents the various ways in which patients can be fed enterally. (The term "enteral nutrition" refers to the administration of nutrients directly into the gastrointestinal tract.)

In our experience the most practical and most common method involves the infusion of a formulated enteral diet with or without the use of a peristaltic pump via nasal fine bore feeding tubes positioned in the stomach or the small intestine. As with other forms of nutritional support, two important objectives of treatment are to improve the nutritional state of the malnourished patient and then to maintain nutritional status while the underlying disease process is treated. It has now become clear that in traumatized and septic hypermetabolic patients even an adequate nutritional intake may not overcome the primary neuroendocrinologic responses to injury, and at least in the early phases, these patients will

53

TABLE 1 Methods of Providing Enteral Nutrition

Oral administration
 Normal food
 Liquefied food
 Palatable liquid supplements

Per nasal tube feeding
 Nasogastric
 Nasoduodenal
 Nasojejunal

Enterostomy feeding
 Cervical pharyngostomy
 Cervical esophagostomy
 Gastrostomy
  Stamm
  Witzel
  Janeway
  Rombeau gastrostomy-jejunostomy
   tube technique
  Percutaneous endoscopic gastrostomy (PEG)

Jejunostomy
 Witzel
 Roux-en-Y
 Needle catheter jejunostomy

remain in overall negative nutritional balance. In other patients, however, negative nutritional balance is more likely to persist on account of inadequate intake.

We have identified a number of factors that are important in optimizing the efficacy of nutritional support provided via the enteral route. These include the correct type of diet adequately formulated, optimally designed enteral feeding tubes, and relatively large volume diet containers. The correct route of administration has to be chosen and appropriate techniques of administration used. Finally, an understanding of the pathogenesis of side effects can lead to better results.

ENTERAL DIETS

Table 2 summarizes the different categories of enteral diets. Until recently, controversy existed as to whether enteral feeds formulated and prepared in the hospital dietetic department should be used in preference

TABLE 2   Classification of Enteral Diets

Type	Comments
Polymeric	Protein nitrogen source. For use in patients with normal or near normal gastrointestinal function.
Predigested chemically defined elemental	Free amino acid or oligopeptide nitrogen source. Small quantities of long chain triglycerides. For use in patients with *severe* gastrointestinal disease.
Disease-specific diets	
Portosystemic encephalopathy	Free amino acid nitrogen source. High branched-chain amino acid content, low aromatic amino acid content. Indications still under discussion.
Stress	Branched-chain amino acid enriched. Indications still under discussion.
Respiratory and cardiac failure	Protein nitrogen source. Reductions in carbohydrate component of energy source.

to their commercially prepared counterparts. Problems with infection have been well documented with "home brew" diets and there is now controlled data to show that the incidence of diarrhea is higher when home brew is used for enteral feeding. We, therefore, recommend the routine use of commercially available diets.

Choice of Diets

Patients with Normal or Near Normal Gastrointestinal Function. In a carefully performed study, Moriarty and colleagues showed that no significant differences occurred in nitrogen balance when patients with normal gastrointestinal function were fed three enteral diets that differed only in nitrogen source, which was composed of whole protein, oligopeptides, or free amino acids. There would thus seem to be no significant advantage in feeding patients with normal gastrointestinal function a predigested, chemically defined diet; a conclusion supported by the results of two controlled clinical trials.

The formulation of polymeric diets is based on our knowledge of the physiology of nutrient absorption and nutrient requirements in health and disease. The composition of the different defined formula diets is summarized in Table 3. Until recently we have recommended the routine use of polymeric diets with an energy density of 1 kcal per milliliter for nonhypermetabolic patients with normal or near normal gastrointestinal function. It has been a clinical observation in our unit that it is often difficult to actually administer more than 2.0 to 2.5 L of enteral diet per day to the routinely ward fed patient. In a recent study, significantly better nitrogen balance was seen when an energy- and nitrogen-dense diet (1.5 kcal per milliliter, 9.4 g N per liter) was administered as compared to either an energy-dense (1.5 kcal per milliliter, 7.8 g N per liter) or a standard (1 kcal per milliliter, 6.3 g N per liter) polymeric diet. As a result of these findings we are now recommending that energy- and nitrogen-dense diets (1.5 kcal per milliliter, 9.4 g N per liter) should be used for routine enteral feeding as they are well tolerated and lead to a greater efficiency of enteral nutrition, at least as far as nitrogen balance is concerned. For very hypermetabolic patients (for example, those with burns and multiple trauma) with normal gastrointestinal function, polymeric diets are available with an energy density of 2 kcal per milliliter and nitrogen content of up to 13 g N per liter. These are hypertonic diets and we have very limited personal experience with them.

It should be borne in mind that there may be a real risk of infusing excess carbohydrate to these patients, some of whom already have insulin resistance. Furthermore, excessive carbohydrate loading could adversely affect respiratory function.

Patients with Impaired Gastrointestinal Function. In those clinical situations where the rate of nutrient absorption is limited by impaired luminal hydrolysis or reductions in mucosal absorption or hydrolytic capacity, the use of enteral diets containing predigested nutrients will result in more efficient nutrient repletion than the polymeric diets discussed previously. In practice, these predigested or so-called chemically defined elemental diets are usually used in patients with severe exocrine pancreatic insufficiency or inadequate or short bowel syndrome. When nutrient assimilation is severely impaired, there are theoretical reasons for believing that nutrients should be presented to the mucosa in the form that results in maximal absorption in normal subjects.

In practical terms it may often be difficult to decide whether a polymeric or a predigested diet should be used. In the author's opinion the assimilatory capacity of the gastrointestinal tract for nutrients is often underestimated. For example, there is no evidence that there is any clinically significant impairment of exocrine pancreatic function or intestinal

TABLE 3 Choice and Formulation of Enteral Diets

	Polymeric Diets for Patients with Normal or Near Normal Gastrointestinal Function			Predigested Diets for Patients with Severely Impaired Gastrointestinal Function
	Nonhypermetabolic to Moderately Hypermetabolic		Hypermetabolic	
	Current	Proposed		
Nitrogen source (g/L)	Protein (5–7)	Protein (9–10)	Protein (11–13)	Purified low molecular weight peptide mixtures (5–10)
Carbohydrate	Glucose polymers	Glucose polymers ± sucrose	Purified glucose polymers (now >10 glucose molecules) ± sucrose	Glucose polymers
Fat source	Long chain triglycerides	Long chain triglycerides	Long chain triglycerides	Medium chain triglycerides linoleic acid
Energy (%)	32–36	32–36	34–41	?
Kcal/ml	1.0	1.5	2.0	1.0
Electrolytes (mmol/L)				
Sodium	30–70	30–70	30–70	70–90
Potassium	30–70	30–70	30–70	30–70
Chlorine	30–70	30–70	30–70	70–90
Minerals (fraction RDA)	1.0	1–1.5	1.5–2.0	1.0–1.5
Vitamins (fraction RDA)	1.0	1–1.5	1.5–2.0	1.0–1.5
Osmolality (mOsm/kg)	300–400	Up to 500	Up to 600	450–650

absorptive capacity in the postoperative period. Moreover, there is no clinical evidence to support the contention that the use of predigested rather than polymeric diets in jejunostomy feeding results in more efficient nutrient repletion.

Patients with Stress. There has been much interest in the role of branch chain amino acids (BCAAs) in the nutritional management of the stress patient. Since in vitro experimental data indicates that leucine specifically increases the rate of protein synthesis and decreases the rate of protein degradation, a special role for BCAAs as anticatabolic amino acids in stress patients has been proposed. It has been argued, however, that the in vitro studies were not physiologic as all preparations were in negative nitrogen balance (degradation > synthesis). On the basis that leucine has no apparent stimulatory effect on muscle protein synthesis in vivo, it would seem hard to justify the use of BCAA-enriched formulations in stressed patients, and only two of nine published studies show any positive effect of BCAA-enriched formulations on nitrogen balance.

TECHNIQUES OF ADMINISTRATION

The administration techniques used during enteral feeding are important. In fact, we believe we have increased the efficacy of enteral nutrition to a greater extent by modifying and improving administration techniques than by altering diet formulation.

Feeding Tube Design and Performance

When wide bore tubes of the Ryle type are used for nasogastric feeding, the size and rigidity of the tubes tend to produce irritation and inflammation of the esophagus with subsequent hemorrhage and stricture formation. Such side effects have not been seen with the new softer and narrower bore tubes now available. We developed a special interest in enteral feeding tube design and performance when the limitations and drawbacks of the early open-ended and unweighted polyvinylchloride fine bore nasogastric feeding tubes were highlighted. Incorporating a weight into the tip of the tube failed to improve performance, and because of disappointment with the overall performance of these early fine bore feeding tubes, a new generation of polyurethane tubes has been developed.

The use of polyurethane has permitted a substantial increase in flow area of the tubes. The interior wall as well as the outside of the tip of the feeding tube is impregnated with a water-activated lubricant, which eases tube insertion and facilitates the removal of the introducer wire. The new tube (Corpak Co., Wheeling, IL), contains a long single wide-necked, smooth and curved edged outflow port that prevents blockage with mucus or curdled diet while facilitating aspiration of gastric contents. The superior performance of these new polyurethane tubes has been confirmed under controlled trial conditions.

Diet Containers

Concern about diet contamination led to the widespread use of 0.5 L diet containers that required changing at least every 6 hours. Recent work has shown, however, that if sterile enteral diets are carefully emptied into diet containers on the ward they remain sterile, whereas if a diet is blended with additives in the diet kitchen it is likely to become contaminated. Consequently, if enteral diets are to be prepared in the diet kitchen then 0.5 L diet containers must be used; if presterilized enteral diets are used without blending, then 1.5 to 2.0 L containers can be used. Our recent work has shown that significantly greater proportions of the daily prescribed diet can actually be administered to the patient from the larger single 2.0 L containers than from four 0.5 L or two 1.0 L containers.

ROUTES OF ADMINISTRATION

Nasogastric versus Nasoenteral Tube Feeding

The main disadvantage of nasoduodenal or nasojejunal feeding is that the pylorus is bypassed. Gastric emptying is mediated by the action of the pylorus, the rate of gastric emptying in turn being governed by entry of gastric contents into the duodenum, the so-called "duodenal brake." The importance of the duodenal brake has often been ignored in enteral nutrition. Abdominal cramping, bloating, and diarrhea may occur when the duodenal brake is bypassed during nasoduodenal or nasojejunal enteral feeding, probably due in part to the rapid secretion of fluid and electrolytes in response to the high osmotic load in nutrients entering the upper small bowel. The duodenal brake will reduce these symptoms if enteral feeds are infused intragastrically. In our experience, using the nasogastric rather than the nasoenteral route reduces the necessity of slowing infusion rates to counteract the development of gastrointestinal side effects.

Although there have been no controlled clinical trials to support the theory, it does seem that regurgitation and aspiration of enteral diets occur more commonly when neurologic patients are fed via the nasogastric route. A case can, therefore, be made to feed this subgroup of patients nasoenterally, and this problem is discussed in more detail in the chapter *Chronic Neurologic Disease*.

Routes for Long-Term Enteral Feeding

On occasion, it might be clear from the outset that a patient requires long-term (> 4 to 6 weeks) of enteral feeding. In such cases consideration should be given to resorting to the surgical creation of a more permanent route of administration. The techniques of surgically creating tube enterostomy feeding routes have been summarized by Rombeau and colleagues (All Suggested Reading). Recently a number of percutaneous endoscopic techniques for fashioning a tube feeding gastrostomy have been described. Experience is being gained with this approach, and it is likely to gain a much wider application in the future, particularly when enterostomy feeding tube design has been improved.

Starter Regimens

Gastrointestinal side effects of enteral nutrition include nausea, abdominal bloating, and pain. Diarrhea, defined as the passage of loose and frequent stools of discomfort to the patient or the nursing staff, has been reported in up to one-fourth of patients receiving enteral nutrition. It has been the prevailing wisdom that these side effects, particularly diarrhea, can be minimized by gradually introducing full-strength feeding over a 3- to 4-day period at the outset of feeding—the so-called "starter regimen" technique. Recent work, however, clearly shows that it is perfectly safe to prescribe full-strength feeding regimens from the outset providing that patients have normal gastrointestinal function and that a polymeric diet is infused continuously over 24 hours via the nasogastric route. Further work has also shown that it is safe to infuse a predigested chemically defined elemental diet by continuous 24-hour infusion via the nasogastric route to patients with acute exacerbations of inflammatory bowel disease. The advantage of not using a starter regimen is that over a 10- to 12-day period of enteral feeding, substantially greater quantities of nutrients can be administered than when starter regimens are used.

TABLE 4 Complications of Enteral Nutrition

Type	Comment	Remedy
Feeding tube related:		
Esophageal inflammation, hemorrhage, or stricture formation	Rare with new fine bore PVC or polyurethane tubes	Prophylactic treatment with H_2 receptor antagonists if wide bore Ryle type tubes have to be used for more than 4 to 5 days
Tube misplacement	Occurs most commonly in unconscious patients	Check position by radiography
Esophageal, nasopharyngeal, or gastric perforation	Rare	Can be treated conservatively
Nausea	Occurs transiently in 5 to 15% of patients; not usually severe	Usually settle spontaneously. Occasionally need to reduce rate of diet infusion.
Abdominal bloating	Probably due to gastric stasis and high osmotic loads of nutrients administered	
Abdominal pain		
Diarrhea	See text	If possible stop antibiotics. Treat with imodium or codeine phosphate.
Biochemical:		
Hyperglycemia	Usually related to insulin resistance	Insulin
Hypokalemia	Related to nitrogen losses or occurs in anabolic phase	Supplements required
Hypophosphatemia	Related to nitrogen losses	Supplements required
Vitamin, mineral, trace element, essential fatty acid deficiencies	Rare. Monitor clinically and biochemically.	Supplements required
Abnormal liver function tests	Causes are multifactorial and related to underlying disease or malnutrition. May in part be due to continuous 24-hour infusion of diet.	In our experience seldom clinically significant. In patients without liver disease, LFTs return to normal after cessation of feeding.

COMPLICATIONS*

In our experience, the efficacy of enteral nutrition can be maintained even when side effects are developing. This is so because once an understanding is gained of the factors involved in its pathogenesis, the necessary steps can be taken to deal with the problem, often without reducing the rate of diet infusion. The common complications of enteral nutrition are summarized in Table 4.

Probably the commonest is diarrhea occurring, as mentioned, in up to one-fourth of patients. A number of factors have been implicated in its pathogenesis, and these include the use of infected feeds, lactose intolerance, intolerance of high osmotic loads, inappropriate release of gastrointestinal polypeptide hormones, concomitant antibiotic therapy, and laxatives. If an unexpected outbreak of diarrhea occurs, the water used for diet dilution or reconstitution of powder should be suspected and cultured. Lactose intolerance is seldom a cause of diarrhea, except in patients who are bolus fed. Few lactose-containing diets are now marketed. It is likely that diarrhea will occur if hyperosmolar diets are infused rapidly into the duodenum or jejunum, on account of the rapid secretion of fluid and electrolytes that occurs in order to render the upper small intestinal content iso-osmotic with plasma. Diarrhea does not occur if a 2.0 to 2.5 L polymeric diet with an osmolality up to 450 mOsm per kilogram is infused continuously over 24 hours into the stomach. To date there is no evidence that the onset of diarrhea during enteral feeding is related to an inappropriate release of gastrointestinal polypeptide hormones. In the majority of patients, diarrhea occurs in association with concomitant antibiotic therapy administered by either the oral or the parenteral route.

* See also page 389.

SUGGESTED READING

Rees RG, Attrill H, Quinn D, Silk DBA. Improved design of nasogastric feeding tubes. Clin Nutr 1986; 5:203-207.

Rombeau JL, Barot LR, Low DW, Twomey PL. Feeding by tube enterostomy. In: Rombeau JL, Caldwell MD, eds. Enteral and tube feeding. Philadelphia: WB Saunders, 1984:275.

Silk DBA. Diet formulation and choice of enteral diet. Gut 1986; 27:Suppl.1:40–46.

TOTAL PARENTERAL NUTRITION

PAUL D. GREIG, M.D., F.R.C.S.(C)

With the recent advances in enteral and parenteral nutrition, it is now possible to completely feed virtually any hospitalized patient. In the patient with a nonfunctioning gastrointestinal (GI) tract, total parenteral nutrition (TPN) can provide all the daily requirements for protein, calories, fluid, electrolytes, trace elements, and vitamins. While specific techniques of administration will vary from center to center, the principles of TPN are universal. Their application at the Toronto General Hospital is presented in this overview.

INITIATING TOTAL PARENTERAL NUTRITION

The decision to begin TPN is based on the clinical setting and the presence or absence of malnutrition. The traditional techniques of nutritional assessment concentrate on measurements of body composition and include anthropomorphic measurements of tricep skin fold thickness and midarm circumference to give estimates of muscle mass and fat stores, creatinine height index as a reflection of muscle mass, and serum albumin or transferrin levels as an estimate of "visceral protein." Absolute lymphocyte count and the presence of anergy in response to delayed cutaneous hypersensitivity testing are affected by malnutrition and reflect a more functional assessment of nutritional status. However, each of these tests suffers from lack of sensitivity and specificity and while each may be helpful, the decision to initiate TPN is usually based on clinical factors. A history of significant recent weight loss or prolonged inadequate intake usually indicates malnutrition, regardless of the results of these other tests. The "subjective global assessment" of the patient appears to be as accurate a predictor of postoperative morbidity and mortality as any combination of the more objective measures of nutritional assessment. While the presence of malnutrition might increase the urgency for beginning TPN, the clinical setting is usually the overriding factor. If it is anticipated that a patient will not be taking a full oral intake within

5 to 7 days of assessment, then nutritional intervention is indicated. If malnutrition exists, then nutritional support should be started sooner.

METHODS OF ADMINISTRATION

In the patient with an intact and functional GI tract, enteral feeding should be employed. Occasionally, if a delay in the tolerance of enteral feeding is anticipated, then supplemental parenteral nutrition (partial parenteral nutrition) may be given while enteral feeding is increased. TPN should never be used as a substitute for enteral feeding in the patient with an intact and functional GI tract.

TPN may be delivered through either a peripheral or a central vein. Peripheral TPN may be considered in a patient with "good" peripheral veins who requires TPN for a short period of time, usually 7 to 10 days. The phlebitis associated with the hypertonic solutions usually limits the use of any single peripheral vein to less than 48 hours. The hypertonicity can be reduced by limiting the glucose concentration of the amino-acid dextrose solution to 10 to 12 percent, keeping the potassium content below 40 mmol per liter and continuously delivering a 10 percent lipid emulsion through a connector that is piggy-backed into the amino-acid dextrose tubing. Despite these techniques, phlebitis often occurs and the intravenous cannula becomes interstitial. This results in frequent interruptions of the infusion, and the patient is left underfed. An "antiplebitic mixture" of neutralization of pH, small doses of heparin, and steroid added to the solutions may enhance the peripheral vein tolerance of these solutions. Long-term peripheral vein access, however, remains the major problem associated with peripheral parenteral nutrition.

For longer term TPN, a central venous catheter is used. The principle of delivering hypertonic solutions into a large central vein is accomplished by a central line whose tip lies in the superior vena cava. The infraclavicular subclavian catheter is the preferred approach to facilitate dressings on the anterior chest wall. The internal or external jugular or supraclavicular subclavian catheters are more difficult to isolate and dress because of neck movement, and are less comfortable for the patient.

The ideal catheter is minimally thrombogenic and floats freely in the superior vena cava with the tip lying at the junction of the superior vena cava and the right atrium. Silastic is an excellent material because of its low thrombogenicity; however, thin-walled temporary silastic catheters are difficult to see in the mediastinum on chest radiography and are difficult to change over a wire. The polyurethane catheters become soft at body temperature and a "hydromer coating" can reduce the thrombogenicity to that of silastic. These lines are easily seen on films and can be changed over a wire. In addition, the permanently attached Luer-lock hub is less liable to become dislodged than the type of hub that is attached after catheter insertion. In patients who will require TPN for months, a Broviac or Hickman catheter, which is used for home parenteral nutrition, may be preferred. These silastic catheters are tunnelled subcutaneously to further reduce line sepsis.

Double and triple lumen catheters should be avoided if possible. Since hub colonization is a major source of catheter sepsis, two or three hubs significantly increase the risk of catheter sepsis with these lines. TPN should be given through a single-channel dedicated subclavian catheter that is not interrupted for medications, blood products, or measurements of central venous pressure.

Placement of the subclavian catheter should be performed by an experienced physician using strict aseptic technique to minimize complications, which include injury to the lung with pneumothorax, injury to the subclavian artery with hemothorax, extrapleural hematoma or intimal dissection, injury to the brachial plexus, air embolism, and malposition of the catheter tip. A portable chest film must be reviewed carefully prior to beginning parenteral nutrition infusion.

An occlusive dressing technique should be standardized for nursing care throughout the hospital. The dressing should be changed weekly, or more frequently if it becomes disturbed. IV tubing and filters are changed every 24 hours. Surveillance of TPN lines by the TPN nurse is important to reduce the incidence of septic complications.

PRESCRIBING TPN

TPN is a complex intravenous preparation, and each of its components—protein, calories, fluid and electrolytes, vitamins, and trace elements—must be individualized for each patient.

The technique for prescribing TPN will depend on the system that has been established within the hospital. The need to prescribe a wide range of protein and calories with variable amounts of electrolytes, trace elements, and vitamins requires a flexible system. This, however, is more labor intensive and less efficient for the pharmacy; a simpler system that makes available only one or two solutions with some flexibility in the electrolytes is often adequate for smaller hospitals. Ideally, the clinician should be able to prescribe the protein and calories to within 10 percent estimated requirements and tailor fluid and electrolytes to the individual. However, the importance of a high degree of precision in these prescriptions has not been proven, particularly in stable patients receiving short-term parenteral nutrition. A pharmacist, with expertise in parenteral nutrition solutions, must check the composition of each order for compatibility of nutrients and/or drugs.

As part of the nutritional assessment, prior to beginning parenteral nutrition, full TPN blood work should include a complete blood count and measurements of electrolytes, creatinine, BUN, albumin, bilirubin, AST, ALP, magnesium, calcium, phosphate, cholesterol, triglycerides, folate, vitamin B_{12}, and iron indices. The additives to the glucose amino-acid solution should be adjusted to these pre-TPN levels. While TPN is underway, serum glucose and electrolytes should be followed daily for a minimum of 3 days. Full TPN blood work should be done weekly.

CONTENT OF TPN SOLUTION

Protein. The crystalline amino acid solutions that are available from different manufacturers vary in the proportions of the individual amino acids. While most are very similar, the newer amino acid solutions contain more cystine, glutamine, and aspartic acid and less glycine and alanine. The solutions of essential amino acids and those enriched in branched-chain amino acids will be considered in the chapters on renal and liver disease, respectively.

The amount of protein and calories to be administered depends on the goals of parenteral nutrition—i.e., either to deliver complete nutritional support (TPN) or to provide only some protein and calories for a short course of "protein sparing" therapy, anticipating oral intake within 5 to 7 days. To meet daily requirements, the amount of protein to be administered will vary with the clinical status of the patient and will range from 0.75 to 1.5 g of amino acids per kilogram per day; this amount will be higher in the hypercatabolic patient and lower in the patient with liver disease or renal failure.

Calories. Nonprotein calories should be given to equal the best estimate or actual measurement of the total energy expenditure. The resting energy expenditure (REE) can be estimated from the Harris-Benedict equation and corrected for "stress factors" of plus 10 to 100 percent and "malnutrition factors" of minus 10 to 25 percent, and then adjusted for activity. Alternatively, the REE can be calculated (using the principles of indirect calorimetry) from measurements of O_2 consumption and CO_2 production made using portable bedside metabolic measurement equipment. This measurement is particularly valuable in the critically ill patient in whom the effect of sepsis or injury on energy expenditure may be quite variable. In general, the nonprotein energy requirements range from 20 to 35 kcal per kilogram per day.

While many patients can tolerate receiving most of their nonprotein calories as glucose, hyperglycemia and insulin requirements can be reduced and a more normal hormonal milieu established by the daily administration of lipid emulsion. A minimum of 100 g of fat emulsion should be given per week to prevent essential fatty acid deficiency. The ideal ratio of fat to glucose for daily administration is not known, however ratios from 30:70 to 70:30 are well tolerated by most patients. Whether to administer 10 or 20 percent lipid emulsion will depend on fluid requirements.

Micronutrients. Amounts of sodium, potassium, bicarbonate, chloride, magnesium, calcium, and phosphate should be based on the patient's pre-TPN levels, with estimates of daily requirements and ongoing losses. In critically ill or edematous patients, sodium restriction (20 to 40 mmol per day) will reduce the refeeding edema associated with TPN. Patients with renal failure should be potassium and phosphate restricted; once dialysis is begun, conventional electrolytes may be given.

Vitamins should be administered daily as recommended by the Nutritional Advisory Group of the American Medical Association (Table 1), although these amounts may be insufficient for many patients on TPN. Standard amounts of trace elements are usually adequate for short-term in-hospital feeding (Table 2). In patients with liver disease, copper and manganese should be omitted from the TPN as they are predominantly excreted in the bile.

FORMULATION

Formulation of TPN solutions is usually performed in the pharmacy in a laminar flow hood, although certain medications may be added by

TABLE 1 Guidelines for Daily Vitamin Dosages

Vitamin	RDA*	NAG†
A (IU)	4000–5000	3300
D (IU)	400	200
E (IU)	12–15	10
C (mg)	45	100
B$_1$ (mg)	1.0–1.5	3
B$_2$ (mg)	1.1–1.8	3.6
Niacin, B$_3$ (mg)	12–20	40
Pantothenate, B$_5$ (mg)	5–10	15
Pyridoxine, B$_6$ (mg)	1.6–2.0	4
B12 (μg)	3	5
Folate (μg)	400	400
Biotin (μg)	150–300	60
K (mg)	–	0.5

*For oral administration.
† For parenteral administration.
(Adapted from Multivitamin preparations for parenteral use. A statement by the Nutritional Advisory Group. JPEN 1979; 3:258–262 and Recommended Daily Allowances, 9th ed. Food and Nutrition Board of the National Research Council, National Academy of Sciences, 1980.)

the nursing staff (Table 3). The amino acid–dextrose solutions containing electrolytes, trace elements, and vitamins may be hung in bags separate from the lipid emulsion bottle; however, the total nutrient admixture system of combining all of the TPN for a 24-hour period in a single bag appears to be safe and well tolerated by patients. While an intravenous pump may be helpful in regulating the rate of delivery, it is not necessary in most patients receiving central TPN.

TABLE 2 Guidelines for Daily Trace Element Dosages

Trace Element	Oral	Parenteral
Chromium (μg)	50–290	10–20
Copper (mg)	1.2–3.0	0.5–1.5
Iodine (μg)	150	50–150
Iron (mg)	6–23	1.2–1.8
Manganese (mg)	0.7–5.0	0.12–2.0
Molybdenum (μg)		20–120
Selenium (μg)		120
Zinc (mg)	10–15	2–4

**TABLE 3   Medications That May Be Added
to Parenteral Nutrition**

Insulin
Hydrocortisone
Cimetidine
Ranitidine
Metoclopramide

THE TPN TEAM

The optimal delivery of TPN requires a multidisciplinary approach that includes the expertise of nurses, pharmacists, dietitians, and physicians. The team approach has been shown to reduce the complications of TPN. Each member of the nutrition support team has an important role, and communication within the team and with the primary attending physician or surgeon is essential.

The nurse's responsibilities begin with recognizing the potential requirement for nutritional intervention in each patient. Once TPN is ordered, the responsibilities range from the addition of medications to the TPN solution to care of the catheter and delivery system and hour-by-hour surveillance of the actual delivery of the nutrients. The nurse must be familiar with the problems of TPN as he or she is often the first to suspect complications. The TPN nurse teacher should see all patients receiving TPN on a regular basis to ensure that nursing standards are maintained and central venous catheter care is immaculate.

The pharmacist has an important role in checking the TPN prescription for compatibility and ensuring that it conforms to the standards of the institution and in overseeing the formulation, storage, and delivery of the solutions. Quality control is critical since the "nutrient broth" of TPN is at significant risk for contamination.

The hospital dietitian is often the person who identifies the need for TPN in the patient with inadequate oral intake. Coordination between enteral and parenteral feeding is important to avoid the complications of under- or overfeeding, particularly as the patient begins oral intake or is switched over to enteral feeding.

COMPLICATIONS*

It is important to watch for the potential complications of TPN, which can be considered as either mechanical or metabolic. The mechanical complications of TPN include all the risks of insertion of the central venous catheter. Immediate complications include pneumothorax, injury to the subclavian artery or brachial plexus, and misdirection of the catheter up the internal jugular vein. Late complications of a central line include air embolism, central venous thrombosis, and sepsis. Using strict aseptic technique, the complication rate of central line placement by the experienced physician should be less than 5 percent. Strict adherence to standards for catheter care should minimize septic complications.

Catheter sepsis should be suspected in any patient who develops a fever while receiving TPN. Appropriate investigation includes inspection of the exit site for erythema or drainage, both peripheral and retrograde blood cultures, and search for other sites of infection. If the patient has no other potential focus of infection, TPN-related catheter sepsis should be assumed. If the patient is in septic shock, the line should be removed and appropriate antibiotics begun. Otherwise TPN should be discontinued, the solution cultured, and the patient monitored closely. If the blood cultures are positive, the line may be changed over a wire if the tunnel and exit site are clean; otherwise it should be removed and replaced by a new catheter. If all cultures are negative or another source of infection is found and treated and fever resolves, TPN can resume using the original catheter.

The metabolic complications of TPN can involve any of the components. Excessive protein administration is associated with increases in BUN, oxygen consumption and resting energy expenditure, and ventilatory drive. Excessive caloric intake, particularly excessive glucose, results in hyperglycemia; increased O_2 consumption, CO_2 production, and resting energy expenditure; and sometimes respiratory distress. Excessive fat administration can result in hyperlipidemia with increased serum cholesterol and triglycerides and decreased immunologic function. Excessive sodium and water administration can result in salt and water overload, manifestations of which may range from peripheral swelling to pulmonary edema. With nutritional repletion hypokalemia, hypomagnesemia and hypophosphatemia must be avoided by the administration of adequate amounts of these elements. Trace element and vitamin deficiencies

* See also page 389.

can be prevented by the daily administration of copper, manganese, iron, selenium, zinc, chromium, and all vitamins.

SUMMARY

Through the administration of TPN, the nutritional support of all hospitalized patients is now possible. The safe delivery of this complex preparation requires the coordinated efforts of all members of the TPN team: nurses, pharmacists, dietitians, and physicians. Parenteral nutrition should be individualized to the protein, calories, fluid, and electrolyte needs of the patient. Well-established hospital-wide standards are important to maintain a low rate of mechanical and metabolic complications. Surveillance during TPN is important for the prevention or early detection of complications.

SUGGESTED READING

ASPEN Board of Directors. Guidelines for use of total parenteral nutrition in the hospitalized adult patient. JPEN 1986; 10:441–445.

Bonadimani B, Sperti C, Stevanin A, et al. Central venous catheter guidewire replacement according to the Seldinger technique: usefulness in the management of patients on total parenteral nutrition. JPEN 1987; 11:267–270.

Brown R, Quercia RA, Sigman R. Total nutrient admixture: a review. JPEN 1986; 10:650–658.

Dempsey DT, Mullen JL, Rombeau JL, et al. Treatment effects of parenteral vitamins in total perenteral nutrition patients. JPEN 1987; 11:229–237.

Detsky AS, McLaughlin JR, Baker JP, et al. What is subjective global assessment? JPEN 1987; 11:8–13.

Faubion WC, Wesley JR, Khalidi N, et al. Total parenteral nutrition catheter sepsis: impact of the team approach. JPEN 1986; 10:642–645.

Goodhart RS, Shils ME, eds. Modern nutrition in health and disease, 6th ed. Philadelphia: Lea & Febiger, 1980.

American Medical Association, Department of Foods and Nutrition. Guidelines for essential trace element preparation for parenteral use: a statement by an expert panel. JAMA 1979; 241:2051–2054.

McCarthy MC, Shives JK, Robison RJ, et al. Prospective evaluation of single and triple lumen catheters in total parenteral nutrition. JEPN 1987; 11:259–262.

Multivitamin preparations for parenteral use. A statement by the Nutritional Advisory Group. JPEN 1979; 3:258–262.

Shils ME. Guidelines for total parenteral nutrition. JAMA 1972; 22:1721–1729.

Traeger SM, Williams GB, Milliren G. Total parenteral nutrition by a nutrition support team: improved quality of care. JPEn 1986; 10:408–412.

Recommended Daily Allowances, 9th ed. Food and Nutrition Board of the National Research Council, National Academy of Sciences, 1980.

HOME PARENTERAL NUTRITION

C. RICHARD FLEMING, M.D.

Since patients were first managed with home parenteral nutrition (HPN) approximately 15 years ago, thousands of individuals have benefited from this major advance in the care of patients with gut failure and malnutrition. Because of the complexity of such care, most centers have concentrated on delivering HPN through multispecialty teams consisting of physicians, nurses, pharmacists, dietitians, and social workers. The involvement of industry as intermediary providers to patients has greatly facilitated the transition from hospital to home and decreased significantly the time required of hospital pharmacists. Although HPN teams and industry have facilitated the management of HPN patients, the major responsibility for the success of HPN resides with patients.

At Mayo Clinic, we first utilized HPN in 1972 when we were confronted with a patient with severe short bowel syndrome who was totally dependent on parenteral nutrition. It was not until 1975 that an organized effort was initiated and the multispecialty team organized. From August 1975 through 1986, approximately 100 patients were trained and discharged on the full complement of HPN. Many other patients have been discharged with instructions to infuse only fluids, electrolytes, and vitamins.

PATIENT SELECTION

Any patient with gut failure is a potential candidate for HPN. However, most patients with bona fide gut failure can be managed with enteral nutrition; 50 percent of patients referred to us for consideration of HPN are fed adequately by other means. We have generally limited HPN to those patients with nonmalignant diseases and gut failure who have proved refractory to all other forms of treatment or for whom other forms of treatment (e.g., surgery) are thought inadvisable at the time. Most patients have severe short bowel syndrome, extensive Crohn's disease, radiation damage to the small intestine, refractory sprue, chronic adhesive obstruction, or a diffuse motility disorder of the gut.

PATIENT TRAINING

The consultant on the Nutrition Consulting Service usually sees patients who are subsequently referred to the HPN team. If HPN is the only alternative, the physician director of the HPN team C. R. Fleming (CRF) evaluates and subsequently follows all patients before and during HPN. If the patient is a candidate and wishes to proceed, he is relocated to one station for gastroenterology patients where the nurses and other staff are familiar with HPN policies. A nurse HPN coordinator initiates a sequence of consultations with the health care members of the HPN team (Fig. 1). A social worker gives an independent assessment of the suitability of the patient (and his family) for a long-term artificial support device. With assistance from a member of the business office, the social worker assures financial coverage of HPN by contacting the in-

HOME PARENTERAL NUTRITION
Team Approach

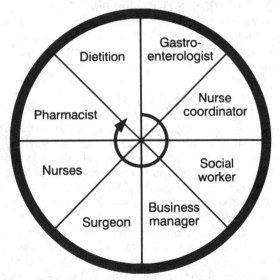

Figure 1 Pie graph showing the usual chronological (clockwise) sequence of involvement by medical and paramedical staff in each HPN patient's care. (From Trans Am Clin Climatol Assoc 1986; 98:199.)

surance company or other third-party sources. A surgeon then inserts a tunnelled subcutaneous catheter in the operating room using general anesthesia. One of the "core" nurses on the gastroenterology floor who is trained in HPN techniques teaches the details of aseptic technique, catheter care, regulation of the intravenous pump, potential complications, and proper responses to the complications; this is supplemented with an HPN training manual written for patients that serves as a reference when they return home. The "core" nurse administers a written evaluation at the end of the teaching session. A pharmacist then teaches the patient about the purpose, stability, and order of mixing of drugs to add to the premixed intravenous solution. In contrast to our first 60 patients, most patients in recent years have accepted offers from pharmaceutical companies to have their solutions premixed prior to bulk delivery at regular intervals. A dietitian meets with the patient frequently to emphasize the importance of enteral nutrition, even if he will receive nearly all nutrients intravenously.

The physician director of the HPN team contacts the local physician regarding the HPN. After discharge, the patient is followed by his local physician at regular intervals. The frequency of returns to see us is inversely proportional to time on HPN and the distance from us. In general, a patient returns on an average of once every 6 to 12 months after stabilization.

VENOUS ACCESS

We continue to be pleased with the single-lumen catheters for delivery of HPN. A nurse member of the HPN team will usually discuss with patients the preferred exit site on the lower anterior chest wall and mark it for the surgeon. It is important that the exit site is low enough on the chest wall that it can be seen easily with the head in the flexed position. If the exit site is too high on the chest wall, patients will often have to use a mirror to perform catheter site care. We also ask patients if they have a preferred side for catheter placement, since some enjoy recreational activities (e.g., hunting) that may add to the risk of catheter displacement or damage. Many patients will have had a temporary central line immediately prior to insertion of the HPN line in which case we try to use the subclavian vein on the opposite side.

NUTRIENTS

Prior to initiation of HPN, basal energy expenditure (BEE) is measured by indirect calorimetry or estimated by the Harris-Benedict equation. The BEE serves as a baseline with which to estimate the necessary caloric intake. If severely malnourished, patients will frequently require 1.5 to 1.7 × BEE until the goal weights are reached. We attempt to achieve an average weight gain of ¼ to ½ pound per day or at the most, 3 to 4 pounds per week. As the patients approach the desired weights, we frequently have to reduce calories to a maintenance level that approximates 1.2 × BEE. These adjustments can usually be made after conversations with the patients and without necessarily requiring a return trip.

The distribution of calories provided in the HPN varies depending on what the patients are eating. If they are eating a generous amount, we may provide intravenous fat calories (500 ml of a 10 percent fat emulsion) only twice weekly. For patients who rely exclusively on HPN, we attempt to provide 20 to 30 percent of nonprotein calories as fat. We have not used the 3-in-1 (fat, carbohydrate, and protein) admixtures for HPN patients because they do not provide the flexibility that each patient's formula requires and there are reports that catheter occlusion occurs more frequently with the 3-in-1 admixtures than when the fat is simply piggybacked in the line.

Special Nutrient Needs (Table 1)

Protein

Before HPN, most patients have marked depletion of their visceral proteins and many with severe Crohn's disease, radiation enteritis, or refractory sprue will continue to have protein-losing enteropathy. All patients should receive at least 0.8 g per kilogram per day of protein and most will receive 1.5 g per kilogram per day. Most amino acid preparations consist of approximately two-thirds nonessential and one-third essential amino acids. These preparations are very efficiently used; the mean nitrogen retention when 1 g per kilogram per day is given is equivalent to high biologic value protein given orally to healthy adults.

TABLE 1 Representative* HPN Formula

Nutrient	Quantity			kcal
Dextrose	20%		400 g	1360
Amino acids	4.25%		85 g	340
Sodium	28 mEq/L = 56 mEq/bag			
Potassium	30 mEq/L = 60 mEq/bag			
Calcium	6.8 mEq/L = 13.6 mEq/bag			
Magnesium	3.75 mEq/L = 7.5 mEq/bag			
Chloride	33 mEq/L = 66 mEq/bag			
Phosphate	11.25 mEq/L = 22.5 mEq/bag			
Acetate	61 mEq/L = 122 mEq/bag			
Trace elements				
Zinc			4 mg	
Copper			1 mg	
Selenium			40 µg	
Patient adds:	10 ml MVC§ 9 + 3/bag			
	5,000 units heparin/bag			
Final volume	2,000 ml each day over 10 hours			
			Total	= 1700

IV Fat

10% Fat emulsion	500 ml	7/week	50g fat	550
Infuses over	8 hours	PB† to HPN		

HPN: 85 g protein 13.6 g N 1360 NP‡ kcal kcal/N ratio 100:1 7/week
HPN + Fat: 1910 NP kcal kcal/N ratio 140:1 7/week

---

* Nutrient needs vary greatly from patient to patient and with time for each patient.
† PB = piggy-back
‡ NP = nonprotein
§ MVC = multivitamin concentrate

Vitamins

Patients receive all necessary vitamins daily in the form of MVI-12 (Armour Pharmaceutical), except for vitamin K. We administer vitamin K orally if the prothrombin time is prolonged. Some of our patients have elevated serum vitamin A levels, in which case we alternate MVI-12 with an intravenous B-complex vitamin preparation on alternate nights.

Trace Elements

Zinc. While patients are in the hospital for HPN training, we measure 24- to 48-hour zinc losses (stool, urine, fistulas) and give as the intravenous replacement of zinc at least 2 mg more than the sum of the losses. Only 2.5 mg of intravenous zinc per day maintains zinc balance in patients without diarrhea, but zinc requirements may increase markedly with increased gut losses and catabolism.

Iron. Iron is not routinely given, but we monitor the complete blood count, mean corpuscular volume, and ferritin levels and give iron when deficiency is evident. A bone marrow examination with iron stains is occasionally necessary. Parenteral iron must be administered as a firmly bound complex, since unbound iron given intravenously that exceeds binding capacity may produce serious side effects. Systemic reactions occur in approximately 10 percent of patients given intravenous iron dextran. Reactions may include fever, flushing, headaches, joint pains, lymphadenopathy, and, rarely, anaphylaxis and death. It may be given as a series of intramuscular injections, but the discomfort and potential soft tissue discoloration often discourage this. Intravenous iron dextran is given as a fractionated dose given daily, not to exceed 100 mg per day, for several days. A test dose of approximately 25 mg intravenous iron should be given before the treatment is started. Iron dextran added to the total parenteral nutrition (TPN) solutions for fractionated-dose replacement remains stable after 18 hours of room-temperature storage. The side effects of iron dextran prompted a search for safer and more effective substitutes. When iron citrate was added to TPN solutions, 74 percent of the iron was available to transferrin and in vivo availability to red blood cell incorporation was 81 percent; adverse reactions did not occur. However, iron citrate has not yet been marketed.

Other Trace Elements. We titrate selenium and copper additives to normalize blood levels; 40 to 80 μg of selenium and 500 μg of copper usually suffice. We do not routinely give chromium, manganese, and iodine.

Minerals

Calcium. Twenty-four hour urinary calcium and serum 25-hydroxy vitamin D levels are used to monitor calcium status. Most patients receive 250 to 400 mg (12 to 20 mEq) of intravenous calcium, and the amount of oral dietary calcium fluctuates greatly. Bone densitometry of the lumbar spine is performed every 1 to 2 years. If the densitometry is normal and the patient does not have symptoms or signs to suggest osteopenia (e.g., long bone pain, fractures), we only monitor with yearly densitometry measurements. If the densitometry is below the "fracture threshold," and especially if there are significant reductions on serial measurements, then a bone biopsy is performed. Measurements of serum and 24-hour urinary aluminum levels have generally been normal or only slightly elevated in our patients, perhaps due to the fact that we use crystalline amino acids and not protein hydrolysates that have elevated levels of aluminum and can cause increased aluminum values in biologic fluids and bone as well as low bone turnover.

Magnesium. Patients with short bowel syndrome are especially susceptible to magnesium deficiency, which can contribute to hypocalcemia and decreased urinary citrate levels. The serum magnesium level is not as reliable as the 24-hour urinary magnesium value in determining magnesium deficiency.

Electrolytes. Patients with short bowel syndrome with an end jejunostomy or proximal ileostomy are susceptible to large volume losses of fluid and electrolytes. Even those patients with approximately 50 percent of a healthy small bowel remaining can usually absorb two-thirds of macronutrients (carbohydrate, protein, and fat) but frequently experience recurrent dehydration. Attempts should be directed at slowing intestinal transit and increasing absorption by using antidiarrheals on a regular basis and, when necessary, adding intravenous fluids to maintain positive fluid balance. "Cholera cocktails" rich in glucose and electrolytes have been shown to contribute to positive fluid balance and to lessen the need for intravenous fluids, especially in patients in whom the small bowel is in continuity with the colon. Other less fortunate patients require supplemental intravenous fluids to replace the large volume ostomy losses. Rather than piggy-back more intravenous fluids during the overnight period (which often contributes to frequent nocturia and sleep deprivation), we encourage patients to give the extra fluids in the mid afternoon. Usually, we use 5 percent dextrose and 0.45 percent saline with 20 mEq of potassium chloride per liter; a liter can be given by gravity drip over 2 hours. Most patients have not been receptive to a portable vest and pump that allows continuous infusion over 24 hours.

With time and gut adaptation, the requirements for extra fluids will frequently lessen. It is very important for the patient to monitor his weight on a regular basis and urine and stool volumes less frequently.

MEDICATIONS

Patients on HPN may require anticoagulation. Although they may have markedly shortened or diseased (or both) small bowels, anticoagulation is very easy with low-dose Coumadin. The absence of vitamin K in commercial vitamin preparations likely explains this observation. There are reports that hospitalized patients on TPN have a lower incidence of venous thrombosis if low-dose heparin is routinely included in the TPN mixture. Therefore, we include 5,000 units of heparin in every 2-liter HPN solution.

Some patients with short bowel syndrome develop gastric hypersecretion that contributes to maldigestion. The intravenous amino acids stimulate gastric secretion to approximately one-third the maximal response to pentagastrin, and its effect can be blocked with cimetidine. For patients with a past or present history consistent with peptic ulcer disease, we add 600 mg to 900 mg of cimetidine to the HPN solution.

Patients with severe Crohn's disease on HPN experience clinical relapses that sometimes require corticosteroids. The absorption of oral corticosteroids is likely suboptimal; therefore, we give intravenous prednisolone as an early morning single bolus dose after the HPN infusion is completed and before heparin is instilled into the catheter.

MONITORING AND QUALITY CONTROL

The frequency of monitoring the patient's hematologic status is inversely related to the duration and stability of the clinical course. Initially, patients are advised to see their local physician for chemistry and hematology profiles every 2 weeks for at least the first 6 weeks. If the results are repeatedly normal and the patient continues to improve, the frequency of tests is decreased. We have many patients who have been on HPN for more than 5 years who have their chemistries checked only every 6 months.

All patients are sent home with a sterile catheter repair kit that can be used by the local physician if the external segment of the catheter cracks. If a crack occurs close to the exit site on the chest wall, the catheter is replaced.

The HPN team meets weekly for several reasons. A summary of developments with patients in the past week is circulated and discussed so that all HPN personnel remain informed. Special problems with patients or technology frequently surface and require more lengthy group discussion. Regular updates are given on clinical investigation involving HPN patients. The HPN nurse coordinator, assisted by contributions from other HPN members, sends our patients an HPN newsletter on a quarterly basis.

Special Complications

Complications of HPN are legion and are discussed in many sources. I bring special attention to an uncommon problem that will eventually occur as one manages more patients. Of our first 88 patients, at least 3 had superior vena cava thrombosis. We have managed each patient successfully by performing a thoracotomy and placing the Hickman catheter directly into the right atrium and downstream from the superior vena caval occlusion. We chose that route rather than the inferior vena cava because of an unproved fear of an increased incidence of catheter infection when catheters exit on the abdominal wall in the vicinity of an ostomy.

SUGGESTED READING

Fleming CR, Beart RW Jr, Berkner S, McGill DB, Gaffron R. Home parenteral nutrition for management of the severely malnourished adult patient. Gastroenterology 1980; 79:11–18.

Fleming CR, Berkner S. Home parenteral nutrition: a handbook for patients. Philadelphia: JB Lippincott, 1987.

Howard L, Heaphey LL, Timchalk M. A review of the current national status of home parenteral and enteral nutrition from the provider and consumer perspective. J Parenter Enter Nutr 1986; 10(4):416–424.

HOME ENTERAL NUTRITION

PEGGI A. GUENTER, R.N., M.S.N., C.N.S.N.
SUSAN JONES, R.D.
JOHN L. ROMBEAU, M.D.

Enteral nutrition is defined as the provision of liquid formula diets either orally or by tube into the gastrointestinal tract. For purposes of this discussion, home is defined as a patient's residence excluding chronic care or extended care facilities. The rationale for provision of enteral nutrition in the home is twofold: (1) reduced costs compared to hospital care and (2) a marked improvement in the psychosocial well-being of the patient. This chapter presents our therapeutic approach to the management of patients requiring home enteral nutrition from admission to the hospital through outpatient monitoring.

INDICATIONS

The general indications for enteral nutrition include malnutrition or potential for malnutrition, a functional gastrointestinal tract that can be used safely, and an inability to ingest all required nutrients. The rationale for enteral nutrition as compared to parenteral nutrition is that it is less expensive and has beneficial effects on gastrointestinal structure and function.

Specific indications for home enteral nutrition are identified in Table 1. The majority of these criteria should be met prior to discharge.

DISCHARGE PLANNING—PATIENT EDUCATION

For the transition from in-hospital to home enteral nutrition to be a successful one, discharge planning must begin as soon as it is anticipated that home therapy is required. A multidisciplinary health care team should be involved throughout the hospitalization with one person acting as coordinator of the discharge planning-teaching process. Very often the primary staff nurse or nutrition support nurse assumes the role

TABLE 1   Home Enteral Nutrition Patient Selection Criteria

Anticipated length of enteral nutrition longer than 2 weeks.

In-hospital care no longer required.

Appropriate enteral access in place.

Patient/family willing to continue enteral nutrition at home.

Demonstration of in-hospital tolerance to enteral nutrition regimen.

Goals of home enteral nutrition formulated by patient/family and health care team.

Available financial support.

Patient/family education provided by knowledgeable health care team members.

Enteral formula and equipment available on an outpatient basis.

Discharge support and monitoring available.

of coordinator. A checklist is used in the patient's medical record to assure that all team members complete their required tasks. Frequent team meetings are held to update members on discharge planning-teaching progress, plans, and problems. Table 2 lists the roles and tasks of the team members in meeting the needs of the patient and family. The basic content of the patient/family education process is listed in Table 3. Patient education booklets with large print and illustrations, slide-tape or video programs, and actual demonstration techniques are helpful. Return demonstration of feeding techniques by the caregiver to the instructor is essential.

ACCESS

Access for feeding is achieved by various methods depending on the patient's disease, motivation, and body image and the anticipated duration of enteral nutrition. Some patients prefer not to have a permanent feeding tube and may self intubate nasoenterically prior to feeding. Short-term home enteral nutrition may simply require a soft, small-bore

**TABLE 2 Roles and Tasks of Health Care Team in Home Enteral
Nutrition Discharge Planning Process**

Team Member	Roles and Tasks
Nutrition support nurse	Coordinator*—Responsible for completion of all tasks.
Primary staff nurse	Continues and reinforces teaching.
Primary physician	Orders appropriate enteral feeding regimen, provides access, monitors and treats complications.
Dietitian	Recommends appropriate formula, performs nutritional assessment and participates in teaching
Pharmacist	Monitors drug-nutrient interactions, participates in metabolic monitoring, and teaches administration of enteral medications.
Social worker	Investigates and arranges financial support with family.
Discharge planning nurse/commercial vendor	Arranges for home nursing services and equipment/formula provision from supplier in the community. Plans follow-up visits with coordinator and team.

* Coordinator can be any one of the members.

nasoenteric tube. Most often, longer term feeding is anticipated and a more permanent access or tube enterostomy is required.

The tube enterostomy is placed either endoscopically or surgically. The percutaneous endoscopic gastrostomy (PEG) is growing in popularity, because it eliminates the need for a laparotomy and general anesthesia. However, patients with esophageal or gastric lesions and those with prior upper gastrointestinal surgery are not good candidates for this technique. These patients require surgical gastrostomy or jejunostomy that can be placed primarily or at the time of concomitant gastrointestinal surgery. The feeding jejunostomy generally decreases the incidence of pulmonary aspiration in those patients at higher risks for this complication.

TABLE 3   Contents of the Home Enteral Nutrition Education Process

Assessment of patient/family understanding of need and motivation for home enternal nutrition.

Type of enteral access and its appropriate care.

Delivery system including bag, tubing, and pump.

Formula and feeding schedule for intermittent, continuous, or cyclic regimens.

Storage and care of formula and equipment.

Recognition, prevention, and treatment of complications.

Arrangement of appropriate follow-up care.

Phone list of health care team members for emergencies.

FORMULA SELECTION

The dietitian performs a nutritional assessment including calculation of nutrient requirements. It is then determined if the patient needs nutritional maintenance or repletion, followed by the selection of the most appropriate formula. If the patient is taking some food by mouth, the required amount of supplemental feeding is determined. Fluid requirements or restrictions, type of enteral access, secondary disease processes, and cost are also considered. Most patients require a prepackaged, commercially available, complete polymeric formula. Some patients may prefer home blenderized diets because of reduced cost or for social-family inclusion at mealtime. Blenderized diets are generally not encouraged because of the possibility of clogging the feeding tube, nutritional inadequacy, and increased preparation time. It is beyond the scope of this chapter to discuss the details of diet selection, which are discussed elsewhere in this book.

DELIVERY METHODS

Delivery depends on the formula, type of access, and patient or family desires. Generally, the intermittent or bolus method is used when the feeding is being delivered into the stomach (nasogastric tube, PEG, or gastrostomy), and the continuous method is used when the feeding is delivered into the small bowel (nasointestinal or jejunostomy tubes). The feeding schedule should allow the patient as much free time and mobility as possible.

Cyclic feeding is delivered usually via a pump for only part of the day. Many patients prefer 12 or 16 hours of feeding during the evening and night to allow for daytime activities. This feeding schedule should be implemented gradually while the patient is still in the hospital. The delivery system should be as simple as possible for the patient and family. Extraneous equipment should be minimized and individualized to the patient's needs. Some patients are unable to read small print on syringes, handle certain clamps, or hear audio alarms on pumps.

SPECIAL CONSIDERATIONS

When preparing for the patient to return home, the family should set aside a place for formula and equipment storage and preparation. Additional considerations include skin care, both of the nose and around a surgically placed tube, daily cleansing with warm water and mild soap, and application of fresh tape or dry dressing to the nose or wound.

Administration of medications through the tube may be a problem. The pharmacist can help by providing medications as elixers and teaching proper administration techniques. Some medications are given with feedings; however, the therapeutic efficacy of other medications decreases when mixed with the formula and must be given separately.

Often patients wish to receive feedings in a nonconventional setting such as while traveling or fishing. A portable, light-weight pump with a long battery life may meet these needs. The feeding bags can be hung from a hook in an automobile, a nail in a tree, or a clothes hanger.

Although not ideal, often it is necessary to initiate home enteral nutrition to a patient in an outpatient clinic. The goal should be to prevent hospital admission if possible. In this situation enteral formula progression is performed in the home, and the role of the home health care professional becomes even more important to reinforce clinic teaching and monitor feeding tolerance. Teaching patients and family in outpatient settings can be successful depending on the patient and the in-home support system; however, some patients may need to be hospitalized despite the best team efforts.

MONITORING

Monitoring and patient follow-up are crucial in the home enteral nutrition process. Follow-up should be conducted in the home to fully assess the transition. Follow-up is indicated in order to judge nutritional efficacy and prevent complications. It can be accomplished in a variety of ways, all of which should complement each other.

Some form of home nursing service is incorporated into the follow-up plan. This is arranged by the discharge planning nurse or nursing services of commercial vendors or "home companies." The home nurse assesses the patient's adaptation to discharge and gives feedback to the in-hospital team as to compliance, feeding tolerance, and complications.

The patient should return to an outpatient clinic for follow-up with the in-hospital team to assess nutritional efficacy of the enteral therapy, complications, and their prevention and treatment. The monitoring process should include objective serial measurements of weight, anthropometrics, visceral protein levels, mineral and electrolyte levels, and oral food intake if applicable. Subjective measurements of compliance and reinforcement of previous education should also be performed. The key to successful outpatient follow-up is good communication between the in-hospital team, the health care professionals visiting the home, and the patient or family.

It is beyond the scope of this chapter to discuss all enteral nutrition–related complications. Mechanical complications occur more often than gastrointestinal, metabolic, or infectious ones, especially if the patient is on a stable regimen in the hospital. The most frequent complications, including their prevention and treatment are listed in Table 4. The patient or family needs to be taught to identify and handle these complications. Those most likely to occur in an individual patient should be particularly emphasized.

Conclusion. Current health care professionals are discharging patients more rapidly, thereby necessitating increased usage of home enteral nutrition, and the health care team must be prepared to provide this service. The management of home enteral nutrition is a rewarding and challenging task. It requires a team approach with special attention to communication and education.

TABLE 4 Complications of Home Enteral Nutrition

Complication	Prevention	Treatment
Mechanical		
Tube clogging/obstruction	Flush often with water	Flush with carbonated beverage
Tube inadvertent removal	Assure tube is taped or sutured	Replace tube immediately
Tube breakage	Avoid angulation or tension on tube	Replace tube or remove broken end and repair with new end-adaptor
Skin or nasal irritation	Daily skin care as outlined	Use of Karaya or Stomadhesive
		Consult enterostomal therapist
Gastrointestinal		
Diarrhea	Use of fiber in diet	Antidiarrheal medications
	Slow formula progression	
	Use clean technique for formula preparation and delivery	
Constipation	Increase water intake	Stool softeners
	Increase patient activity	
Metabolic		
Hyponatremia	Serial blood chemistries	Add salt
	Assure that formula includes enough sodium	Restrict water
	Monitor intake and output	
Infectious		
Aspiration	Elevate head of bed	Antibiotics
	Provide access distal to pylorus	
	Monitor gastric residuals	

SUGGESTED READING

Folk CC, Courtney ME. Home tube feedings: general guidelines and specific patient instructions. Nutr Supp Serv 1982; 2:18–22.

Nelson JK, Palumbo PJ, O'Brien PC. Home enteral nutrition: observations of a newly established program. Nutr Clin Prac 1986; 1:193–199.

Standards for nutrition support—home patients. Silver Spring, MD: American Society for Parenteral and Enteral Nutrition, 1985.

NUTRITION AND GASTROINTESTINAL DISEASE

ESOPHAGEAL DISEASE

DANIEL W. MURPHY, M.D.
DONALD O. CASTELL, M.D.

Nutritional considerations may play an important role in many esophageal abnormalities. Physician-directed changes in diet are integral in the *management* of gastroesophageal reflux disease, while attention to the timing and nature of the patient's changes in diet may be critical in the *diagnosis* of obstructive esophageal lesions and motility disorders. This discussion is primarily concerned with outlining and exploring the rationale for the dietary modifications recommended in the treatment of gastroesophageal reflux disease (GERD).

GERD is defined as the abnormal movement of gastric contents into the esophagus, resulting in symptomatic or asymptomatic injury to the esophageal mucosa (esophagitis). A detailed discussion of the pathogenesis of GERD is beyond the scope of this chapter. The major antireflux mechanism is generally considered to be the level of pressure and therefore competence of the lower esophageal sphincter (LES). This simplification is particularly germane to this discussion, since the rationale for dietary modifications is largely based on the effect of foods on the competence of the LES.

RATIONALE FOR DIETARY MODIFICATIONS IN THE TREATMENT OF GERD

Heartburn and regurgitation, the symptoms of gastroesophageal

TABLE 1   Foods Most Commonly Implicated as Producing Heartburn*

Food	Daily Heartburn	Infrequent Heartburn
	(% of patients)	(% of patients)
Tomatoes	76	37
Oranges	72	24
Orange juice, grapefruit juice	76	31
Coffee	68	31
Candy (chocolate)	40	12
Alcohol (whiskey, etc.)	60	62
Fried food	88	56
Spicy food	88	80
Hot dogs	68	62

* Results of a survey of 25 patients with daily heartburn and 292 patients with infrequent symptoms (weekly or monthly). Numbers listed represent the percentage of patients reporting that the foods listed precipitate symptoms. A more complete list is detailed in Nebel et al. Am J Dig Dis 1976; 21:953–956.

reflux, are typically postprandial events and are often related to specific foods. Patients will often avoid or at least regret having eaten those foods that precipitate symptoms. A survey of more than 1,000 individuals, including patients and otherwise healthy subjects, demonstrated that there are specific food groups that more often cause heartburn and regurgitation. These include hot dogs, tomatoes, citrus juices, alcohol, fried foods, and spicy foods. Table 1 lists some of the foods evaluated and their potential to produce heartburn. This information raised questions about how these foods cause symptoms. Two general mechanisms have been theorized to account for postprandial symptoms: (1) a weakening of the antireflux barrier by a direct lowering of the LES pressure, and (2) a direct irritative effect of certain foods on the esophageal mucosa.

Food Influence on LES Tone

Many foods have been tested to determine their possible effect on LES tone. Carminatives were actually the first food products shown to have an effect on LES tone. These are substances that by strict definition cause one to expel gas from the stomach. The term "carminative" is usually applied to volatile oil extracts of plants used for flavoring food and includes oil of spearmint, peppermint, garlic, and onion. Oil of peppermint has been shown to significantly lower LES pressure in a group

TABLE 2   Foods Known to Effect LES Pressure

Carminatives	↓
Chocolate	↓
Fat	↓
Protein	↑
Carbohydrate	no change
Alcohol	↓
Coffee	↓ ↑

of normal volunteers, and that action has been generalized to carminatives.

The basic biochemical food groups (fat, protein, and carbohydrates) were individually tested in equicaloric quantities with the following results: (1) fats decreased LES pressure, (2) protein increased LES pressure, and (3) carbohydrate ingestion produced no change in LES pressure.

Chocolate syrup has been shown to decrease LES tone in a dose-dependent fashion, producing immediate and sustained effect of 60 minutes duration. This effect was seen after ingestion of as little as 10 cc of chocolate syrup. Likewise, intravenous and enterally administered alcohol were shown to significantly decrease LES pressure. Inference would lead to the impression that the traditional after-dinner drink and chocolate mints represent a boon to late-night over-the-counter antacid sales. Known food effects on LES pressure are summarized in Table 2.

Food Irritants to Esophageal Mucosa

The information above fits the hypothesis that food-induced heartburn results from food-induced decrease in LES pressure with resultant reflux of stomach contents. However, foods well known to cause heartburn, such as orange juice and tomato juice, fail to cause a significant decrease in LES tone. Doctors and patients alike often point to the acid content of these foods as causing a direct irritating effect on sensitive esophageal mucosa. In actuality, these foods are not very acidic (relative to gastric acid), and their ability to cause heartburn occurs even when their acidity is adjusted to a neutral pH. The chemical characteristic of orange juice, tomato juice, and coffee that results in the sensation of heartburn appears to be their high osmolality. Acid-sensitive patients also developed heartburn with esophageal exposure to hyperosmolar solutions of saline and sucrose. In the studies performed, these solutions had osmolarities in the 600 to 700 range, very similar to the osmolality of commercial orange juice concentrates, tomato products, and coffee.

Coffee was initially thought to cause reflux symptoms secondary to a decrease in LES pressure. As mentioned, coffee has a high osmolality and in "acid-sensitive" individuals, exposure of the esophageal mucosa to coffee reliably results in heartburn. It has been shown that this effect can be blocked by cimetidine (a potent acid inhibitor) but not by placebo, despite the fact that coffee in this setting had no significant effect on LES pressure. Coffee caused only minimal increases in gastric acid secretion in the cimetidine-responsive group. Whether coffee produces heartburn by direct irritative effect or by secondary reflux on stomach contents, or both, remains controversial.

Individuals who report the largest number of foods precipitating reflux symptoms have, as a group, lower LES pressures than individuals who have fewer food intolerances. This is demonstrated in Figure 1, which plots the LES pressure of 25 patients with daily symptoms and 25 patients with monthly symptoms, and in Figure 2, which shows that these

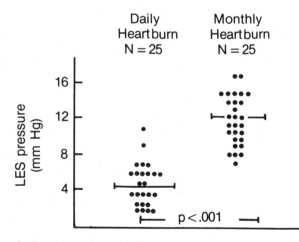

Figure 1 Lower esophageal sphincter (LES) pressures in patients with daily and monthly symptoms of heartburn. (Adapted from Nebel et al. Am J Dig Dis 1976; 21:953–956.)

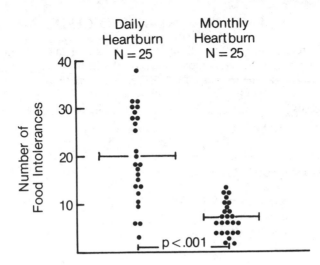

Figure 2 Number of food intolerances cited in patients with daily and monthly symptoms of heartburn. (Adapted from Nebel et al. Am J Dig Dis 1976; 21:953–956.)

same patients with daily heartburn cite a greater number of foods that cause symptoms than do those patients with infrequent heartburn.

Additionally, there appears to be an inverse relationship between the number of foods that precipitate symptoms and the LES pressure, i.e., people with daily heartburn and low LES pressures as a group cite more foods that cause heartburn. The correlation coefficient between increasing numbers of food intolerances and increasing LES pressure is $r = -0.48$, $p < 0.01$.

While LES pressure is an imperfect measure of the antireflux barrier, epidemiologic data such as this supports a role for food-induced decrease in LES pressure in causing symptoms.

It is interesting to note also in Table 1 that those individuals with daily heartburn, and therefore those most likely to have esophageal mucosal damage, are more likely to report symptoms after ingestion of the "irritative foods" (juice, coffee, etc.) while both groups report a high incidence of symptoms after ingesting foods that are thought to act primarily on the LES.

DIETARY APPROACH TO GERD

Therefore, if a patient with reflux disease knows that specific foods cause symptoms, we recommend that those foods be avoided. Likewise, as the end-organ damage of reflux disease (esophagitis) can occur with or without symptoms, we make the following recommendations to individuals with chronic GERD whether the below-listed foods exacerbate symptoms or not:

1. High-protein, low-fat diet
2. Avoid: chocolate
   alcohol
   carminatives
   citrus juices
   tomato products
   coffee

Additionally, we ask these patients to avoid lying down for 3 to 4 hours after eating, as the supine position makes reflux more likely. We prefer that they eat three or four small meals a day, as opposed to one or two large meals, since increased gastric volume also makes reflux more likely. Obesity appears to worsen reflux, probably as a result of increased abdominal pressure associated with increased abdominal girth. Accordingly, we ask these patients to attempt to attain ideal body weight.

These recommendations, in addition to antacids or Gaviscon as needed, constitute the first phase of the treatment of GERD, and these modifications alone will often provide satisfactory symptomatic relief and prevent exacerbation in reflux-prone individuals.

SUGGESTED READING

Cohen S. Pathogenesis of coffee-induced gastrointestinal symptoms. N Engl J Med 1980; 303:122–124.

Nebel OT, Forms MF, Castell DO. Symptomatic gastroesophageal reflux: incidence and precipitating factors. Am J Dig Dis 1976; 21:953–956.

Price SF, Smithson KW, Castell DO. Food sensitivity in reflux esophagitis. Gastroenterology 1978; 75:240–243.

Richter JE, Castell DO. Drugs, foods, and other substances in the cause and treatment of reflux esophagitis. Med Clin North Am 1981; 65:1223–1234.

PEPTIC ULCER DISEASE

JAMES D. WOLOSIN, M.D.
JON I. ISENBERG, M.D.

Peptic ulcer disease represents a group of diseases that result in the formation of a break, or hole, in the gastrointestinal mucosa extending through the muscularis mucosa. In simple terms, this is due to an imbalance in the so-called "aggressive" versus "defensive" factors. The pathogenesis remains incompletely understood despite decades of research, largely into the aggressive factors. Whereas gastric acid and pepsin secretion are required for the formation of peptic ulceration, it is clear that other modulating factors are important. For example, there are some patients with the Zollinger-Ellison syndrome and massively increased basal secretion who have no ulcer. Therefore, acid-pepsin secretion alone is not responsible for ulcer formation in each patient. Duodenal ulcer patients have a tendency towards higher gastric acid secretory rates, but there is a large overlap between normal subjects and ulcer patients; approximately two-thirds of duodenal ulcer patients have normal gastric acid secretory rates. Although the incidence of duodenal ulcer in males has declined during the past 30 years, the lifetime incidence of duodenal ulcer in males remains high (5 to 10 percent). The economic costs, both direct plus indirect, are enormous and have been estimated to approach 3 billion dollars each year in the United States.

The therapeutic options available to the clinician have changed dramatically since the mid 1970s when the first clinical trials demonstrated a clear superiority of high-dose antacids to placebo in the healing of duodenal ulcer. Regarding the physiology and treatment of ulcer disease, many basic questions remain unanswered. What is the basic defect allowing for disruption of the mucosal barrier? Can the natural history of chronic, recurrent peptic ulceration be modified? What is the role of the newer, more potent antisecretory agents in the treatment of routine ulcer disease? How much acid suppression is necessary to allow for healing of an active ulcer? The primary goals of therapy in peptic ulcer disease are fourfold.

1. Expedient Healing. Rapid healing of peptic ulcers is presumed to decrease pain and, more importantly, the incidence of complications. The development of fiberoptic endoscopy has permitted many large, randomized, double-blind clinical trials in which ulcer healing has been objectively measured. The effectiveness of therapy must be compared to placebo controls, which may heal up to 60 percent of duodenal ulcers in 8 weeks and 70 percent of gastric ulcers in 12 weeks. Multiple clinical trials have confirmed the superiority of antacids, histamine H_2 receptor antagonists, and sucralfate over placebo in the healing of gastric and duodenal ulcers; no superiority has been clearly documented for one over the other.

2. Relief of Symptoms. Symptom relief is difficult to assess because of inter- and intra-patient and variability, as well as imprecise methods for the quantitation of pain. Rapid improvement in symptoms has been noted in most trials with both active therapy and placebo. Much of the current data is conflicting; some studies indicate equal efficacy of placebo and active drug, whereas others suggest that active therapy is superior to placebo.

3. Prevention of Recurrence. Prospective studies of ulcer patients have demonstrated a high rate of recurrence following initial healing of the ulcer (both duodenal and gastric). Relapse rates are, for the most part, similar following healing by H_2 receptor antagonists, antacids, and sucralfate. Chronic treatment with H_2 receptor antagonists or sucralfate significantly decreases relapse rates in both duodenal and gastric ulcer. Recently, a single study indicated that antacid tablets taken twice daily also prevent duodenal ulcer recurrences. Although the efficacy of maintenance therapy in duodenal ulcer has been demonstrated, the defined patient population and timing remain less clear.

4. Prevention of Complications. The complication rates for gastric and duodenal ulcers are low, and the effects of long-term medical treatment on complication rates have been difficult to measure. Multiple clinical trials have failed to demonstrate any effect of medical therapy on gastrointestinal bleeding, the most common complication of peptic ulcer disease. However, many of these studies were less than optimally controlled. Complication rates in placebo-controlled prospective ulcer trials have not been systematically assessed.

MEDICAL THERAPY

Medical therapy for peptic ulcer disease can be divided simplistically into those agents that reduce gastric acidity and those that may enhance mucosal defense (Table 1). Prior to 1977, no controlled clinical trials in peptic ulcer disease had been performed, and treatment was empiric with dietary modification, antacids, and anticholinergics. In 1977, Peterson et al demonstrated the superiority of high-dose liquid antacids over placebo in the healing of duodenal ulcer. Since that time, cimetidine, ranitidine, and sucralfate have been introduced in the United States, and multiple controlled trials have demonstrated their efficacy. The phy-

TABLE 1 Drugs Utilized in the Treatment of Peptic Ulcer Disease

Drugs	*Mechanisms*
Agents that reduce gastric acidity:	
Antacids	Neutralization of gastric acid
$AlOH_3$	
$MgOH_2$	
Antisecretory agents:	Suppression of gastric acid and
Histamine H_2 receptor antagonists	pepsin secretion
Cimetidine, ranitidine, famotidine	
Anticholinergic agents	
Probanthine, hyoscyamine, pirenzepine, and others	
Tricyclic antidepressants	
H^+/K^+ ATPase inhibitors	
Omeprazole	
Prostaglandins	These also may enhance mucosal bicarbonate and mucus secretion
Agents that do not alter gastric acid or pepsin secretion:	Multiple mechanisms reported include coating of ulcer crater, binding of bile acids and pepsin, increased mucosal prostaglandin production
Colloidal bismuth compounds	Coating of ulcer crater, suppression of *Campylobacter pyloridis*

sician now has a wide variety of medications with which peptic ulcer disease can be effectively treated.

Drug Therapy

Agents that Reduce Gastric Acidity

These agents form the mainstay of ulcer therapy. They can be further subdivided into those that neutralize acid (i.e., antacids) and those that reduce or inhibit acid and pepsin secretion. At appropriate doses, these have all been shown to have equivalent efficacy in the healing of acute peptic ulcer (Table 2). Pepsinogens are activated as gastric acidity increases (i.e., pH decreases). Therefore, agents that reduce gastric acidity cause a secondary, pH-mediated inhibiton of gastric pepsinogen.

Antacids. Most antacids available today are based on aluminum or magnesium hydroxide or calcium carbonate as their active ingredient.

TABLE 2 Approximate Healing Rates as Determined Endoscopically in Duodenal and Gastric Ulcer Patients

	Daily Dose		Healing Rate (%) At 4 weeks	At 8 weeks
Duodenal ulcer:				
Cimetidine	1.2	g	65–80	80–90
Ranitidine	300	mg	65–80	80–90
Antacids	210	ml	60–75	—
Sucralfate	4	g	60–75	—
Pirenzepine	50	mg	70	—
Colloidal bismuth	20	ml or 4 tab	60–100	80–100
Prostaglandins E_2	400	mg	70–90	—
Omeprazole	20	mg	90–100	—
Placebo	—		20–75	—
Gastric ulcer:				
Cimetidine	1.2	g	50–70	85
Ranitidine	300	mg	40–90	85
Antacid	60	ml	40	70
Sucralfate	4	g	30–60	70
Colloidal bismuth	20	ml or 4 tab	—	61–100
Placebo	—		20–45	55

Their buffering capacity lowers intragastric hydrogen ion concentration, thereby raising gastric pH. Peterson et al demonstrated in 1977 that high-dose antacid therapy (1,008 mEq per day: 30 ml, equivalent to 144 mEq of neutralization, 1 and 3 hours after meals and at bedtime) resulted in superior healing rates over identically appearing placebo. After 4 weeks of treatment, 78 percent of antacid-treated patients' duodenal ulcers had healed versus 45 percent of placebo-treated patients. Unfortunately, these high antacid doses resulted in diarrhea in about 25 percent of patients. In practice, compliance tends to be poor due to untoward side effects as well as the inconvenience of carrying around large quantities of liquid antacid. High doses of aluminum-containing antacids may result in constipation as well as hypophosphatemia.

Berstad et al, Weberg et al, Lam et al, and others have recently examined the dosage and formulation of antacid necessary to promote ulcer healing. They noted that doses much lower than originally tested are equally efficacious. In Hong Kong, doses as low as 120 mEq per day in tablet form produced 4-week healing rates of almost 80 percent, equivalent to those seen with the H_2 receptor antagonists (Fig. 1). Evidence is now

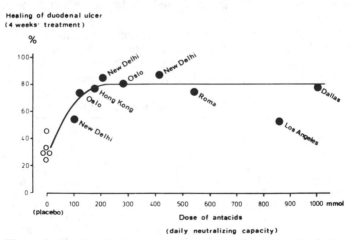

Figure 1 Relationship between percentage healing of duodenal ulcer after 4 weeks of treatment and daily dose of antacids expressed in acid neutralizing capacity in prospective studies in seven different cities worldwide. (Reprinted with modification, with permission from Berstad A, Weberg R. Antacids in the treatment of gastroduodenal ulcer. Scand J Gastroenterol 1986; 21:385–389.)

accumulating that tablet antacids may have a longer duration of action than liquids, probably due to their particulate structure and slower gastric emptying. Many antacid preparations are now available that have low sodium content and high acid buffering capacity (i.e., greater than 5 mEq per milliliter). The cost of a full 6-week course of high-dose antacid therapy may be greater than a course of cimetidine (Table 3).

Histamine H_2 Receptor Antagonists. Receptors for histamine are present on the basal surface of the parietal cell and, when stimulated, result in acid secretion via intracellular cyclic adenosine monophosphate, (Fig. 2). In 1972, Black and his associates developed the first H_2 receptor antagonists, a development that has had a profound effect on the management of peptic ulcer disease. Cimetidine was the first such agent approved for clinical use. It has a structure based on an imidazole ring and closely homologous to histamine. Ranitidine was the second antagonist approved for use; it contains a furan rather than an imidazole ring. Cimetidine, in an oral dose of 300 mg, reduces basal acid output by 95 percent and meal-stimulated acid output by 75 percent. Seventy to ninety percent of duodenal ulcers treated with cimetidine will heal after 4 to 6 weeks of therapy compared to a placebo healing rate of 30 to 60 percent (see Table 2).

The dose of cimetidine used in most clinical trials has varied from 400 mg twice a day to 300 mg four times a day. Recent studies have examined a single dose of 800 mg at bedtime. The healing rates on each of these regimens is equivalent. Therefore, suppression of acid secretion

TABLE 3   Costs of Antiulcer Therapy*

Drug	Dose		Regimen	Cost to Patient for 30-Day Course
Cimetidine	300	mg	q.i.d.	$51 (44–62)
Ranitidine	150	mg	b.i.d	$60 (54–70)
Sucralfate	1	g	q.i.d.	$54 (38–61)
Mylanta II	144	mEq	1 & 3 hr pc + hs	$73 (21–114)
	72	mEq	1 & 3 hr pc + hs	$37 (11–57)
	30	mEq	1 hr pc and hs	$15 (4–24)
Mylanta II tablets	23 mEq/tab		2 tabs 1 hr pc + hs	$13 (10–16)
Maalox Plus tablets	8.5 mEq/tab		2 tabs 1 hr pc + hs	$11 (10–11)

* Costs compiled from five San Diego pharmacies in September 1986.

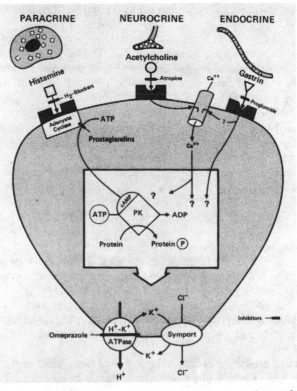

Figure 2 Model representing the secretagogue pathways for stimulation of the parietal cell. Note that there are specific receptors and inhibitors located on the basolateral membrane for the three agonists: histamine, acetylcholine, and gastrin. Also, note that the final step of hydrogen ion secretion involves a H^+/K^+ exchange inhibited by substituted benzimidazoles (e.g., omeprazole). (PK = protein kinase.) (Reprinted with permission from Olson C, Soll AH. The parietal cell and regulation of gastric acid secretion. View Dig Dis 1984; 16(Suppl 1):1–4.)

during the night is of greatest importance. Ranitidine is five to seven times more potent than cimetidine in suppression of gastric acid secretion. It is prescribed as a single 300 mg dose at bedtime or as 150 mg twice daily. No significant difference has been detected between these two drugs in regard to healing.

Side effects with cimetidine occur in less than 4 percent of patients and have generally been mild and reversible. The most significant of these has been mental confusion, especially with intravenous administration, in elderly patients and those with hepatic or renal dysfunction. Inhibition of the hepatic cytochrome P_{450} system by cimetidine may decrease the metabolism of various drugs (e.g., theophylline, warfarin, diazepam, propranolol, and phenytoin), leading to increased blood levels and potential toxicity. In addition, impotence, gynecomastia, and interstitial nephritis have been reported on rare occasions. Ranitidine does not cross the blood-brain barrier and is only infrequently associated with mental confusion or headache. It has a much smaller effect on the cytochrome P_{450} system than cimetidine. Mild alterations in liver function tests have been reported with ranitidine, especially when administered by the intravenous route.

Famotidine, a third H_2 receptor antagonist, was recently approved for use by the Food and Drug Administration. It contains a thiazole ring structure and is 20 times more potent than cimetidine and 7.5 times more potent than ranitidine. Oral doses of 20 mg twice daily or 40 mg once daily at bedtime lead to healing rates for gastric and duodenal ulcer equivalent to those of other H_2 receptor antagonists. Side effects are rare and include rash, headache, and dizziness. Hepatic drug metabolism is not affected.

Anticholinergic Agents. These agents were used in the past for the treatment of peptic ulcer because of their modest effects on gastric acid secretion. There is little data to suggest that these agents are useful as single agents for ulcer healing. Tricyclic antidepressants may exert their antiulcer effect via their specific anticholinergic properties. The routine use of anticholinergic agents is often limited by side effects, including dry mouth, blurred vision, and urinary retention. Pirenzepine, a selective antagonist of the muscarinic M_1 receptor located on the parietal cell is effective in peptic ulcer therapy with fewer side effects. It is not approved for use in the United States.

Omeprazole. Omeprazole, a newly developed substituted benzimidazole compound, is an extremely potent inhibitor of parietal cell

H^+/K^+ ATPase, the final enzyme responsible for gastric acid secretion. Even at low doses, prolonged inhibition of gastric acid secretion is produced. This leads to hypergastrinemia, and after prolonged therapy in animals, gastric endocrine cells as well as the gastric mucosa undergo hyperplasia. In rats, carcinoid tumors of the stomach have developed. Nevertheless, this agent may prove to be useful in the treatment of refractory hypersecretory states such as the Zollinger-Ellison syndrome and in patients with severe peptic ulcer disease. It is currently available in the United States only on an investigational basis.

Prostaglandins. Prostaglandins have broad effects on the gastrointestinal tract. Since they protect the gastroduodenal mucosa from damage, the prostaglandins may be a factor in the pathogenesis of peptic ulcer. Those of the A and E class inhibit gastric acid secretion. In animals, and in some preliminary human studies, natural prostaglandin E and some of its synthetic analogues protect the gastroduodenal mucosa against injury. However, the naturally occurring prostaglandins are rapidly metabolized and relatively ineffective inhibitors of acid secretion when given orally. Several synthetic prostaglandins have been developed that are resistant to degradation in acidic gastric juice and inhibit gastric acid output. In addition, the prostaglandins of the A and E class also stimulate gastroduodenal bicarbonate secretion, thereby increasing mucosal resistance. In initial double-blind prospective studies, synthetic analogues of prostaglandin E have a beneficial effect on the healing of duodenal ulcer. The healing rates at 4 weeks for duodenal ulcer are about 70 percent and at 8 weeks for gastric ulcer about 90 percent, quite similar to those for antacids and histamine H_2 receptor antagonists. In the United States, prostaglandins are available only on an experimental basis.

Drugs that Do Not Alter Acid or Pepsin Secretion

Sucralfate. Sucralfate is the dissacharide sucrose that contains eight aluminum hydroxide sulfate residues. It is approved for use in the United States for treatment of gastric and duodenal ulcers. Its mechanism of action is not fully understood. At a pH of less than 3 to 4, the aluminum hydroxide residues dissociate and become negatively charged. They then may bind to the ulcer base. In experimental studies, sucralfate also binds to bile acids and pepsin. Moreover, recent animal studies suggest that sucralfate stimulates gastroduodenal prostaglandin production.

Sucralfate, when given orally in 1-gram doses four times a day, has produced healing of gastric and duodenal ulcers at rates equal to those for the H_2 receptor antagonists, i.e., about 60 to 75 percent at 4 weeks for duodenal ulcer and 70 percent at 8 weeks for gastric ulcer. However, most trials with sucralfate have allowed the patients to use antacids as needed for relief of pain, which may effect the results, especially in light of recent data indicating that low doses of antacids may expedite healing of duodenal ulcers. It has been suggested that sucralfate should be taken on an empty stomach as food proteins neutralize gastric acid and may bind the sucralfate, thereby rendering it inactive. The major advantage of sucralfate over the H_2 receptor antagonists is its very limited systemic absorption as well as its lack of major side effects. Constipation may occur in 3 to 4 percent. Some medications (e.g., phenytoin, tetracycline, digoxin, and cimetidine) taken at the same time as the sucralfate may be bound to the molecule, thereby decreasing their absorption.

Environmental Manipulations

Diet

Although once heralded as a crucial factor in the treatment and prevention of peptic ulcer disease, there is no evidence that dietary manipulations are of therapeutic benefit in either the acute or the chronic management of patients with peptic ulcer. In fact, over 15 therapeutic trials have failed to reveal a difference in healing rates with bland versus regular diets. In the 1930s through the 1950s, patients were commonly advised to drink milk on an hourly basis and to eat multiple, frequent, small, bland meals for the treatment of peptic ulcer. Milk is actually a very potent stimulus for gastric acid secretion due to its protein and calcium content. In one study, 240 ml of milk, equivalent to one glass, produced an acid secretory response similar to the maximal acid response to pentagastrin. In addition, although milk, like other proteins, has a buffering effect, it leaves the stomach promptly and elevated acid secretion persists. Despite the theoretical disadvantages of milk intake (high lipid content and acid stimulatory effect), many ulcer patients report relief of dyspepsia following milk ingestion.

Bland or soft diets with frequent small feedings have been advocated as well. There is no evidence to suggest that coarse or rough food, high in fiber, abrades or irritates the active ulcer base. Recent studies by Rydning, Berstad, and others have shown that a low-fiber diet may be associated with a greater ulcer relapse rate than a high-fiber diet; no significant advantage was shown for a high- or low-fiber diet in the treatment of acute gastric or duodenal ulcer.

Alcohol and coffee, both caffeinated and decaffeinated, are potent stimulants of gastric acid secretion but have not been shown to retard ulcer healing. Interestingly, whiskey (80 proof) diluted 1:2 (therefore 20 percent alcohol) does not increase gastric acid secretion. However, both white and red wine are very potent stimulants of gastric acid secretion as well as gastrin release; acid stimulation is similar to that with a protein meal or a maximal dose of pentagastrin. The constituent(s) in wine responsible for gastrin release and the marked secretory response is as yet undefined. Furthermore, epidemiologic studies do not indicate that people who ingest moderate amounts of alcohol or coffee have any greater incidence of ulcer disease than those who avoid these substances. Excessive alcohol ingestion can damage the gastrointestinal mucosa, but there is no evidence to demonstrate that small amounts of alcohol impair ulcer healing. A single study involving college students suggested that long-term intake of coffee (and soft drinks) might lead to an increased incidence of peptic ulcer at a later date. While strict avoidance of coffee and alcohol is not necessary for healing of peptic ulcer, they should be avoided in those patients in whom they aggravate symptoms.

Geographic variations in the incidence of peptic ulcer disease have been evaluated in an attempt to correlate dietary patterns with ulcer, but no consistent pattern has emerged. A report from India failed to demonstrate a difference in gastric acid secretion in those patients who resided in an area of increased incidence of peptic ulcer and whose diet consisted primarily of rice compared to a population in southern India who had a lower incidence of ulcer and consumed a diet high in flour.

Thus, there is no clear-cut evidence that dietary manipulation is useful in the management of peptic ulcer disease. It is best that patients avoid those foods that aggravate their symptoms. Night-time snacks should be avoided as these stimulate nocturnal acid secretion. Peptic ulcer patients should not be placed on severely restrictive diets but should be encouraged to eat sensibly and in moderation.

Smoking

Abundant data exist demonstrating that cigarette smoking increases the incidence of ulcers, impairs ulcer healing, and increases relapse rates.

In a 1-year prospective follow-up of 370 patients with healed acute duodenal ulcer, 72 percent of smokers and 21 percent of nonsmokers on no maintenence therapy experienced a relapse, a highly significant difference. Cimetidine prophylaxis decreased the relapse rate to 34 percent in smokers and 18 percent in nonsmokers. These results would suggest that prophylactic therapy is valuable for smokers with duodenal ulcer disease.

Analgesic Medications

Aspirin and other nonsteroidal anti-inflammatory medications are potent inhibitors of prostaglandin synthesis and can damage the gastric and duodenal mucosa. Recent studies have indicated that nonsteroidal analgesics may decrease gastroduodenal bicarbonate secretion, thereby leading to increased susceptibility to the damaging effects of gastric acid. While these agents clearly have been implicated in the pathogenesis of gastric ulcer (i.e., chronic aspirin users have a significantly increased incidence of gastric ulcer), the evidence is less conclusive in regard to duodenal ulcer. Preliminary information indicates that inhibition of gastric acid secretion may lessen the damaging effects of nonsteroidal analgesics.

Stress

Conflicting information is available regarding the influence of stress on peptic ulceration. Severe, overwhelming physiologic stress as is encountered with catastrophic illness, burns, or major surgery is associated with a high incidence of acute erosive gastritis. The influence of daily routine psychologic stress on peptic ulcer diathesis has not been clearly defined. This may be a reflection of the difficulties encountered in the objective measurement of stress. Sedative medications are of no benefit in the routine treatment of peptic ulcer disease.

Initial Therapy

Duodenal Ulcer

Following the diagnosis of ulcer on endoscopy or upper gastrointestinal series, medical treatment is initiated and continued for 4 to 6 weeks. Healing rates of 70 to 90 percent can be anticipated with either cimetidine, ranitidine, antacids, or sucralfate. The cost of each of these medications is nearly identical (see Table 3). Choice of a particular agent is somewhat arbitrary; a 6-week course of either cimetidine or ranitidine is most commonly recommended. Since cigarette smoking is particularly detrimental for ulcer subjects, discontinuation of cigarette smoking is advised. If feasible, discontinuation of nonsteroidal analgesic use is encouraged. Moderation of alcohol and coffee intake seems sensible. If the patient is symptom free at the end of 6 weeks, the medication is discontinued. There is no need to routinely repeat diagnostic studies to document duodenal ulcer healing.

If the patient fails to respond to therapy completely, it is important to consider why. Factors such as noncompliance, nonsteroidal analgesic use, cigarette smoking, and the possibility of Zollinger-Ellison syndrome should be considered. Increasing the dosage of the current medication or changing to another medication may prove useful in this situation. However, there are no data to indicate that combining two different antiulcer medications is better than a single agent. Perhaps in the future omeprazole will be useful for those patients with refractory ulcer disease. If symptoms persist or a complication develops, then repeat endoscopy should be performed.

Recurrent Duodenal Ulcer. In the patient with an acute duodenal ulcer that heals with therapy, there is approximately an 80 percent chance of recurrence in the ensuing year. Twenty to thirty percent of these will be asymptomatic. Relapse rates are similar following healing by H_2 receptor antagonists, antacids, and sucralfate. However, there are preliminary data suggesting that ulcers healed by the colloidal bismuth compounds (not available in the United States) may have a lower rate of relapse. It is curious that *Campylobacter pyloridis*, a bacteria implicated in the etiology of peptic ulcer, is killed by this compound. Cigarette smoking is associated with higher recurrence rates. Long-term maintenance therapy with H_2 receptor antagonists has been shown to lower the relapse rate in patients with healed duodenal ulcer; 70 to 90 percent will have a recurrence within 1 year on placebo therapy as compared to 10 to 30 percent of patients on maintenance treatment. However, as is the case with initial duodenal ulcers, approximately 80 percent of ulcers will heal within 4 to 6 weeks with reinstitution of the standard acute therapy. Unfortunately, once long-term prophylactic therapy is discontinued, duodenal ulcers recur at a rate equal to that in patients who were never placed on maintenance therapy.

What to do in the individual duodenal ulcer patient? This is not totally clear. However, it makes sense to just treat the acute ulcer for 6 to 8 weeks in the patient with a first episode of duodenal ulcer. In the patient who experiences two or more recurrences of duodenal ulcer within a short period of time (i.e., 1 year), maintenance therapy with cimetidine (400 mg at bedtime) or ranitidine (150 mg at bedtime) makes good sense. If recurrent symptoms or ulceration develop on this regimen, long-term treatment with full doses of H_2 receptor antagonists may be in order. Also, consideration of surgical intervention is appropriate.

Gastric Ulcer

The therapeutic approach for gastric ulcer differs from that for duodenal ulcer in that a small but significant risk exists for malignancy at the ulcer site. Approximately 4 percent of benign appearing ulcers may contain cancer. Therefore, endoscopy and multiple (at least six) biopsies from the ulcer margin are routinely performed at the time of diagnosis and also following 8 weeks of therapy. Acute benign gastric ulcer responds equally well to therapy with H_2 receptor antagonists, antacids, or sucralfate (see Table 2). A recent controlled clinical trial demonstrated healing rates with cimetidine of 53, 86, and 89 percent at 4, 8, and 12 weeks, respectively. Large and small ulcers heal at approximately 3 mm per week. Nonsteroidal anti-inflammatory medications are probably the most common inciting agents in gastric ulcer. Our initial approach to gastric ulcer is to discontinue nonsteroidal analgesics (if at all possible), cigarettes, and excess alcohol consumption. Cimetidine or ranitidine is prescribed in full dose (i.e., 300 mg four times daily or 150 mg twice a day, respectively) for 8 weeks followed by repeat endoscopy to assess healing and to rebiopsy unhealed ulcers. If the ulcer has completely healed, therapy is discontinued and the patient followed at regular intervals for symptom recurrence. If the ulcer has not healed, therapy is continued for another 4 weeks and endoscopy is repeated. If the ulcer has still not healed at that time, surgical intervention is usually warranted. Surgery for gastric ulcer is highly effective and associated with a very low (less than 3 percent) postoperative recurrence rate.

Recurrent Gastric Ulcer. The role of maintenance therapy in prevention of recurrent gastric ulcer has recently been studied. Up to 70 percent of patients with acute gastric ulcer will relapse within 1 year. A recent prospective 1-year follow-up study of healed gastric ulcers from our group revealed recurrence in 34 percent, many of which were asymptomatic. Since gastric ulcer tends to occur in patients 10 to 20 years older (about 50 to 70 years old) than the average duodenal ulcer patient, since the recurrence rate is high, and since complications (particularly gastrointestinal bleeding) carry a high risk of morbidity and mortality, we tend to place gastric ulcer patients on chronic long-term treatment.

SURGICAL THERAPY

Duodenal Ulcer

Surgery in duodenal ulcer patients is generally reserved for those with hemorrhage, perforation, penetration, obstruction, or intractability. The latter has become unusual since the development of the H_2 receptor antagonists. Surgery provides the most reliable method of control of chronic ulcer diathesis at the expense of potential chronic morbidity. While less extensive operations, such as proximal gastric vagotomy, are complicated by chronic morbidity in less than 14 percent of patients, the ulcer recurrence rate may be as high as 10 to 15 percent (Table 4). Vagotomy and antrectomy provide a lower ulcer recurrence rate of 0 to 3 percent, but are complicated by long-term morbidity in up to 35 percent. For those patients undergoing elective surgery, proximal gastric vagotomy is the most reasonable procedure unless gastric outlet obstruction is present. The success of this procedure is very much dependent on the experience of the surgeon.

Gastric Ulcer

The indications for surgery in gastric ulcer include those listed for duodenal ulcer. The usual procedure is antrectomy alone or antrectomy plus vagotomy. Gastric ulcers that do not heal should be surgically removed and examined histologically to exclude cancer. Many centers have recommended surgical intervention after two or more recurrences of gastric ulcer. The indications for elective surgery in patients with gastric ulcer include lack of complete healing after 12 weeks of acute therapy, recurrence while on chronic therapy, and recurrence in the noncompliant patient.

In summary, the treatment of peptic ulcer disease continues to evolve as new therapeutic approaches are developed. The widespread availa-

TABLE 4 Approximate Frequencies of Complications due to Surgical Treatment of Peptic Ulcer Disease

| | Operative Mortality | | Late Postoperative Complications | | | | | |
| | | | Dumping | | Diarrhea | | | Incidence of |
	Elective	Emergent	Mild	Severe	Mild	Severe	Weight Loss	Recurrent Ulcers
Subtotal gastrectomy	1%	10%	60%	5%	15%	0%	+++	8%
Truncal vagotomy and pyloroplasty	1%	7%	20%	2%	20%	2%	+	8%
Truncal vagotomy and antrectomy	1%	9–15%	30%	2–5%	20–30%	2%	++	1%
Proximal gastric vagotomy	0.1%	1%	0.5%	0%	1–2%	0%	0	10%

* With permission from Thirlby RC. Surgical therapy. In: Wyngaarden JB, Smith LH, eds. Cecil textbook of medicine. Philadelphia: WB Saunders, 1986:691.

bility of endoscopy and endoscopic biopsy have refined diagnostic and therapeutic capabilities. Current therapy available in peptic ulcer disease is safe and effective. We now have the capacity to induce nearly complete achlorhydria with medications such as omeprazole and to heal ulcer craters rapidly. But how important is near total achlorhydria in the treatment of routine duodenal or gastric ulcer? Probably not terribly important. Higher potency preparations may be unnecessary for the average ulcer patient in whom adequate healing may be achieved with low-dose antacid tablets or nocturnal H_2 receptor antagonist therapy alone. We have rapidly gone from a time when no effective antiulcer medication was available to a period with a surplus of effective drugs. Over the next 10 years, new antisecretory agents and drugs that strengthen the defensive factors may become available. The major goal will be to modify the long-term natural history of peptic ulcer disease and thereby prevent the complications and recurrences that are associated with patient suffering, high economic costs, morbidity, and mortality.

SUGGESTED READING

Isenberg JI, Johansson C. Peptic ulcer disease. Clin Gastroenterol 1984; 13:287–654.

Legerton CW. Management of the ulcer patient: therapeutic advances. Am J Med 1984; 77:1–122.

McArthur K, Hogan D, Isenberg JI. Relative stimulatory effects of commonly ingested beverages on gastric acid secretion in humans. Gastroenterology 1982; 83:199–203.

Peterson WL, Barnett C, Walsh JH. Effect of intragastric infusions of ethanol and wine on serum gastrin concentration and gastric acid secretion. Gastroenterology 1986; 91:1390–1395.

Peterson WL, Richardson CT. Pharmacology and side effects of drugs used to treat peptic ulcer. In: Sleisenger MH, Fordtran JS, eds. Gastrointestinal diseases: pathophysiology, diagnosis, and management. 3rd ed. Philadelphia: WB Saunders, 1983:708.

Richardson CT. Gastric ulcer. In: Sleisenger MH, Fordtran JS, eds. Gastrointestinal diseases: pathophysiology, diagnosis, and management. 3rd ed. Phildelphia: WB Saunders, 1983:672.

Soll AH, Isenberg JI. Duodenal ulcer disease. In: Sleisenger MH, Fordtran JS, eds. Gastrointestinal diseases: pathophysiology, diagnosis, and management. 3rd ed. Philadelphia: WB Saunders, 1983:625.

Walker CO. Complications of peptic ulcer disease and indications for surgery. In: Sleisenger MH, Fordtran JS, eds. Gastrointestinal diseases: pathophysiology, diagnosis, and management. 3rd ed. Philadelphia: WB Saunders, 1983:725.

GASTRIC SURGERY

JERRY RADZIUK, M.D., Ph.D., C.M.
DON C. BONDY, M.D., F.R.C.P.

PRINCIPLES OF GASTRIC SURGERY

A number of surgical procedures for the treatment of peptic ulcer dis-' ease, reflux esophagitis, and neoplasia are associated with clinical nutritional problems. The surgical procedures most commonly used in the treatment of peptic ulcer disease have as their goal the reduction of gastric acid secretion. Either the nervous phase of gastric secretion (by vagotomy) or the hormonal phase (by partial gastrectomy) are attacked. In this context, the common operative procedures are vagotomy and pyloroplasty (or gastrojejunostomy) and subtotal gastrectomy (including antrectomy) with or without vagotomy. With the subtotal gastrectomy there are three common methods of anastomosis of the remaining stomach to the intestine: gastroduodenostomy (Billroth I, Bl), gastrojejunostomy (Billroth II, B2), or less commonly, to a surgically created side limb of the jejunum (Roux-en-Y procedure).

For some patients with stomach cancer a total gastrectomy may be the required treatment. For patients with severe reflux esophagitis who develop such complications as hemorrhage, stricture or pulmonary disease, or who do not respond to intensive medical management, surgical treatment may be considered. Recent surgical techniques are aimed at creating an intra-abdominal segment of the esophagus by means of various fundoplication operations (Nissen, Hill, or Belsey) that are designed to prevent gastric acid reflux into the esophagus.

EFFECTS OF SURGERY ON GASTRIC SECRETION

One might think that operations designed to decrease gastric acid secretion would be associated with significant metabolic or nutritional disturbances arising from the achlorhydria produced by these procedures. Gastric acid does reduce the number of microorganisms in the stomach and small intestine. Colonization of the upper small intestine by bacteria would be expected to cause significant malabsorption, but such malabsorption is in fact uncommon. Bacterial metabolites such as N-nitroso

112

compounds may be carcinogenic. The question of an increased incidence of carcinoma following subtotal gastrectomy remains a matter of some controversy. Retrospective studies suggested an incidence of carcinoma of up to 16 percent of these patients, but subsequent prospective studies reduce this estimate to 3 percent of patients 20 years or more after the surgery. The need for and frequency of screening assessments in this patient population have not been well established. The loss of gastric intrinsic factor might be expected to lead to the development of pernicious anemia, but again this is uncommon.

EFFECTS OF SURGERY ON GASTRIC MOTILITY

There are profound changes in gastric motility as a result of gastric surgical procedures; in general, these operations lead to dramatic increases in the gastric emptying of both liquids and solids. Our own work has shown that for a 100 g load of 50 percent glucose, nearly half of the ingested glucose is emptied from the stomach of patients with gastric surgery within 10 minutes, whereas in normal subjects only 25 g of this load is emptied after 1 hour. This rapid gastric emptying is seen after partial gastrectomy with or without vagotomy and after vagotomy with pyloroplasty or gastrojejunostomy. What is responsible for the increased gastric emptying?

Vagotomy

There are three types of vagotomy: the traditional truncal vagotomy in which the nerve trunks are divided with loss of nerve supply to the stomach and other abdominal organs; total gastric or selective vagotomy with division of the nerves supplying the stomach but not those supplying other viscera; and proximal gastric or superselective vagotomy with division of the branches of the vagus to the upper stomach only. Each of these procedures affects the upper stomach similarly. With swallowing there is a normal vagally mediated response of relaxation of the proximal stomach as it fills with food. This "receptive relaxation" keeps intragastric pressure low. Gastric accommodation or compliance is also vagally mediated. After all types of vagotomy the proximal stomach develops higher pressures and empties more quickly. Inhibitory reflexes mediated by the vagus are also affected; fatty meals are less effective in slowing emptying and the stomach now empties more rapidly in the upright position with loss of some neural reflexes. Antral peristalsis is either reversed or ineffective after truncal or selective vagotomy; gastric stasis and vomiting develop. Because of this stasis these two procedures must be accompanied by a separate drainage operation. Because superselective vagotomy does not affect antral peristalsis, no drainage procedure is necessary.

Gastric Resection

Distal gastric resection and total gastric resection are followed by rapid emptying of large solid particles. The loss of the pylorus also allows reflux of bile from the intestine; to prevent reflux the Roux-en-Y anastomosis was developed. With this procedure gastric emptying remains rapid but less so than with B1 or B2 anastomoses and reflux is prevented. The rapid emptying is observed when these operations are done with or without an added vagotomy.

PHYSIOLOGIC CHANGES

After most forms of gastric surgery large quantities of food are emptied from the stomach with much of the meal still in the form of large particles, which are poorly digested. With many of these operations the food is passed into the small intestine distal to the biliary and pancreatic secretions, which enter the intestine in the duodenum. There is poor mixing of food and digestive juices. The duodenum is a major source for the enteric hormones stimulating digestive secretions; food entering the jejunum as in a B2 anastomosis would provoke a weaker and less prompt digestive response. Our studies indicate that the small intestine is able to absorb glucose at a maximum rate of about 1 g per minute. The rapid emptying of carbohydrate meals easily saturates the absorptive capacity with unabsorbed, osmotically active carbohydrate passing through the small intestine to the colon. The presence of carbohydrate in the distal small intestine causes peptides such as neurotensin and nonpancreatic glucagon to appear in the blood. When undigested carbohydrate reaches the colon, colonic bacteria may produce large amounts of gas from this substrate.

Carbohydrate metabolism is profoundly affected in these patients. Our observations revealed that only 60 percent of a glucose load was absorbed (normal 92 percent), and absorption took place over only 100 minutes because of the rapid emptying as opposed to a normal interval of 220 minutes. Glucose clearance from the circulation remained unchanged, peaking at 130 minutes after absorption had ceased in these patients. This mismatch between the rate of absorption and the rate of clearance of glucose resulted in hypoglycemia. We were able to duplicate these observations in normal patients by infusing glucose into the duodenum at the same rapid rate as was observed in the patients who had had gastric surgery. We therefore believe that the rapid gastric emptying and the resulting decrease in absorption following these surgical procedures are the principal sources of the complications of gastric surgery. Their circumvention forms the rationale for treatment.

CLINICAL COMPLICATIONS

It must be stressed that about 75 percent of patients undergoing gastric surgery have an excellent result with minimal complications. The remaining 25 percent have a number of clinical problems: early satiety, reduced dietary intake, weight loss, steatorrhea, diarrhea, nutritional deficiencies, anemia, lactose intolerance, bone disease, dumping syndrome, late dumping or hypoglycemia, and bile gastritis. Following the fundoplication operations for reflux esophagitis, some patients develop a gas-bloat syndrome. Although we have emphasized the importance of rapid gastric emptying as the usual result of these operations, a few patients will instead have delayed gastric emptying and phytobezoar formation.

Postprandial Abdominal Discomfort

A variety of postprandial complaints are voiced by these patients. Symptoms may include early satiety, abdominal cramps, and vomiting. At times these symptoms may be so severe as to leave the patient literally afraid to eat, and it is not surprising that decreased dietary intake and weight loss follow. In our experience this has been much more common with partial gastrectomy than with vagotomy and pyloroplasty. If the patient has a job requiring physical exertion he may be forced to seek other employment when these symptoms prevent food intake sufficient to meet energy requirements. As many as 10 percent of postgastrectomy patients may have that outcome. Many patients will attribute their symptoms to various foods and eliminate them until they finally arrive at a nutritionally deficient "tea and toast" type of diet. As discussed, these symptoms can obviously be attributed to decreased gastric accommodation and gastric incontinence, which result in the entry of food into the jejunum at a rate exceeding absorptive capacity. Painful distention of this organ results.

Therapy. The obvious treatment for this problem is to take frequent small feedings of up to six meals daily. A dietary history should be obtained; we recommend a food diary for 3 days with subsequent analysis by a dietitian. The dietitian and the patient together can work out an adequate diet taking into account the patient's needs, daily schedule, and personal preferences. Usually a satisfactory dietary intake can be obtained within the year following the surgery.

Dumping Syndrome

When the symptoms of postprandial discomfort are associated with a feeling of weakness, a desire to lie down, and such vasomotor disturbances as flushing, sweating, tachycardia or hypotension, that clinical complex is termed the dumping syndrome. Again, rapid gastric emptying and decreased absorption are the underlying causes. The discomfort is due to jejunal distention: the jejunal absorptive mechanisms are saturated, with the result that the small intestine contains osmotically active particles. Fluid drawn into the intestine to restore normal osmolarity comes from the vascular volume causing hypovolemia and explaining, in part, the weakness, tachycardia, and hypotension. As mentioned, a number of enteric peptides such as neurotensin, glucagon, bradykinin, serotonin, gastric inhibitory polypeptide (GIP), and vasoactive intestinal polypeptide (VIP) are present at abnormally high levels. Since some of these are vasoactive they may contribute to the problem. Again their presence is linked to abnormal patterns of absorption (e.g., increased ileal absorption).

Therapy. The aim of therapy remains the decrease of the osmolar load in the small intestine. This can be achieved by slowing gastric emptying and/or increasing the consumption of complex carbohydrates. General principles of the physiology of gastric emptying suggest that solid meals are emptied more slowly than liquids, that after vagotomy emptying is slower in the supine position than in the upright, and that fat or hyperosmolar solutions will inhibit gastric emptying. The application of these principles leads to the following approaches:

1. Prefeeding fat or such hypertonic solutions as sweetened orange juice 15 to 30 minutes before the meal. Reflexes will be activated and enteric hormones released, thus potentially slowing gastric emptying by the time the meal is consumed.
2. Dry meals. Liquids are withheld until 1 hour after the meal.
3. Frequent small meals to prevent jejunal overloading.
4. Avoidance of simple sugars, with the dietary carbohydrate supplied primarily as starches in an attempt to decrease the osmolarity if rapid emptying develops.
5. Having the patient lie down for a half hour or so immediately after eating when possible.

Other therapeutic agents, including anticholinergics and serotonin antagonists, have been used. An interesting recent approach has been the use of agents that increase viscosity and slow gastric emptying. Pectin and guar gum are two such agents, the usual dose being of the order of 10 to 15 g with each meal. Inhibition of glycoside-hydrolase activity decreases the osmolarity within the intestine by preventing complete breakdown of carbohydrate to monosaccharides. Acarbose, the first such agent to be used experimentally and to be marketed, has been found to improve clinical symptoms. Evidently since it decreases absorption there will be some compensating increase in the osmotic load. However, our own studies have shown that the decrease in absorption is dose dependent, while there is a significant lengthening of the period of absorption even at the lowest doses. It is thus likely that low doses of Acarbose would decrease the osmolar load, slow transit, and in an apparently paradoxical fashion, even increase the amount of carbohydrate absorbed. A suggested starting dose is 50 mg before meals, which can be titrated to improve symptoms.

Most patients with the dumping syndrome will improve considerably within a year of beginning treatment. About 1 percent of all postgastric surgery patients may suffer with prolonged dumping syndrome that is unresponsive to therapy.

Diarrhea, Steatorrhea, Malabsorption, and Maldigestion

As outlined above, the causes of diarrhea following gastric surgery also relate to rapid gastric emptying, absorptive and digestive capacities that are consequently overwhelmed, and poor mixing of food and digestive juices. The release of large solid particles resistant to digestion by the postoperative stomach is also contributory. As before, water is drawn into the intestine to counter the osmotic load, with resultant volume loading. This leads to rapid transit through the small bowel. Previously undocumented lactose intolerance may appear as lactase is stripped from the luminal wall by the rapid passage of large fluid volumes. This will obviously aggravate the problem.

Diarrhea is a common and troublesome sequel to gastric surgery affecting up to 25 percent of patients. It is seen least often after superselective vagotomy without a drainage procedure.

Therapy. All of the above-mentioned efforts to decrease the intestinal osmotic load apply. If lactose intolerance is a problem, lactase may be added to milk or ingested in tablet form with the milk (Lactaid).

Should dietary measures prove ineffective cholestyramine 4 g with meals, codeine 15 mg or diphenoxylate 5 mg 30 minutes before meals, or loperamide 2 to 8 mg twice a day can be used. On a cost basis codeine is preferable. The opiate agents codeine, diphenoxylate, and loperamide have little potential for addiction, particularly if their use is reserved for important social engagements when diarrhea would be embarrassing.

The steatorrhea and maldigeston are usually not of clinical importance and do not require pancreatic enzyme replacement. When steatorrhea is significant, a search for the usual causes such as celiac disease or pancreatic insufficiency is mandatory.

Anemia

Patients who have had a B2 partial gastrectomy are particularly susceptible to the development of anemia over a period of years. Inadequate dietary folate, malabsorption of iron, and decreased intrinsic factor, or more likely inadequate digestion of bound vitamin B_{12}, are factors leading to folate, iron, and vitamin B_{12} deficiency anemias. Iron deficiency is the most common type of anemia. Therapy is by replacement of the deficient nutrient.

Late Dumping or Hypoglycemia

As described earlier this is another sequel to rapid gastric emptying and inappropriate absorption patterns. Hypoglycemia appears 2 hours after a meal as a result of an imbalance between intestinal absorption and clearance of glucose from the circulation.

Therapy. Frequent, small, low-carbohydrate meals with some portion of the meal withheld to be consumed 90 minutes later are usually all that is required to control this complication. Acarbose with or without pectin or guar gum is also effective. When the symptoms are intractable and follow vagotomy and pyloroplasty, a take-down of the pyloroplasty with restoration of the pylorus has been done with some success.

Bone Disease

Both osteoporosis and osteomalacia may develop when patients have inadequate intake of calories, calcium, or vitamin D after gastric surgery. In our experience this is most often observed in patients who have undergone a partial gastrectomy and gastrojejunostomy. Treatment is primarily preventive, i.e., ensuring that nutrition is adequate. Replacement of calcium and vitamin D is necessary if bone disease develops.

Phytobezoar Formation

In the less common situation where poor or incomplete gastric emptying of solids follows gastric surgery, undigested plant material may collect as a yellow-green mass. Anorexia, nausea, vomiting, and abdominal pain then follow. Very rarely, the bezoar may pass into and obstruct the small intestine.

In our experience these phytobezoars disappear after 1 or 2 weeks of a liquid diet without requiring endoscopic disruption with a snare, cellulase therapy, or surgical removal. Once the bezoar has been dissolved or removed, recurrence can be prevented by the use of the prokinetic agents metoclopramide or domperidone 10 to 20 mg, 30 minutes before meals.

Gas-Bloat Syndrome

After fundoplication some patients experience postprandial discomfort, bloating, and distention. They feel that if they could belch the sensation would be relieved, but the fundoplication prevents this. In our experience, it occurs in those patients who preoperatively had some symptoms of dyspepsia suggestive of delayed gastric emptying in addition to the symptoms of esophagitis. We have had some modest success with the use of prokinetic agents before meals, but in a few patients the symptoms have been so troublesome that a revision of the fundoplication was necessary.

Bile Reflux Gastritis

Significant reflux of bile is seen often with both gastric resections and pyloroplasty. The gastric mucosa may be inflamed or coated with exudate or bleed easily. Clinical correlation is poor in that severe gastritis may not be associated with any symptoms while severe bilious vomiting and epigastric pain may occur with less obvious gastritis.

While treatment with cholestyramine has not been successful and the use of cytoprotective agents such as sucralfate or misoprostil has not been clearly established to be of benefit, the prokinetic agents may offer some relief. Relief from severe bile reflux can be obtained in up to 70 percent of patients with conversion to a Roux-en-Y anastomosis.

SUGGESTED READING

Becker HD. Hormonal changes after gastric surgery. Clin Gastroenterol 1980; 9:755–771.

Creutzfeldt W. Acarbose, effects on carbohydrate and fat metabolism. Excerpta Medica, International Congress Series 594, 1982.

Radziuk J, Bondy DC. Abnormal oral glucose tolerance and glucose malabsorption after vagotomy and pyloroplasty. Gastroenterol 1982; 83:1017–1025.

CELIAC DISEASE

LYN J. HOWARD, M.A., B.M., B.Ch.(Oxon), F.R.C.P.(UK),
F.A.C.P.(USA)
SHARON A. ALGER, M.D.

DIAGNOSIS

Gliadin, a polypeptide component of wheat, rye, barley, and oat flour, has been identified as the etiologic agent in celiac disease. An antigenic response is triggered through the binding of gliadin to a receptor protein at the enterocyte surface, resulting in inflammatory mucosal changes, especially within the proximal small bowel. Suppression of this destructive process is dependent on elimination of gluten from the diet. The implications for life-long dietary restriction, along with an associated risk of autoimmune disorders and malignancy, necessitates diagnostic accuracy.

Jejunal biopsy has been the traditional method of detecting the villous blunting and enhanced crypt mitoses characteristic of celiac disease. Since similar findings are seen in other inflammatory bowel disorders, such as severe viral gastroenteritis, giardiasis, cow's milk allergy, and hypogammaglobulinemia, a triple biopsy approach has been recommended in an effort to enhance diagnostic specificity. Biopsy specimens are taken at the time of initial diagnosis, after gluten withdrawal, and once again following gluten challenge. Although an initial biopsy remains essential in the evaluation of celiac disease, other tests have been described that offer less invasive monitoring options and may obviate the need for a subsequent in vivo gluten challenge. Table 1 lists the tests that are usually abnormal in celiac disease and also references several new tests that have potential for use in long-term patient surveillance as well as diagnosis.

The "sugar tests" (see Table 1) are based on the observation that patients with villous atrophy have decreased absorption of monosaccharides secondary to the damaged brush border, while at the same time exhibiting an increased permeability to larger polar molecules; this perhaps reflects widened interepithelial cell junctions. A ratio expressing the urinary excretion of two types of sugars, a mono- and polysaccharide, has been shown to provide a sensitive and specific method for distinguishing gluten sensitivity from other malabsorptive syndromes. The

TABLE 1 Initial Assessment and Diagnosis of Celiac Disease

Routinely Available Tests	Special Tests
Anthropometric measurements	Cellobiose/mannitol 5-hr excretion ratio[*] ⎫ "sugar tests"
72-hour fecal fat	Lactulose/L-rhamnose 5-hr excretion ratio[†] ⎬
RBC folate	[51]Cr EDTA absorption test[‡]
D-Xylose absorption	α-Gliadin antibody[§]
Serum carotene	In-vitro mucosal culture and assessment
Breath hydrogen	of alkaline phosphatase with and without
Radiography: barium meal	gliadin in the growth medium[#]
Jejunal biopsy	

With permission from

[*] Cobden I, Rothwell J, Axon ATR. Intestinal permeability and screening tests fro celiac disease. Gut 1980; 21:512–518.

[†] Menzies IS, Pounder R, Heyer S, et al. Abnormal intestinal permeability to sugars in villous atrophy. Lancet 1979; 2:1107–1109.

[‡] Bjarnason I, Peters TJ. A persistent defect in intestinal permeability in coeliac disease demonstrated by a ^{51}Cr-labelled EDTA absorption test. Lancet 1983; 1:323–325.

[§] O'Farrelly C, Kelly J, Hekkens W, et al. α-Gliadin antibody levels: a serological test for coeliac disease. Br Med J 1983; 286:2007–2010.

[#] Katz AJ, Falchuk ZM. Definitive diagnosis of gluten sensitive enteropathy. Gastroenterology 1978; 75:695–700.

presence of increased mucosal permeability in celiac patients is also shown by the enhanced absorption of ^{51}Cr EDTA and excretion of radioactivity in the urine. This test accurately distinguishes celiac patients from controls. Celiac patients in complete remission, as demonstrated by lack of symptoms and a normal biopsy, are still mildly abnormal by this test, which suggests the possibility of a primary defect of the mucosal structure that may predispose the patient to an exaggerated immunologic response from enteral antigenic stimulation. This test may be useful in screening high-risk populations, such as asymptomatic relatives of celiac patients, for evidence of subclinical mucosal abnormalities.

Cultures of small bowel biopsies have demonstrated in vitro changes in enterocyte alkaline phosphatase enzyme levels between celiac and control tissue cultures, exposed to a gluten-containing medium. This test holds potential for avoiding the in vivo gluten challenge and rebiopsy.

CLINICAL MANIFESTATIONS

The clinical presentation of celiac disease covers a wide spectrum. Patients may be asymptomatic with abnormalities evident only through laboratory data (anemia, mineral and vitamin deficiencies) or they may present in a severe malabsorptive state, exhibiting life-threatening fluid and electrolyte losses. The extent of mucosal damage may range from a small area of the proximal jejunum to involvement of the entire small bowel.

Severe disease is more common in infants less than 9 months and develops shortly after the introduction of solid food, classically gluten-containing cereals. The presentation typically includes diarrhea, weight loss, and growth arrest. The child is usually whiny and irritable and may exhibit evidence of abdominal distention. Fifteen percent of children present primarily with vomiting, which may be projectile. The term "celiac crisis" refers to the severely dehydrated state that may arise from combined emesis and diarrhea, often precipitated by an underlying infection. Abdominal radiography reveals large dilated loops with air fluid levels, suggestive of paralytic ileus.

In older children and adults, the symptoms are more variable. Chronic diarrhea, growth failure, and anemia refractory to iron are common presenting symptoms. More insidiously, the clinical picture may reflect chronic malnutrition with edema, bone pain due to osteomalacia and secondary hyperparathyroidism resulting from calcium and vitamin D malabsorption. Table 2 lists laboratory tests that are helpful in evaluating and managing celiac disease. The list includes tests for many potential mineral and vitamin deficiencies that may arise as a result of severe malabsorption and that can be scaled down in patients with minimal evidence of malabsorption.

DIETARY MANAGEMENT

Acute and chronic dietary modification in the management of celiac patients is best addressed through division into various age categories:

Infants (3 to 12 months)

Dietary management for this age group consists of:

1. Assessment and repletion of fluid and electrolytes
2. Correction of acidosis
3. Evaluation and stabilization of Ca^{++} and Mg^+ levels
4. Caloric repletion
5. Vitamin and mineral supplementation

TABLE 2 Laboratory Tests for Evaluation and Management of Celiac Disease

Laboratory Assessment	Normal Values	Deficiency
Serum Fe/ferritin	Iron >60 µg/dl Ferritin >30 mg/dl	Iron <50µg/dl Ferritin <12 mg/dl
Serum folate	Serum 3–9 ng/ml RBC folate 150–600 ng/ml	Serum <3 ng/ml RBC folate <100 ng/ml
Vitamin K evaluation, PT ratio	1.0–1.2	>1.3
$Na^+/K^+/Cl^-/HCO_3^-$	Na 135–145 mEq/L K 3.5–4.0 mEq/L Cl 98–106 mEq/L	Na <130 mEq/L K <3.5 mEq/L Cl <85 mEq/L
Magnesium—serum and 24-hr urine collection	Serum 1.3–2.5 mg/dl Urine 8 mEq/day (96 mg/day)	Serum <1.0 mg/dl Urine <4 mEq/day (<50 mg/day)
Calcium	Serum 8.6–10.8 mg/dl	<8.5 mg/dl with normal albumin
Albumin	>3.5 g/dl	<3.0 g/dl
Vitamin A	25–60 µg/dl	<20µg/dl
Vitamin E (α-tocopherol)	0.8–1.2 mg/dl	<0.5 mg/dl
Vitamin D (25-OH-D)	10–80 ng/ml	<5 ng/ml
Zinc	70–120 µg/dl	<50 µg/dl with albumin normal
Copper	90–130 ng/dl	<50µg/dl
Vitamin B_{12} (cobalamin)—if terminal ileum involved	200–900 pg/ml	<150 pg/ml

With permission from Howard L, Michalek A. Home parenteral nutrition. Ann Rev Nutr 1984; 4:78–81.

Young infants are most at risk for severe dehydration, and they frequently have marked electrolyte imbalances. These problems must take first priority in treatment. Calcium and magnesium may fall to dangerously low levels, and infants have presented with seizures as a result. It is important to recognize that hypomagnesemia can contribute to the hypocalcemia and hypokalemia of steatorrhea. Magnesium is the metallo-cofactor for both hydroxylation steps of vitamin D (25 [OH] vitamin D formed in the liver, and 1:25 Di [OH] vitamin D formed in the kidney). Dihydroxyvitamin D is required for calcium absorption from the gut and calcium reabsorption in the kidneys. Magnesium is also involved in the release and function of parathormone and resorption of calcium from bone. Magnesium is the metallo-cofactor for the chief membrane Na/K adenosinetriphosphatase (ATPase), which pumps potassium into cells and pumps sodium out. With magnesium deficiency, potassium leaks out of cells into the extracellular fluid and the urine. Correction of hypocalcemia and hypokalemia is only temporarily achieved by exogenous supplementation unless hypomagnesemia is also corrected. Magnesium is poorly absorbed from the gut, and massive doses exacerbate diarrhea; thus acute replacement is best achieved parenterally (deep intramuscular injection or slow intravenous drip), providing 1 to 2 mEq magnesium per kilogram over 24 hours. Once these concerns have been addressed, attention can be focused on the need for dietary modifications.

With severe diarrhea, especially in young infants, therapy should begin with a trial of a defined formula diet, starting one-half strength to avoid a high osmotic load. Clinical severity may dictate continuous nasogastric drip. Studies suggest that protein is best provided as di- and tripeptides, not as free amino acids, since small peptides have enhanced ability to traverse damaged gut mucosa. A lactose-free carbohydrate source is necessary initially, and a large percentage of fat calories should be provided as medium-chain triglycerides (MCT). An example of such a formula is Pregestimil (Mead Johnson).

In severe cases where vomiting and diarrhea persist despite a defined diet, a short course of parenteral nutrition may be necessary. This option should be strongly considered for infants presenting in celiac crisis. Clinical improvement commonly begins within 2 to 3 days. The child becomes less irritable and starts sleeping well. As the diarrhea subsides on parenteral feeding, a slow nasogastric drip of enteral formula is started and then incrementally shifted to full volume over 3 to 5 days as parenteral infusion is decreased. If the progress is maintained, the infant is switched to bolus and then oral feeds. After the infant has been doing well on this regimen for several weeks, a more polymeric lactose-free formula can be substituted. After 2 to 3 months, lactose is gradually reintroduced, and rice cereal, fruit, and vegetables are added (Table 3). Mineral and vitamin supplementation should be provided at twice the daily requirement until growth is fully restored.

Young Children (Toddlers aged 1 to 3 years)

Dietary management for this age group consists of:

1. Fluid/electrolyte repletion
2. Caloric repletion
3. Vitamin and mineral supplementation

In cases of severe diarrhea, both gluten and lactose should be eliminated from the diet. A high degree of fat malabsorption as determined by 72-hour fecal fat may warrant the use of medium-chain triglyceride oils as a supplemental fat and calorie source until steatorrhea decreases. This oil may be substituted for other oils in frying and baking. Toddlers will tolerate rather monotonous dietary regimens, and therefore, it is most efficacious to simply provide the family with a list of a few foods within the various food groups that can be safely consumed and that form a balanced diet. A sample list of ten allowable foods is presented in Table 3.

Older Children and Adults

Dietary management for this age group consists of:

1. Caloric repletion
2. Mineral and vitamin supplementation

The introduction of MCT oil is helpful in the initial stages when there is significant intolerance of long-chain triglycerides. The temporary restriction of lactose during the early stages of gut healing helps to eliminate excessive bloating and cramping. The diet should provide protein, carbohydrate, and fat calories in the ratio of 20:50:30, respectively. The total caloric intake should be increased to one- and one-half times

TABLE 3 Feeding Guide for Recovered Gluten-Sensitive Enteropathy Children

Infants (6–12 months)	Toddlers (1–3 years)	10 "Safe Foods"
Breast milk or up to 32 oz Fe-fortified formula	3 servings milk/milk products*	Hard cheese/milk*
8–10 tbsp Gerber's dry rice cereal Heinz/Beechnut rice cereal	2 servings meat or meat substitute	All plain fresh meat/poultry
Daily servings fruit/vegetable ad lib	3–4 servings fruit/vegetables/fruit juice	All fresh fruit/vegetables
Teething foods—gluten-free rice wafers and table food	3 servings gluten-free bread or cereal	Eggs
		Rice cakes/flour/cereal (Sugar Pops, Puffed Rice)
		Jif or Skippy peanut butter
		Oscar Mayer hot dogs and bologna
		Jello pudding*
		Homemade ice cream *
		Corn tacos

* Omitted while diet is lactose free; Lact-Aid milk can replace regular milk. With permission from Weiss M, Davis J, Smith A. Pointers for parents coping with celiac sprue. Chicago: Children's Memorial Hospital, 1982.
With permission from Flock M. Nutrition and diet therapy in gastrointestinal disease. New York: Plenum, 1981.

maintenance in patients recovering from severe cachexia. After a month, the reintroduction of lactose should begin with partially fermented products, such as hard cheese, yogurt, and buttermilk. A slow progression to other lactose-containing foodstuffs is then attempted, with final return to ingestion of all dairy products.

The total elimination of gluten requires a high degree of patient and family education. Wheat is used as an extender in many foodstuffs, including ice cream and salad dressing, and in ingredients as ubiquitous as "hydrolyzed vegetable protein." It is also found in many commonly prescribed drugs including Dyazide (SK&F), Dexedrine (SK&F), Tagamet (SK&F), Xanax (Upjohn), and Ibuprofen (Kenral). It is helpful to provide patients with a list of local and national celiac support groups and references on gluten-free cooking (Table 4). The celiac support groups assist patients in keeping abreast of commercially available gluten-free products.

It is recommended that initially patients be seen by a nutritionist twice monthly and keep a 7-day diet diary prior to each session. Clinical signs of malabsorption can then be carefully correlated with dietary intake. In children, lack of growth may be the only manifestation of persistent malabsorption. It has been found that 80 percent of patients will respond to a gluten-free diet over a 2 to 3 month trial period.

The proximal small bowel is the normal absorptive site of most

TABLE 4 Resources for Patients with Celiac Disease

Reference Books	Support Groups
Lawson L, Garst P (eds). Living with celiac sprue: the gluten free diet, 1983.	National Celiac Society 5 Jeffrey Road Wayland, MA 01778
Requests: M. Stevens Agency PO Box 3006 Frankfort, KY 40603	Gluten Intolerance Group Elaine Hartsook Ph.D., R.D. PO Box 23053 Seattle, WA
Wood M. Gourmet food on a wheat free diet. Wood M. Delicious and easy rice flour recipes.	Midwestern Celiac Sprue Association PO Box 3554 Des Moines, IA 50322

Requests: Charles C Thomas, Publisher
301–327 E. Lawrence Avenue
Springfield, IL 62717

essential nutrients, with the exception of cobalamin. There is evidence that many vitamins and minerals play a vital role in the immunologic response. Since gliadin is believed to exert its adverse effect through antigenic stimulation of T and B lymphocytes, the pathologic mechanism may be significantly affected by vitamin and mineral status during both deficiency and supplementation. Table 5 lists the common micronutrient deficiency states, their clinical and immunologic consequences, and recommendations for supplementation.

REFRACTORY DISEASE

Patients who have been given a 2 to 3-week trial of gluten elimination yet continue to exhibit clinical symptoms pose several challenges. The first line of investigation involves careful scrutiny of the diet to rule out any "hidden" sources of gluten. Second, some patients have been noted to exhibit cramping abdominal pain secondary to intestinal spasm exacerbated by a high-fiber diet. Symptomatic relief may be obtained through temporary reduction of dietary fiber. A third possibility is the presence of other food intolerances. In 1982, a study was done of 113 children diagnosed with celiac disease by biopsy and responsive to a gluten-free diet. Through a retrospective survey, many were found to have intolerance of several non–gluten-containing foodstuffs, which could also precipitate abdominal pain, cramping, nausea, vomiting, and diarrhea (Table 6). Multiple food sensitivities are more common in young children, and their management requires a more extensive elimination diet in which the patient is allowed only the least allergenic foods, (lamb, rice, green beans, pears). Foods are added one at a time, with observation for recurrence of symptoms. Severe cases may require hospital admission for parenteral or enteral feeding prior to the gradual reintroduction of foodstuffs.

It has been estimated that 20 percent of patients will not respond to gluten elimination within 2 to 3 months. Assuming that gluten elimination is complete and associated food intolerances have been excluded, a trial of steroids is warranted. The recommended dosage is 40 to 60 mg daily for adults and 2 mg per kilogram for children, with a gradual taper over 4 to 6 weeks. In nonresponsive patients other diseases also merit consideration. Sprue may be associated with intestinal lymphoma and carcinoma. Lymphoma patients tend to have fever, increased abdominal pain, and radiographic evidence of a small bowel infiltrative lesion.

TABLE 5 Common Micronutrient Deficiency States: The Clinical, Immunologic, and Treatment Implications

Deficiency	Clinical Signs	Immunologic Effects	Treatment Adult	Treatment Children
Iron	Anemia (microcytic)	↓ Lymphocyte response to antigen	Fe sulfate 325 mg t.i.d. Fe gluconate 600 mg t.i.d.	3 mg/kg/day elemental Fe
Folate	Anemia (macrocytic), neuropathy	↓ Lymphocte response to antigen ↓ Phagocytosis ↓ Leukocytes	5 mg/day	1–5 mg/day
Vitamin B₁₂	Anemia (macrocytic), neuropathy		1,000 µg IM monthly	500 µg IM monthly
Vitamin B₆	Anemia (microcytic), neuropathy	↓ Synthesis of arachidonic acid from linoleic acid ↓ Level of cellular/humoral response ↓ Antibody response to antigen	50–100 mg/day	50–100 mg/day
Vitamin K	Hemorrhage, petecchiae		10 mg IV over 10 min	1–3 mg IV over 10 min
Vitamin D	Bone pain, osteomalacia, tetany, secondary hyperparathyroidism	↓ Neutrophil motility ↓ Phagocytosis	Calcium 4 g/day Vitamin D 25–50 µg/day	Calcium 2–4 g/day Vitamin D 25 µg/day

Vitamin A	Night blindness, follicular hyperkeratosis	Maintains anatomic barrier	Water-soluble vitamin A 3,000 μg/day	Water-soluble vitamin A 3,000 μg/day
Vitamin E	Neuropathy, ↓ proprioception, spinocerebellar ataxia	↑Lipid peroxidation	Water-soluble vitamin E 50–100 mg/day	Water-soluble vitamin E 25–50 mg/day
Magnesium	Cramping, tetany, persistent hypokalemia	↓ Antibody response to antigenic stimulation	30 mEq/day IV	10–20 mEq/day IV
Zinc	↓ Taste, dermatitis, hyperkeratosis, ↓ disaccharidase	↓ T helper and killer cell function	50 mg/day	10–25 mg/day
Selenium	Proximal muscle weakness, fatigue, hemolytic anemia	↑Lipid peroxidation ↓T cell activation	100 μg/day (dependent on intake of polyunsaturated fats/vitamin E)	

Adapted from the following sources:
Walker AW, Watkins JB. Nutrition in pediatrics. Boston: Little, Brown, 1986; Recommended dietary allowances, 9th ed. Washington, DC: National Academy of Sciences, 1980; Corman L. Effects of specific nutrients on the immune response. Med Clin North Am 1985; 69:4:759–791; Lebenthal E. Total parenteral nutrition. New York: Raven Press, 1986; Sleisenger MH, Fordtran JS. Gastrointestinal diseases, 2nd ed. Philadelphia: WB Saunders, 1978.

TABLE 6 Percent of Children with Celiac Disease Found to Have Other Food Intolerances*

Lactose intolerance	50%
Fat intolerance	20%
Sugar intolerance	12%
Citrus fruit	10%
Eggs	10%
Tomatoes	6%
Soybeans	5.3%
Nuts	4%
Seafood/corn	3.5%

* Data from a 1982 study of 113 children with biopsy-diagnosed celiac disease responsive to a gluten-free diet. Garst PM, Larson L (eds). Living with celiac sprue. Des Moines: Midwestern Celiac Sprue Association, 1983:168.

The incidence of neoplasm depends upon the population studied, with values ranging from 1 to 20 percent. Ulcerative jejunitis is sprue complicated by severe intestinal bleeding, stricture formation, and a risk of perforation and peritonitis. Two rare refractory subtypes include collagenous and amitotic sprue. There is no known effective primary therapy for these disorders.

Dermatitis herpetiformis, a pruritic pattern of recurrent blisters, primarily over the elbows and knees, is an extraintestinal manifestation of celiac disease. It responds to gluten elimination and sulfa antibiotics; however, the response is slow, with up to 6 months of dietary restriction required before the lesions disappear.

Celiac patients also appear to have an increased risk of diabetes, thyroid disease, rheumatoid arthritis, ulcerative colitis, and even schizophrenia.

SURVEILLANCE

Since histologic abnormalities can continue despite improvement in clinical symptoms, some authorities believe that repeat jejunal biopsies are necessary to rule out the development of lymphoma and intestinal carcinoma in celiac patients. It has also been documented that 5 to 10 percent of asymptomatic relatives of celiac patients have changes within the gut mucosa and are perhaps also at risk for these associated complications. A schema for long-term monitoring, employing several of the previously outlined methods of evaluation, is proposed (Fig. 1).

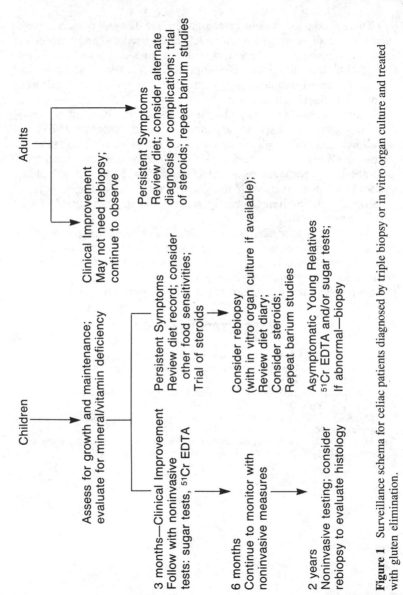

Figure 1 Surveillance schema for celiac patients diagnosed by triple biopsy or in vitro organ culture and treated with gluten elimination.

Children

Assess for growth and maintenance; evaluate for mineral/vitamin deficiency

3 months—Clinical Improvement
Follow with noninvasive tests: sugar tests, ^{51}Cr EDTA

Persistent Symptoms
Review diet record; consider other food sensitivities;
Trial of steroids

Consider rebiopsy
(with in vitro organ culture if available);
Review diet diary;
Consider steroids;
Repeat barium studies

6 months
Continue to monitor with noninvasive measures

2 years
Noninvasive testing; consider rebiopsy to evaluate histology

Asymptomatic Young Relatives
^{51}Cr EDTA and/or sugar tests;
If abnormal—biopsy

Adults

Clinical Improvement
May not need rebiopsy;
continue to observe

Persistent Symptoms
Review diet; consider alternate diagnosis or complications; trial of steroids; repeat barium studies

There is no good evidence that a gluten-free diet will reduce the concurrence of malignancy or autoimmune disease in adults, and many celiac adults do knowingly cheat and live with a degree of cramping and diarrhea. In children, a more careful approach is advised, since they may have an improved prognosis with early detection and strict elimination of further antigenic stimulation.

There is controversy in the literature about temporary gluten sensitivity. It is fairly common to see apparent clinical improvement with gluten withdrawal in a child with chronic diarrhea but subsequent tolerance of gluten after 3 to 6 months. Such children should be kept on the restricted diet until their growth rate has normalized and then challenged with gluten and followed at intervals with absorption tests. In most series, only 25 percent of such children ultimately relapse and show evidence of sustained gluten sensitivity.

As the etiologic mechanism for celiac disease becomes more clearly defined, noninvasive tests may achieve greater acceptance in the detection and management of these patients. Improvements in the methods of evaluation, along with dietary education, offer success at long-term suppression of symptoms and hope for decreased morbidity and mortality.

SUGGESTED READING

Cole SG, Kagnoff MF. Celiac disease. Annu Rev Nutr 1985; 5:241–266.

Corman Lourdes C. Effects of specific nutritions on the immune system. Med Clin North Am 1985; 69(4):759–791.

Garst PM, Lawson L, (eds). Living with celiac sprue: the gluten free diet. Des Moines: Midwestern Celiac Sprue Association, 1983.

Patel DG, Krogh CME, Thompson WG. Gluten in pills: a hazard for patients with celiac disease. Can Med Assoc J 1985; 133:114–115.

Trier JS, Falchuk ZM, Carey MC, Schreiber DS. Celiac sprue and refractory sprue. Gastroenterology 1978; 75:307–316.

SHORT BOWEL SYNDROME

KHURSHEED N. JEEJEEBHOY, M.B., B.S., Ph.D., F.R.C.P.(C)

Small-intestinal resection is necessary in various conditions, including congenital abnormalities, trauma, inflammation, vascular insufficiency, and tumors. In young people the reason for bowel resection is often Crohn's disease, and in the elderly, intestinal infarction. When more than 50 percent of the bowel has been resected, impairment of absorption tends to be long term or permanent despite the intestinal reserve and adaptation. The degree of malnutrition that results from bowel resection thus depends on several factors, and functional disability cannot be predicted exclusively from the extent of the resection.

THE NORMAL SMALL INTESTINE

Motility

Ingestion of nutrients, especially fat, inhibits gastric emptying, and the bigger the meal the longer the emptying. Studies of small-bowel transit show a pronounced ileal effect in slowing transit. The marker traverses the first 50 percent of the bowel in a third of the time it takes to pass through the next 30 percent. The ileocecal valve and the colon also figure significantly in slowing overall intestinal transit.

Even during fasting, the stomach and small bowel become active during the periodic interdigestive migratory myoelectrical complexes. Up to 30 percent of the maximum secretions of bile and pancreatic juice occur then.

Secretion and Absorption of Fluid and Electrolytes

The small bowel receives 5 to 6 L of endogenous secretions per day—about 1 L each of saliva and bile and 1.5 to 3 L of gastric and pancreatic juices. All but 1 L is absorbed from the small intestine. The site of absorption depends on the nature of the meal: after meat and salad most absorption occurs high in the jejunum, whereas after milk and donuts there is greater water secretion into the bowel and more distal absorption.

The absorption of fluid and electrolytes differs significantly in the jejunum, ileum, and colon. The differences depend on the nature of the electrolyte transport processes and on the permeability of the intercellular spaces, and thus the particular part resected is important.

Water absorption is generally a passive process resulting from the active transport of nutrients and electrolytes. Sodium transport is mainly responsible for the creation of an electrochemical gradient across the mucosa and for driving the uptake of sugars and amino acids. However, the net effect of transport on intraluminal contents depends not only on absorption, but also on back diffusion through the intercellular junctions. In the jejunum, back diffusion occurs readily, so the jejunal contents remain isotonic; the ileal and colonic intercellular junctions become progressively "tighter." Thus the intraluminal contents become concentrated with respect to plasma, and fluid from the lumen is conserved by the body. In addition to fluid and electrolytes, the intestine absorbs nutrients. In health this is completed within the first 150 cm of the bowel, so very little nutrient reaches the ileum.

Functions of the Ileum

The ileum alone absorbs vitamin B_{12} and bile salts, and ileal resection consequently disrupts this process. Malabsorption of bile salts results in altered digestion and absorption of fat in the jejunum. Normally the demand for bile salts exceeds synthesis and is met by ileal reabsorption of bile salts, which are recycled into the jejunum. After ileal resection, they are no longer recycled and synthesis never increases sufficiently to meet needs. Thus the bile-salt pool is depleted, and fat is malabsorbed. In addition, nutrients in the ileum slows the motility of the upper gastrointestinal tract.

EFFECTS OF INTESTINAL RESECTION

Motility

As would be expected, small-bowel resection increases the rate of gastric emptying. Since motility is rapid in the jejunum and slow in the distal ileum, proximal bowel resection does not raise the rate of intestinal transit, in contrast to ileal resection. The colon has the slowest motility of the intestine, so distal resections involving the colon increase the rate of transit.

Absorption of Fluid and Electrolytes

If the colon is intact, fluid and electrolyte losses are not excessive, unless the fluid load exceeds the colon's reserve capacity of about 5 L per day or the contents of the small intestinal dejecta inhibit colonic absorption. Bile salts and free fatty acids alter the ability of the colon to absorb water and sodium. Ileal malabsorption of bile salts and accumulation of deoxybile acids in the colon reduce absorption of sodium and water and cause fluid secretion. Also certain vegetable residues and carbohydrates can be degraded by colonic bacteria to fatty acids that increase the osmotic load and water output.

Thus proximal resection results in little diarrhea because the ileum can reabsorb the increased fluid and electrolyte load, and any remaining excess is taken up by the colon. In contrast, after ileal resection the colon receives a large isotonic fluid load with unabsorbed bile salts. Thus substances (bile salts themselves, fatty acids, unabsorbed carbohydrates) that reduce the reabsorption of water and electrolytes reach the colon, causing diarrhea.

If both ileum and colon are resected, the remaining bowel cannot concentrate luminal contents. In such patients, isotonic water and salt loss is severe, resulting in dehydration, hypokalemia, and hypomagnesemia—the so-called end-jejunostomy syndrome.

Nutrient Absorption

After resection, the remaining small intestine hypertrophies and also increases its absorptive function. Flint calculated that the observed increase in villus height after small-bowel resection in human beings increased the absorptive surface area fourfold, and other studies have confirmed this. When the jejunum alone is removed, the ileum takes over the absorptive function and there is little malabsorption, whereas ileal resections of only 100 cm cause steatorrhea. The degree of malabsorption rises with increasing length of resection, and a variety of nutrients are malabsorbed. In general, resections up to 33 percent result in no malnutrition and those up to 50 percent can be tolerated without special aids. However, when resection exceeds 75 percent of the bowel, nutritional status cannot be maintained without special help. If only a few centimeters of jejunum remain, the number of patients surviving is limited and most suffer nutritional depletion.

TREATMENT OF INTESTINAL RESECTION

Control of Diarrhea

Diarrhea results from increased secretions and motility and from osmotic stimulation of water secretion due to malabsorption of luminal contents. Initially, diarrhea may be controlled by giving the patient nil per os to reduce the osmotic stimulus. With massive resection, however, there may be substantial fluid losses due to gastric hypersecretion and malabsorption of endogenous secretions stimulated by interdigestive migratory myoelectric complexes. H_2 blockers can reduce secretion, especially gastric secretion. I prefer to give the H_2 blocker initially as a continuous intravenous infusion (cimetidine 300 mg over 6 hr) rather than as a bolus, because of its short half-life. In addition, opioids help in slowing intestinal propulsion and in increasing ion transport. Loperamide, which acts locally, may be tried in increasing doses and if it is ineffective, codeine or Lomotil (diphenoxylate hydrochloride) plus atropine sulfate may be tried.

Oral Feeding

The rigor of any restrictive dietetic measure depends upon the length of bowel resected. In patients who have more than 60 to 80 cm of the small bowel remaining, refeeding should be progressive with a view to achieving a normal or modified oral diet. In patients with only the duodenum remaining, the initial target should be small feeds of isotonic fluids containing carbohydrates and electrolytes. For patients with intermediate lengths of bowel, progressive feeding should begin with isotonic flavored carbohydrate-electrolyte feeds, containing 3.4 percent Caloreen, 85 mmol per liter sodium, 12 mmol per liter potassium, 9 mmol per liter bicarbonate, and 109 mmol per liter chloride, which are well absorbed by patients with massive resection who were previously dependent on intravenous fluids. If the patient has more than 60 to 80 cm of small intestine, an oral diet of natural ingredients should be tried. When trying such feeds, the patient should take dry solids, with isotonic fluids 1 hr after the meal. The separation of solids from liquids is important because of the faster rate of gastric emptying after resection, and it must be carefully explained to the patient.

The type of diet to be fed has been a subject of controversy. Traditional teaching has been to use a low-fat diet with medium-chain triglycerides. This arose from the finding that long-chain fatty acids can cause colonic water secretion, which led to the hypothesis that malabsorbed fat may cause steatorrhea in patients with short bowel. Until recently, this hypothesis had not been carefully tested.

In a carefully controlled trial, we found no differences between high-fat and high-carbohydrate diets with respect to loss of water, electrolytes, or even total calories in stools in patients with a greater than 50 percent bowel resection. The absorption of protein and carbohydrate was no better than that of fat. Thus, the nature of the diet made no difference to the diarrhea or to total malabsorption in patients with massive resection. Other studies have shown that high-fat diets may even be beneficial.

In patients who cannot tolerate a normal diet and those with very short bowel, a constant infusion of defined-formula diet should be tried. Controlled, well-modulated rates of infusion are important, starting with 25 ml per hour, gradually increasing to full strength infused at 100 to 125 ml per hour. This procedure ensures that the intestine receives an osmotic load at a constant rate. If the rate is adjusted to bowel tolerance, patients who would otherwise need intravenous feeding can be managed entirely by the oral route.

PARENTERAL NUTRITION

Initially all patients need intravenous replacement of fluid and eletrolytes, especially sodium, chloride, potassium, and magnesium. These are infused so as to achieve a urine flow exceeding 1 L per day and to maintain normal serum electrolyte levels, central venous pressure, and blood pressure. There should be no postural fall in blood pressure if hydration is adequate. The intravenous infusion is gradually reduced as oral intake increases, but several weeks of adaptation may be needed before oral feeding alone is adequate.

Parenteral nutrition should be started to avoid the development of malnutrition while oral feeding is being attempted. Many patients progress, as oral intake increases, to needing only electrolytes parenterally, while other nutrient requirements can be met orally. The provision of trace elements in parenteral nutrition is often neglected. In patients with a small bowel resection and severe diarrhea, the need for zinc increases to 12 to 15 mg per day because of endogenous losses. These may be estimated by measuring the volume of intestinal fluid lost per day with the patient fasting and adding 12 to 13 mg zinc for every liter of fluid lost.

Long-Term Nutritional Support

The aim should be to progress as the patient adapts from parenteral nutrition with variable oral intake, through oral diet with parenteral fluids and electrolytes, through defined-formula diets on an ambulatory basis, to a normal or modified oral diet, *separating solids from liquids.* However, it is important that the patient be able to maintain a normal nutritional status while also remaining free of serious diarrhea, so that occupational and social rehabilitation are possible. Ten to twelve meals a day and a similar number of bowel movements, including nocturnal movements, do not constitute a desirable quality of life. The options of home enteral and parenteral nutrition have revolutionized the outlook for such patients. Those with less than 60 cm of small bowel remaining will need parenteral nutrition at home on an indefinite basis. The infusion rate and caloric intake are gradually reduced as the patient becomes able to maintain his weight on an oral diet. The decision to reduce intravenous feeding is made from the observation that weight gain is occurring beyond desired limits and that reduced infusion does not result in electrolyte and fluid imbalance.

In contrast to patients with massive intestinal resection, those with more limited ileal resection may have so-called cholereic diarrhea which is best managed with cholestyramine, or fatty-acid diarrhea and steatorrhea in which a fat-restricted diet is also useful. Cholestyramine is helpful in patients with hyperoxaluria caused by excess colonic oxalate absorption induced by bile salts. Vitamin B_{12} absorption should be studied and patients with deficiency should be given 200 μg parenteral vitamin B_{12} per month.

SUGGESTED READING

Hofmann AF, Poley JR. Role of bile acid malabsorption in the pathogenesis of diarrhea and steatorrhea in patients with ileal resection. I. Response to cholestyramine or replacement of dietary long chain triglyceride by medium chain triglycerides. Gastroenterology 1972; 62:918-934.

Hylander E, Ladefoged K, Jarnum S. Nitrogen absorption following small intestinal resection. Scand J Gastroenterol 1980; 15:853-858.

Jeejeebhoy KN, Zohrab WJ, Langer B, et al. Total parenteral nutrition at home for 23 months, without complication and with good rehabilitation. A study of technical and metabolic features. Gastroenterology 1973; 65:811-820.

Wolman SL, Anderson GH, Marliss EB, Jeejeebhoy KN. Zinc in total parenteral nutrition: requirements and metabolic effects. Gastroenterology 1979; 76:458-467.

Woolf GM, Miller C, Kurian R, Jeejeebhoy KN. Diet for patients with a short bowel: high fat or high carbohydrate? Gastroenterology 1983; 84:823-828.

Woolf GM, Miller C, Kurian R, Jeejeebhoy KN. Nutritional absorption in short bowel syndrome. Evaluation of fluid, calorie, and divalent cation requirements. Dig Dis Sci 1987; 32:8-15.

COLONIC DISEASE

STEVEN M. FOWLIE, M.B., M.R.C.P.(UK)
MARTIN A. EASTWOOD, M.B., M.Sc., F.R.C.P.(Edin)

The association between diet, nutrition, and diseases of the colon has long been the subject of debate. This review focuses on the increasingly important role of nutrition and nutritionists in the treatment of diseases of the large bowel. The principal conditions that will be discussed are constipation, diverticular disease, irritable bowel syndrome, and cancer of the colon. Inflammatory bowel disease is dealt with elsewhere.

Defecation is the most commonly appreciated function of the large bowel. The left side of the colon is central to the act of defecation and to the maintenance of continence. The right side of the colon and cecum can be thought of as a fermenting vessel into which the small bowel delivers undigested food, mucus, and bile. Fiber is probably the most important dietary constituent so delivered. The products of the fermentation in the right side of the colon include gaseous methane and hydrogen and volatile fatty acids that are now recognized as having an important role in overall colonic function.

Normal feces are 75 percent water; the remaining dry material is largely bacteria and unfermented fiber in roughly equal proportions. Stool weight in a group of normal, asymptomatic subjects varies considerably between 50 g and 300 g daily. There is almost as great a day-to-day variability in individuals. Fiber—plant cell wall, cell sap, polysaccharides, and lignin—is the only element of the diet known to increase stool weight. Two mechanisms are involved: First, fiber has water-holding capacity and acts like a sponge, increasing the bulk and the water content of the stool. Cereal fiber, especially wheat bran, predictably increases stool weight by effecting an increase in the water content of the feces. The coarser the wheat bran, the greater the water-holding capacity and hence the potential to increase stool weight. Milling and cooking reduce this effect considerably. This explains the very modest stool weight increases obtained by the addition to the diet of whole meal bread and other products in which the fiber is refined and of small particular type. Second, fiber can act as a substrate for the anaerobic bacterial fermentation processes in the cecum. Stool weight increases are unpredictable and less marked with fiber derived from fruit and vegetables, which is mediated through a proliferation of bacteria capable of fiber fermentation in favorable nutritional conditions.

CONSTIPATION

Constipation is an abnormal bowel habit characterized by difficult and/or infrequent defecation. Defecation may be difficult because of abnormal anorectal function or because the stool itself is unusually hard. Reduced frequency of defecation is usually the result of slowed colonic transit. However there is considerable overlap; for example, increasing colonic transit time allows greater resorption of fecal water, which results in a harder stool.

Simple constipation is often a consequence of a diet deficient in fiber. If so, it is usually relieved by simple dietary modification such as the addition of a handful of cereal bran as a breakfast cereal and at least two pieces of fresh fruit daily (apples and oranges are particularly recommended). The bran can be taken as uncooked coarse wheat bran, which has the disadvantage of being relatively unpalatable but is highly effective at a modest intake of 10 to 15 g a day. It is not necessary to alter the diet radically to a whole food diet, and such a dramatic change is unlikely to be sustained unless the individual is so inclined and motivated. The simple regimen explained above has the merit of being understood by, and acceptable to, the intellectually unendowed, the elderly, the frail, and the excessively anxious. The increased stool weight that this regimen effects is usually sufficient to alleviate constipation and to relieve the patient's symptoms. In order to minimize the chances of constipation, we aim to achieve a daily intake of 30 g fiber, half as cereal bran and half from fruit and vegetables. In individuals accustomed to taking considerably less fiber, such quantities may produce abdominal distension and discomfort, borborygmi, and increased flatus. Patients should be warned of these potential effects and advised to persevere—they usually diminish to acceptable levels within a few weeks. It has been suggested that high-fiber diets may contribute to mineral deficiencies, particularly of calcium and zinc. Although there is a theoretical basis for such concern, it is unlikely to be of any clinical significance unless the diet is in some other way extraordinary.

Further supplementation is required in some cases, and here proprietary fiber preparations may be useful, even though weight-for-weight they produce smaller increases in stool bulk. Moreover, some patients find such formulations more palatable than unrefined cereal bran. All Bran should be used with caution in the elderly and in patients with potential problems of fluid retention (e.g., congestive heart failure) because of its substantial salt content. The isphagula (psyllium seed) fecal bulking agents have the important disadvantage of increasing intracolonic pressure, which may be a factor in the development of colonic diverticula, so while they are very effective they too have to be used with caution. Stimulant laxatives are inappropriate in constipation due to fiber deficiency and may eventually precipitate an atonic, nonfunctioning colon as well as causing hypokalemia in a substantial proportion of patients. Fecal softeners have a limited role but are useful when constipation is accompanied by painful anorectal conditions such as hemorrhoids or anal fissure. Prolonged use can cause fat-soluble vitamin deficiency.

In some patients, however, constipation is clearly not simply the result of fiber deficit. With advances in understanding and assessment of anorectal and colonic function, we are increasingly recognizing patients in whom severe intractable constipation (often with associated fecal incontinence) is, at least in part, secondary to disordered neurologic control of the left side of the colon. The lumbosacral outflow to the rectum and descending colon may be subject to a variety of insults such as stretching during difficult or prolonged childbirth, traction during pelvic operations, direct trauma to the lumbosacral spine, and congenital abnormalities of the spine including spina bifida occulta. Long-term laxative abuse and prolonged straining at stool may damage the myenteric plexus in the colonic wall itself. Dietary manipulation plays but a small part in the management of these patients. Indeed, fiber may exacerbate the problem, as fecal bulking may do in other circumstances in which a small-volume stool can be an advantage.

A surgical approach may offer hope of improvement, but this option is appropriate only after careful evaluation, including anorectal manometric studies. Hemicolectomy, ileorectal anastomosis, and even colostomy may afford individual patients significant benefits, but such operations should be contemplated only by specialized units with full investigatory facilities. These operations can be of great relief to a limited number of patients but can aggravate the problems of emotionally compromised individuals.

COLONIC DIVERTICULOSIS

Like much constipation, colonic diverticulosis is probably a consequence of a diet lacking in fiber. The colon accomodates to a small, firm stool by generating contractions of greater strength. Where intracolonic pressures are increased, the viscoelastic properties of the bowel wall may be overwhelmed and small mucous membrane pouches may herniate to form diverticula. The causative relationship between elevated intracolonic pressures and diverticular disease is not universally accepted, and abnormalities of colonic motility may also be important. The colonic tensile strength and expansibility deteriorate with age and are lowest in the distal colon where diverticula are most commonly found. Colonic diverticulosis is a common, essentially benign condition that is increasingly prevalent with advancing age. Often found by chance on a barium enema examination, the condition is of no consequence in itself. The majority of individuals with colonic diverticulosis pass through life with no undue consequences accruing from this byproduct of the aging process.

A minority of individuals with colonic diverticula will become symptomatic. Common symptoms include pain in the iliac fossa (typically, but not exclusively, on the left side), the passage of broken or pellety stool, and relief of pain with defecation. Blood in the stool is very rarely caused by diverticula, and its occurrence suggests the presence of carcinoma, which may coexist with the diverticula. Diverticular disease is associated with increased pressures within the sigmoid colon, and its symptoms are due to spasm and hypertrophy of the colonic musculature.

Increasing dietary fiber is the mainstay of treatment and often produces symptomatic improvement. Certainly, the increased stool bulk so produced ameliorates the increased intracolonic pressure associated with symptomatic colonic diverticula. We recommend a regimen similar to that outlined for constipation such that the daily intake of fiber is of the order of 30 g. In diverticular disease isphagula agents with their tendency to increase intracolonic pressures are in our view contraindicated. Elderly patients often find it difficult to change lifelong eating habits and frequently do better with proprietary fiber products. The importance of taking an adequate quantity of fluid with the increased fiber diet cannot be overstressed, particularly in these patients in whom fecal bulking without sufficient fluids may precipitate intestinal obstruction. In the few patients in whom these modest dietary manipulations fail, the diagnosis must be challenged. Carcinoma must be further considered and sought by flexible endoscopic examination of the descending colon. The patient may be depressed and the symptoms a consequence of the state of mind. If after rigorous reassessment the diagnosis remains one of diverticular disease, resection of the sigmoid colon may be a useful procedure.

Colonic diverticula can be complicated by perforation, bleeding, fistula formation, and true diverticulitis including pericholangitis and subphrenic abscess formation. Such conditions are not to be treated other than in a hospital surgical unit. In such complicated diverticular disease, the nutritional state of the patient may rapidly become compromised by the complication or its treatment. In a few cases, nutritional support is appropriate, delivered enterally or even parenterally.

IRRITABLE BOWEL SYNDROME

Irritable bowel syndrome (IBS) describes a heterogeneous group of conditions characterized by abdominal pain often relieved by defecation, variable bowel habits, and abdominal distension. Patients frequently describe passing a pellety or ribbony stool accompanied by mucus but never blood. This so-called irritable bowel syndrome of constipated type is often due to reduced fiber content in the diet. An increase in dietary fiber intake may relieve the constipation, and consequent upon this, the other features may improve. Other patients have a diarrheal form of the irritable bowel syndrome. Here the diagnosis is often more difficult to reach. In particular, the symptoms may be early manifestations of Crohn's disease.

However, the multifactorial nature of irritable bowel syndrome, both constipated and diarrheal, is demonstrated in the failure of dietary manipulations to effect lasting symptomatic relief in a substantial proportion of irritable bowel sufferers. The symptom complex is greatly influenced by psychologic stress, anxiety, and personality conflicts. The problems besetting the patient with the irritable bowel syndrome derive from disordered motility characterized by spasm that occurs along the whole intestine but particularly in the colon. The approach we find most useful is to view this spasm and the symptom complex as being caused by a combination of three agents, each of which is represented by the corner of a triangle.

One corner contributes to symptoms through physical causes, most notably insufficient dietary fiber. Disease states such as Crohn's disease and lactase deficiency must be excluded from this point of the triangle by careful history-taking and appropriate examinations. Dietary fiber insufficiency is assessed by a diet history.

The second corner of the triangle represents stress and life events. A sequence of events may occur that starts with social and domestic difficulties but that ultimately leads to feelings of hopelessness and entrapment. This causes anxiety that is infectious, upsetting the patient, the family (if they care), and the clinicians looking after the patient. This anxiety makes seeking an elusive diagnosis attractive to the physician, and such a search has the great attraction to the patient of not having to square up to the root cause of the symptoms, for which reason this (further investigation) is often counterproductive and dangerous.

The apex of the triangle is formed by the personality and psychiatric status of the patient. An abnormal personality or an excessively troubled person will run from doctor to doctor, alternative treatment to alternative treatment, until the underlying problem is resolved either through the passage of time or a chance encounter with a wise clinician of whatever clinical persuasion. Sadly, these patients sometimes come across radical cures that compound their difficulties.

When faced with a patient with irritable bowel syndrome, the first step is to establish the diagnosis. Unfortunately, IBS is a diagnosis of exclusion, always an unsatisfactory situation, and the presence of IBS does not rule out the coexistence of other gastrointestinal disease. Overenthusiastic investigation can be as damaging as underinvestigation; where to draw the line is a clinical judgment, unique to each individual, for which strict guidelines are inappropriate. Our second step is to define the shape of the triangle for that patient. It is often useful to demonstrate the concept of the triangle while exploring the presence of stress and assessing the role of life events, personality, and mental state.

Usually, and always in constipated IBS and where dietary fiber deficiency is established, the fiber content of the diet should be increased to about 30 g daily following the simple regimen described for constipation. In suitable cases, antispasmodics, anxiolytics, or antidepressants may prove useful, and in many cases an approach combining such pharmacologic maneuvers with dietary fiber supplementation gives the best symptomatic improvement.

It has been argued that much irritable bowel syndrome is a manifestation of food allergy. Advocates of this proposition advise exclusion diets with gradual reintroduction of identified foods in an effort to pinpoint the dietary constituents responsible for the symptoms. We have not found this approach helpful in dealing with the vast majority of patients with irritable bowel syndrome whom we see. There may be a subgroup for whom it is appropriate, but at present identification of patients within that group is not possible. The majority of irritable bowel patients, particularly those whose symptoms have been present for some time, have high anxiety levels, and placebo effects can be dramatic given the psychologic profile of the group. The increasing advocacy of odd diets and dietary restrictions for this condition and others in which psychologic factors are important, if not paramount, is a worrisome trend. Some such advice seems to be a recipe for malnutrition, particularly mineral and vitamin deficiency or, in some extreme examples, vitamin toxicity. In our view such an approach to irritable bowel syndrome is not justified on the basis of the available evidence; nor do we think it likely to prove the answer for the great majority of our patients.

NUTRITION AND THE PREVENTION OF COLONIC DISEASE

Some authors have suggested that substantial fiber content in the diet is protective against the development of appendicitis, colonic diverticular disease, and cancer of the colon. Populations in whom these conditions have a high incidence certainly have reduced stool volumes when compared with populations in which such diseases are less common, and patients frequently have a history of constipation. Fiber may be protective against colonic carcinoma by a purely dilutional effect; increasing stool volume reduces the concentration of potential carcinogens, notably fecal bile acids. It has been suggested that dietary calcium and vitamin D may be protective against colonic cancer by encouraging the formation of insoluble soaps, thereby reducing the carcinogenic potential of free bile acids. The indole content of vegetables may also be protective against carcinogenesis. In addition to the effect on bile acids, high-fat diets induce changes in the colonic bacterial flora that may increase the carcinogenic potential of the fecal mass.

Increasing the fiber content of the diet is a harmless way of altering the diet that will certainly avoid constipation and reduce energy intake and may also, as an as yet unproved bonus, prevent the development of cancer of the colon, as may reductions in the amount of red meat and fat eaten. Such modifications form part of an evolving picture of what is regarded as a prudent, health-promoting diet. It is important to stress that such dietary recommendations concern average intakes over a period of time, so that beef and fat need not be excluded completely but should be enjoyed less often or in less quantity. Moderation in all things, including fiber, seems to be the recipe for colonic good health.

SUGGESTED READING

National Research Council. Diet, nutrition and cancer. Washington: National Academic Press, 1982.

Trowell H, Burkitt D, Heaton K, eds. Dietary fibre, fibre depleted foods and disease. London: Academic Press, 1985.

Vahouny GV, Kritchevsky D, eds. Dietary fiber basic and clinical aspects. New York: Plenum, 1986.

INTESTINAL PSEUDO-OBSTRUCTION

KHURSHEED N. JEEJEEBHOY, M.B., B.S., Ph.D., F.R.C.P.(C)

Intestinal pseudo-obstruction is a syndrome characterized by signs and symptoms of bowel obstruction without a mechanical cause. It may be acute and self-limited or chronic. The chronic form consists of recurrent attacks of abdominal distention, colicky pain, nausea, and vomiting, aggravated by eating. Patients often have diarrhea because of small intestinal bacterial overgrowth, but patients with colonic involvement may have severe constipation. In order to minimize their symptoms, patients restrict their intake of food and consequently become malnourished.

Regardless of whether chronic pseudo-obstruction is primary (idiopathic) or secondary to an underlying disease such as scleroderma, the gastrointestinal symptoms and radiologic features are the same. In either case, the cause appears to be a motility disorder of all or part of the gastrointestinal tract.

CLINICAL MANIFESTATIONS

Pseudo-obstruction presents in a variety of ways. The presentation, severity of the problem, and the presence or absence of any precipitating factors will dictate the nutritional management of the patient.

Upper Gastrointestinal Symptoms. The patients complain of epigastric fullness, early satiety, and heartburn. They find that solids, high-fat foods, and fiber cause discomfort, and consequently they stop eating and lose weight. These patients may also vomit after large meals.

Small Bowel Symptoms. Recurrent attacks of colicky pain, abdominal distention, diarrhea, and episodes of small bowel obstruction may be the presenting symptoms.

Colonic Symptoms. Patients may have chronic constipation, which is difficult to distinguish from simple constipation. They complain of infrequent bowel movements, marked abdominal distention, and flatulence. Unlike patients with benign obstipation, they cannot eat and rapidly lose weight.

Severity of Disease. Patients with mild disease have a waxing and waning course, with periods of normal eating and other periods of obstruction. Others have progressive symptoms that result in almost continuous obstruction, distention, and pain. Associated problems, consisting of dysphagia due to abnormal esophageal motility, recurrent urinary tract symptoms associated with megaureter and atonic bladder, and ptosis may occur in patients with myopathy. Those with neuropathy may present with peripheral muscular wasting and cerebral calcification.

DIFFERENTIAL DIAGNOSIS

Pseudo-obstruction may be primary due to a myopathic or neuropathic process involving the bowel or secondary to drug intake, chronic systemic disease affecting the bowel, or local bowel disease.

Primary Pseudo-Obstruction

This is the diagnosis if pseudo-obstruction is observed without an underlying cause. It is supported by associated smooth muscle disorders such as megaureter or by the presence of neuropathy.

Drug-Induced Pseudo-Obstruction

It is important to exclude chronic ingestion of opiates or opiate-like drugs as the cause of the problem. The usual history is one of chronic abdominal pain that is alleviated by taking opioid analgesics on a regular basis. The patient claims that the analgesic is crucial to pain relief, and the diagnosis of opiate addiction has to be excluded to confirm pseudo-obstruction. This cause should be suspected in patients who need analgesics even after decompression with nasogastric suction or enemas and being kept NPO. They also rarely lose weight despite vociferous complaints.

Secondary Pseudo-Obstruction

This is most commonly due to systemic sclerosis. The patient usually has a severe motility disorder involving the esophagus. Diabetic neuropathy is another cause of gastric atony. In addition, pseudo-obstruction may follow bowel resection and may be seen in patients with short bowel syndrome and Crohn's disease.

MANAGEMENT

In intermittent and minimal disease, the objective is to prescribe a low-fat diet that does not slow intestinal motility and to combine it with a motility-enhancing drug such as metoclopramide, domperidone, or cisapride. If a solid diet is associated with obstructive symptoms, then a liquid enteral diet may be tried. However, in the author's opinion, once the symptoms are established, they progress so that even liquid formula diets are not tolerated unless the patient has relatively mild and non-progressive disease.

If oral intake is not sufficient to maintain body weight and is associated with constant abdominal pain, then the patient has to be restricted to minimal oral intake and placed on home parenteral nutrition (HPN). In a series of 10 patients treated with HPN and restriction of oral intake, there was significant nutritional benefit.

Home Parenteral Nutrition

Effect of HPN on Nutritional Status and Symptoms

In patients with primary pseudo-obstruction total body weight (mean ± SE) expressed as a percent of ideal body weight rose from 74.7 ± 2.9 percent before HPN to 93.5 ± 3.7 percent. Furthermore, the anthropometrically estimated lean body weight rose from 78.4 ± 6.5 percent ideal to 92.7 ± 2.6 percent. Body fat rose from 57.1 ± 8.8 percent before HPN to 83.8 ± 8.2 percent.

Serum albumin was normal in all cases before HPN (38 ± 1 g per liter) and was unaffected by HPN (39 ± 1 g per liter). Total iron-binding capacity (TIBC) was similarly unaffected, with a baseline of 255 ± 25 μg per deciliter and a value after HPN of 284 ± 30 μg per deciliter. Creatinine-height index rose from 67 ± 22 percent to 78 ± 25 percent. Total body nitrogen (TBN) rose from 66.8 ± 13.7 percent expected TBN (calculated as a function of sex and height) to 78.0 ± 7.1 percent. Total body potassium (TBK) rose from 68.8 ± 13.1 g to 80.5 ± 10.7 g.

In addition to nutritional benefit, patients become mildly symptomatic and most returned to work. About one-third were eventually able to discontinue HPN.

Rationale for HPN

Although patients with chronic intestinal pseudo-obstrucion are usually most troubled by abdominal bloating and discomfort, the most serious manifestation of the disease is severe weight loss and malnutrition. Treatment strategies generally aim to "correct" somehow the motility disorder so that the patient can eat without symptoms. Such intervention causes at best a transient improvement that may simply reflect the natural history of the disease.

Long-term HPN combined with minimal oral intake is an excellent solution to these patients' problems as it both relieves symptoms by resting the bowel and restores nutrition to an adequate state. The largest series of patients with pseudo-obstruction treated with HPN reported in the literature is that of Schuffler, whose 10 patients on HPN had been followed for up to 4 years as of November 1981. He indicated that the patients' nutritional status was restored to normal but did not document the data. In addition, because his patients almost certainly continued to eat (as they were not instructed to refrain from eating), they all remained symptomatic and two continued to have intermittent episodes of severe obstructive symptoms.

We have documented in detail that 9 of our 10 patients had significant malnutrition that improved with HPN. Body weight, lean body mass, body fat, and TBK, which were low before HPN began, increased significantly with HPN. Our patients' symptoms were dramatically improved by HPN due to the fact that they refrained from eating. All patients were able to tolerate at least small volumes of liquid with impunity and could lead a normal life, including full-time employment for the majority.

It is of interest that even after years of persistent symptoms, some patients go into a sustained spontaneous remission and are able to tolerate a full diet. Because the presence of a permanent HPN line can be a cause of morbidity, such patients should have their line removed. However, obstruction may recur on an intermittent basis, requiring use of HPN at sporadic intervals. One way of dealing with this problem is to implant a permanent silastic catheter in the superior vena cava with a subcutaneous injection reservoir. Such a catheter can stay in place between attacks but is far less likely to be a source of recurrent sepsis. We have recently begun to use such catheters for our home HPN patients, but longer follow-up is needed to evaluate their efficacy.

SUGGESTED READING

Jeejeebhoy KN, Cohen Z, Kennedy G, et al. Total parenteral nutrition in the hospital and at home. Boca Raton, FL: CRC Press, 1983.

Jeejeebhoy KN, Langer B, Tsallas G, et al. Total parenteral nutrition at home: studies in patients surviving four months to five years. Gastroenterology 1976; 71:943-953.

Mernagh J, McNeill KG, Harrison JE, et al. Effect of total parenteral nutrition in the restitution of body nitrogen, potassium and weight. Nutr Res 1981; 1:149-157.

Schuffler MD. Chronic intestinal pseudo-obstruction syndromes (Symposium on motility disorders). Med Clin North Am 1981; 65:1331-1358.

Schuffler MD, Rohrmann CA, Chaffee RL, et al. Chronic intestinal pseudo-obstruction: a report of 27 cases and review of the literature. Medicine 1981; 60:173-196.

INFLAMMATORY BOWEL DISEASE

RICHARD V. HEATLEY, M.D., M.R.C.P.

Although many physicians and surgeons are concerned about malnutrition in inflammatory bowel disease (IBD), the problem is seldom addressed in its entirety in individual patients. There are likely to be many reasons for this but difficulties in recognizing the extent of the problem, except in the most extreme cases, and a lack of evidence that giving nutritional treatment actually affects the outcome of the disease in the long-term are undoubtedly important considerations.

A wide range of nutritional disturbances can occur in patients with IBD, and these may significantly affect the general management of many patients. Although any patient with either ulcerative colitis (UC) or Crohn's disease (CD) can become severely wasted during an acute, unremitting attack of disease, chronic undernourishment more commonly accompanies CD. In contrast, while few patients with UC, except those with persistently active disease, suffer severe widespread nutritional depletion, deficiencies of minerals, especially iron, are not infrequent. The pattern is usually most complicated in patients with chronic active CD in whom multiple deficiencies are commonplace.

The causes of undernourishment in many patients with IBD are generally ill understood; in most, it is probably multifactorial. Furthermore, the extent of nutritional impairment is not usually well recognized and the consequences are poorly documented, and there are few clear guidelines about which patients are particularly at risk. As more sophisticated tests become available to measure vitamin and trace element deficiencies, these are being recognized as complications of IBD, in particular CD.

It is important to identify nutritional deficiencies at an early stage, and to initiate appropriate treatment, otherwise many patients may suffer unnecessarily from the consequences of deprivation of vital nutrients (Table 1). Apparently well-nourished patients can become deficient in one or more nutrients and yet may remain otherwise in good health. Undernourished individuals, however, are usually at risk for multiple deficiencies and these shortfalls can complicate and add to the problems en-

155

TABLE 1 Nutritional Deficiencies and Possible Consequences in Inflammatory Bowel Disease

Nutrient	Likely Outcome
Generalized undernourishment	Growth retardation Weight loss and emaciation Poor wound and fistula healing Impaired immunity Slow resolution of infections Increased morbidity
Vitamin B_{12}	Anemia: subacute combined Spinal cord degeneration
Folic acid	Anemia
Iron	Anemia: thrombocytosis
Albumin	Edema
Potassium	Weakness; lethargy; ileus
Magnesium	Nonspecific malaise Muscle weakness
Calcium	Osteomalacia; tetany; ? Osteoporosis
Tryptophan	? Organic depression
Vitamin B complex	Pellagra
Vitamin C	Scurvy
Vitamin A	Impaired night vision
Vitamin D	Osteomalacia
Vitamin K	Hematuria: gastrointestinal hemorrhage
Zinc	Poor taste; impaired growth; acrodermatitis

countered in clinical practice (Table 2). Unfortunately, in many patients treatment is usually started late, is often empirical and based upon a paucity of scientifically derived guidelines, and consequently is not infrequently directed at the wrong patients (Table 3).

PATIENT SELECTION

It is usually not difficult to identify patients who are severely undernourished, which should prompt full nutritional assessment, but identification may be much more difficult in those with lesser degrees of

TABLE 2 Nutritional Consequences of Active IBD

Means of Detection	Nutrient Depletion and Effects	Occurrence in CD	UC
Anthropometry	Weight loss	+	+
	Reduced muscle bulk	+	+
	Diminished subcutaneous fat	+	+
Anemia	Iron deficiency	+	+
	Folate deficiency	+	±
	Vitamin B_{12} deficiency	+	−
Protein status	Hypoalbuminemia	+	±
Electrolytes and minerals	Sodium loss	+	+
	Potassium loss	+	+
	Other minerals	+	−
Vitamins	Water and fat-soluble vitamins	+	−

nutritional depletion. One of the most striking nutritional consequences of active IBD that attracts both the patient's and the clinician's attention is weight loss. This is often, however, only an outward sign of nutritional disturbance that, especially in those with CD, can be much more widespread. Consequently, one of the simplest screening tests is measurement of body weight in comparison with previous records and standard tables, provided the patient is free of edema. Other tests of value include the hemoglobin level, full blood count, and measurement of serum proteins. Abnormalities detected should lead to further assessments, including serum vitamin B_{12}, folate, iron, ferritin, and iron-binding capacity, and red-cell folate levels (Table 4). In chronic, active CD, many of these parameters are likely to be abnormal for a variety of reasons, not necessarily principally nutritional. Varying degrees of mineral and vitamin depletion occur in patients with CD, but isolated abnormal serum values do not necessarily imply that the patient is poorly nourished. Patients who are obviously undernourished though are commonly deficient in a variety of micronutrients.

A simple, readily applicable and reproducible method of identifying those patients most at risk of undernourishment is the measurement of the midarm circumference on the nondominant upper limb. These measurements correlate well with body weight in patients with IBD, avoiding the necessity for using comparative tables of ideal weight. Midarm circumference measurements require only a tape measure, and readings

TABLE 3 Guidelines for Nutritional Assessment
and Treatment in Crohn's Disease

Patient Status	Criteria
Active disease	Abdominal pain; diarrhea; generalized ill health; complications; abdominal mass
	Elevated ESR; acute phase proteins (orosomucoids); platelet count; reduced serum albumin
Diffuse small bowel disease	Radiologic and/or surgical evidence
Postoperative recurrent disease	Based on radiology rather than symptoms
Reduced anthropometric measurements	Midarm circumference <90% ideal

are expressed as a percentage of ideal value: the 90 percent of ideal standard (giving absolute measurements in adults of 26.4 cm in males and 25.7 cm in females) is a useful reference point in patients with CD. In our patients with CD, of those with midarm circumference measurements below these values, half were more than 10 percent below ideal body weight. These individuals are also most at risk for many other consequences of undernutrition, having reduced serum albumin, prealbumin and hemoglobin values, and immunologic parameters. These anthropometric measurements tend to be normal overall in patients with chronic UC. Apart from these simple indicators, the patients with CD who are especially at risk of undernourishment and who should be closely supervised are those with active, extensive small intestinal disease and particularly those with postoperative disease recurrence (Table 3).

TREATMENT

Treating the Disease

Most of the acute nutritional problems that occur in patients with IBD are associated with increased inflammatory activity. Consequently, undoubtedly the most successful method of overcoming nutritional depletion is to treat the disease with either drugs or surgery. With effective treatment, most nutritional problems will resolve. Steroid therapy in CD

TABLE 4 Assessment Criteria for Nutritional Status in IBD

	Screening Tests	More Detailed Investigation
Crohn's disease	Body weight	Serum vitamin B_{12}
	Midarm circumference	Serum and red cell folate
	Hemoglobin and full blood count	Iron, total iron binding capacity (TIBC), ferritin
	Urea and electrolytes	Serum magnesium, zinc, vitamin levels
	Serum proteins	
	Serum alkaline phosphatase	
	Serum calcium	
Ulcerative colitis	Body weight	Serum iron, TIBC, ferritin
	Hemoglobin and full blood count	Serum folate
	Serum proteins	

often results in improved well-being and increased appetite but has little measurable effect on fecal nitrogen loss. Surgical treatment, however, has been clearly demonstrated to promote linear growth in children with growth retardation. Surgery usually improves nutrition despite increasing the risks of malabsorption.

Dietary Modification

It has been reported that in the long-term support of patients with UC, a diet totally free of milk products will clinically benefit about 20 percent. It is certainly not my usual practice to advise all patients with UC to abstain from milk. However, in those with troublesome disease in which inflammatory activity has not been suppressed by conventional treatment, I discuss this with patients and arrange a milk-free diet for a 3-month trial period in the first instance.

Patients with CD may find a low-fat diet or cholestyramine of value to reduce stool frequency, but in my experience, patients often opt to tolerate such symptoms rather than adopt either of these treatment approaches. Care must be exercised with cholestyramine, since it may interfere with the absorption of vitamin D metabolites bound to bile acid complexes, which could lead to osteomalacia. In order to supplement caloric intake, the addition of medium-chain triglyceride oil to the diet may be of some benefit. This compound is readily absorbed and oxidized in the liver, and its unpleasant taste can be disguised by using it in flavored drinks, salad dressings, or cooking. Caution is advisable in its initial use, since some patients experience abdominal pain. It has now been largely superseded by many of the currently available oral nutritional supplements because of its lack of palatability and poor tolerance by patients and the need to supply additional phospholipid and essential fatty acids in the long term.

It has been suggested that a high-fiber diet may be of some value in the management of patients with CD by maintaining remission of disease. This finding has not, however, been widely confirmed, and I do not encounter many CD patients enthusiastic for this approach. A high-fiber diet does not generally confer any particular benefit in maintaining remission for patients with UC, although in those with distal proctitis and associated constipation I often find it a helpful adjunct.

High recorded sugar intake and the reported precipitation of symptoms by individual food items have led to suggestions that dietary exclusions may benefit patients with IBD. Lactase deficiency has certainly been reported in these patients, but there is no evidence that it occurs more frequently than in the population at large. I have not found the evidence for exclusion diets convincing in patients with IBD, and apart from the occasional exception, nor have the limited number of patients I have encountered who have tried this approach; consequently, it is not my current practice to recommend this form of treatment.

Mineral and vitamin supplements should be given to some patients with IBD, especially those with CD. Careful monitoring of blood tests and serum levels of folate, vitamin B_{12}, and ferritin, and perhaps also iron and total iron-binding capacity (TIBC), will act as a guide for replacement therapy; serum calcium and alkaline phosphatase levels, although poor overall indicators, may be of some value in the detection of osteomalacia.

I believe that all patients with significant small intestinal or proximal colonic Crohn's disease or who have had previous distal ileal surgery should be started on parenteral vitamin B_{12} therapy in normal replacement dosages and this should be continued for life. Most patients with radiologic evidence of intestinal involvement in either CD or UC require either repeated courses or small continuous doses of oral iron; ferrous sulfate in normal therapeutic dosages is adequate for most. I think that one can also make a case for giving many patients with extensive small intestinal CD regular oral folate supplements in normal therapeutic dosages (provided the vitamin B_{12} status is satisfactory) and perhaps also small, regular doses of calcium and vitamin D (500 units daily of vitamin D). Although a variety of other vitamin and mineral deficiencies has been described in patients with CD, significant shortfalls tend to occur only in those with extensive active disease. There is no evidence to suggest that patients should regularly receive any form of mineral or vitamin supplement other than those previously mentioned, unless specific clinical needs so indicate.

Most oral vitamin and mineral supplements will fail to correct deficiency states while the disease remains active and are generally more effective during periods of remission. Some agents, such as oral iron, may aggravate diarrhea.

Patients with IBD tend to consume the same amount of calories and protein as the general population. It appears, however, that these quantities are inadequate in some patients, thus exposing them to undernourishment. We have previously shown in a controlled clinical trial that undernourished patients with CD who received additional oral supplementation (to 3,000 cal per day) with a polymeric liquid food preparation showed improvement in a number of nutritional parameters, resulting in a significant increase in body weight and anthropometric measurements and improvement in biochemical and immunologic test results. We used "Ensure Plus" (Ross/Abbott Laboratories) in these studies and have found this entirely satisfactory for nutritional supplementation in patients with CD.

Elemental Feeding

Because of the good theoretic basis for their use and numerous short-term studies enthusiastically claiming benefit from elemental (chemically defined) diets, these have been widely used in CD. They have been tested in controlled trials as primary therapy for CD, giving comparable remission rates to those from steroids. There is little doubt that treatment with an elemental diet can improve nutrition in some patients with CD, and this in itself appears to be associated with some diminution of disease activity in certain patients. The long-term effects on maintaining remission are unproved though, and these diets are poorly tolerated by many patients, may cause diarrhea, and are expensive, making them unsatisfactory for general use. There is little evidence that these preparations are of more benefit than ordinary food, which is of course more palatable, pleasant, and inexpensive.

Intravenous Nutritional Therapy

During acute, severe attacks of IBD, dehydration, usually associated with sodium, chloride, and potassium depletion, is common and should be rectified if necessary by intravenous replacement. Intensive treatment regimens for acute, severe attacks of colitis, which include the provision of intravenous nutrients, achieve excellent results in inducing remission. Similarly, numerous enthusiastic reports have appeared in recent years advocating the treatment of acute inflammatory attacks of CD with intravenous feeding together with total bowel rest and anti-inflammatory treatment, and there are many good theoretical reasons for this form of therapy. It has even been suggested as a possible form of primary therapy for patients with severe IBD, especially those with active fistulas, and as a method of preparing patients for surgery. There are several types of patients with chronic CD, such as growth-retarded children and those with a short bowel, in whom weight gain and improved well-being have been documented with intravenous feeding; these results appear promising, but numerically, these represent very small groups of patients.

Most of the studies have, unfortunately, been uncontrolled and few are prospective, but many show an encouraging initial response to total parenteral feeding, with induction of short-term disease remission and healing of some intestinal fistulas. It may well be helpful, together with more specific treatment modalities, in certain patients with acute small intestinal CD, especially those with associated inflammatory masses, in a limited number of patients with Crohn's colitis, in preparing some patients for surgery, and in the postoperative healing of high small intestinal fistulas due to CD. However, long-term results, for maintenance of disease remission and fistula healing have been generally disappointing. For instance, although temporary closure of fistulas occurs in about 40 percent, long-term healing rates are lower. There has been no good controlled trial showing clinical benefit for total parenteral nutrition as primary treatment in acute CD or UC, and the evidence that does exist is conflicting. Until proof of its value accrues, the widespread use of intravenous feeding is to be discouraged. It can be anticipated, however, that total parenteral nutrition will be used to provide nutrition to replace that not taken orally to prevent the starvation that otherwise might occur in some patients.

Because of this, quantities of intravenous nutrients, if given, should be titrated to the individual patient. Ideally, assessment should be made of the patient's calorie, nitrogen, and fluid and electrolyte requirements. In the absence of this, a TPN regime daily consisting of approximately 2,000 to 3,000 kcal as carbohydrate (glucose), with some fat emulsion included, 10 to 12 g of nitrogen, together with normal quantities of minerals and electrolytes in a fluid volume of about 3 liters, is usually an adequate starter regimen. Subsequent changes can be made depending on the patient's progress.

To conclude this discussion, nutritional depletion is a frequent accompaniment of IBD, particularly active CD. Most patients with IBD will at some time develop a shortfall of one or more nutrients. Although the classic manifestations of severe nutritional deficiencies are uncommon, laboratory investigations confirm that subclinical deficiencies are by no means rare and are likely to contribute significantly to the morbidity of the disease. Each period of inflammatory activity can aggravate the patient's sometimes precarious nutritional state and contribute to general debility and, occasionally, cachexia.

On clinical grounds, it certainly can be difficult to recognize the patients most at risk, although in CD those with active, diffuse small intestinal disease or postoperative recurrence appear to have a greater tendency to develop nutritional problems. We all, however, see the occasional patient with severe colonic disease associated with considerable nutritional depletion.

Measurement of midarm circumference is a useful indicator to identify patients with CD who are most likely to have significant nutritional disturbances and would benefit from more detailed nutritional assessment. Using this criterion in our unselected outpatient population, between 20 and 40 percent of patients had some evidence of undernourishment. Furthermore, when oral nutritional supplementation was given, there was marked improvement in a variety of nutritional parameters, suggesting that nutritional impairment was significant.

The most effective therapy for nutritional depletion in IBD is treatment of the underlying disease whenever possible, and simply concentrating on overcoming the nutritional problem is no substitute for this. If it is not possible to achieve adequate control of the disease process, careful nutritional supplementation when appropriate with hematinics, vitamins, electrolytes, fluid, calories, and protein may be prudent to prevent or correct specific nutritional defects (Table 5). In some circumstances, judicial oral or intravenous feeding support may be advantageous

TABLE 5 Summary of Nutritional Guidelines in IBD

Route	Form of Treatment	Methods
Oral	Dietary advice	Well-balanced, nutritionally adequate diet
		Consider high-fiber, milk-free diet for patients with continuing symptoms
	Minerals and vitamins	Iron (most patients with any significant disease)
		Consider folate (provided vitamin B_{12} status is satisfactory)
		Vitamin B_{12} (CD patients with distal small intestinal disease)
		Consider calcium and vitamin D (in patients with extensive small intestinal CD)
	Nutritional supplements	Polymeric diet in undernourished patients
Intravenous	Fluid and electrolytes	Water, sodium, and potassium during acute, severe attacks
		Consider minerals and vitamins
	Nutrition	Consider IV feeding in some patients with severe, active disease, high small intestinal fistulas, or preoperatively if not responding to alternative measures or to prevent starvation if oral intake is inadequate

but should not be embarked upon lightly, since it is unlikely to have any significant influence on the course of the disease itself over the long term and is accompanied by its own limitations. Attention to the nutritional consequences of IBD is important, since the adoption of these approaches may help to improve the well-being and outlook of many patients suffering from these chronic, often debilitating and unpredictable diseases.

SUGGESTED READING

Harries AD, Heatley RV. Nutrition in inflammatory bowel disease. In: Heatley RV, Losowsky MS, Kelleher J, eds. Clinical nutrition in gastroenterology. Edinburgh; New York: Churchill Livingstone, 1986:146.

Harries AD, Heatley RV. Nutritional disturbances in Crohn's disease. Postgrad Med J 1983; 59:690–697.

Heatley RV, Harries AD. Nutritional support in inflammatory bowel disease. Surv Digest Dis 1984; 2:60–72.

GROWTH RETARDATION IN INFLAMMATORY BOWEL DISEASE

RICHARD J. GRAND, M.D.
KATHLEEN J. MOTIL, M.D., Ph.D.

Chronic inflammatory bowel disease encompasses two intestinal disorders of childhood: ulcerative colitis and Crohn's disease. These diseases are characterized by intermittent, recurrent exacerbations and remissions of gastrointestinal manifestations with or without systemic complications. These entities share many common clinical features and may also masquerade as juvenile rheumatoid arthritis, anorexia nervosa, collagen vascular disease, acute rheumatic fever, primary growth hormone deficiency, or appendicitis before the correct diagnosis is made. The protean manifestations of these diseases account for errors and delays in diagnosis. Careful studies of growth and body composition identify growth retardation in 20 percent of children with ulcerative colitis and 20 to 40 percent of those with Crohn's disease. Impairment of linear growth, lack of weight gain, retarded bone development, and delayed onset of sexual maturation are clinical reflections of chronic malnutrition. Combined height and weight deficits occur in nearly half of children and adolescents with inflammatory bowel disease. Midarm circumference and arm muscle area measurements are less than the 5th percentile in approximately 20 percent and triceps skinfold thickness is reduced in 5 percent of the patients.

DEFINITION OF GROWTH RETARDATION

For clinical purposes, growth retardation is defined as cessation of linear growth for more than 6 months, a decrease of one standard deviation in height percentile, or a bone age delay of greater than 2 years. Physicians responsible for the care of patients with inflammatory bowel disease should be aware of this complication and should be prepared to institute therapy for growth retardation when it is recognized.

NUTRITIONAL ASSESSMENT

Recognition of growth retardation is obviously the first step in defining the clinical problem. Growth data may be obtained from the clinical history and from assessment of growth and developmental milestones, as well as family history, particularly in relation to parental height. Pediatrician's records or school data may be an important source of growth information, and yearly heights and weights should be plotted on an appropriate growth chart to assess the characteristics of growth prior to and subsequent to the onset of inflammatory bowel disease.

Furthermore, nutritional assessment both at the time of diagnosis and subsequently is necessary to assess the initial impact of nutritional failure on the child and also to measure the success of therapy over time.

TABLE 1 Evaluation of Nutritional Status

History:
> Appetite, extracurricular activity
> Type and duration of inflammatory bowel disease, frequency of relapse
> Severity and extent of current symptoms*
> Medications

Three-day diet record

Physical examination:
> Height, weight, arm circumference, triceps skinfold measurements
> Loss of subcutaneous fat, muscle wasting, edema, pallor, skin rash, hepatomegaly

Laboratory tests:
> Complete blood count and differential, reticulocyte and platelet count, sedimentation rate, urinalysis
> Stool guaiac, cultures for bacteria, smears for ova, parasites, and fat
> Serum total proteins, albumin, transferrin, retinol-binding protein, orosomucoid, immunoglobulins
> Serum electrolytes, calcium, magnesium, phosphate, iron, zinc
> Serum folate, vitamins A, E, D, B_{12}

Special tests:
> Xylose absorption, 72-hour fecal fat, fecal, alpha$_1$-antitrypsin, lactose breath test, Schilling test

Radiology:
> Upper gastrointestinal series with small bowel follow-through
> Air contrast barium enema

Colonoscopy with biopsies

---

* Crohn's Disease Activity Index (Gastroenterology 1976; 70:439) or Lloyd Still Clinical Scoring System (Dig Dis Sci 1979; 24:620) may be useful in the assessment.

The evaluation of nutritional status in children with inflammatory bowel disease is shown in Table 1. The use of this sequential assessment allows the clinician to maintain close surveillance not only over nutritional status but also over measurements of linear growth and weight. Alterations in therapy must be made to achieve and maintain normal expected growth rates. Carefully maintained growth and nutritional data are mainstays of treatment.

CLINICAL CHARACTERISTICS OF GROWTH RETARDATION

Certain clinical features of growth retardation are important to remember when caring for children and adolescents with inflammatory bowel disease (Table 2). Growth retardation may precede clinical illness, often by years. Furthermore, growth failure may occur when clinical disease is quiescent. Under these circumstances, it must be assumed that the chronic demands placed on the body by the presence of undiagnosed inflammatory bowel disease account for chronic nutritional debility. Growth retardation is rarely if ever associated with endocrine abnormalities. Tests of hormonal function have generally been normal. However, recent reports have demonstrated that some children with growth retardation due to inflammatory bowel disease have low serum somatomedin-C levels. Somatomedins are dependent on protein intake, and serum levels rise quickly after repletion of protein nutriture. Thus, somatomedin-C levels further identify patients with nutritional failure.

TABLE 2   Clinical Characteristics of Growth Retardation

Growth retardation a common complication of inflammatory bowel disease

May precede clinical illness by months or years

May occur when clinical disease is quiescent

Associated with malabsorption or nutritional deficiencies in some patients

Rarely, if ever, associated with endocrine abnormalities

May occur in the presence or absence of steroid therapy

Reduced energy intake a major factor in poor growth

Adequate nutritional repletion can reverse malnutrition and stimulate growth

Growth retardation may occur in the presence or absence of steroid therapy; thus, it appears that active inflammatory disease has a greater impact on growth than corticosteroid therapy. Furthermore, a single morning dose of steroids appears to affect linear growth less than multiple dose schedules. Reduced energy intake is certainly a major factor in growth retardation. In addition, it is clear that adequate nutritional repletion can reverse malnutrition and stimulate growth in these patients.

CAUSES OF MALNUTRITION IN INFLAMMATORY BOWEL DISEASE

Malnutrition in patients with inflammatory bowel disease is a multifactorial problem and generally cannot be ascribed to a single event. The major factors include inadequate dietary intake, excessive gastrointestinal losses, malabsorption, and increased nutritional requirements (Table 3).

TABLE 3   Causes of Malnutrition in Inflammatory Bowel Disease

Inadequate dietary intake:
Anorexia
Altered taste
Abdominal pain
Diarrhea
Early satiety

Excessive intestinal losses:
Protein-losing enteropathy
Hematochezia
Bile-salt–losing enteropathy

Malabsorption:
Protein
Carbohydrate (xylose, lactose)
Fat
Minerals (Ca, Mg, Fe, Zn)
Vitamins (folate, B_{12}, D, K)
Bacterial overgrowth
Drug inhibiton (folate)

Increased requirements:
Fever
Fistulas
Repletion of body stores
Growth

Inadequate dietary intake may occur as a result of anorexia associated with chronic illness or recurrent bouts of inflammatory activity. Patients refuse to eat because of increased diarrhea or abdominal pain associated with ingestion of food. Early satiety may be a reflection of delayed gastric emptying. Excessive losses of nutrients may originate from the gastrointestinal tract, including protein-losing enteropathy, hematochezia, and increased fecal losses of cellular constituents as a consequence of chronic damage to the intestinal mucosa. Bile salt-losing enteropathy may result from ileal disease, resection, or fistulas. Large doses of corticosteroids or the stress-induced response to acute inflammation may also lead to urinary nitrogen and mineral losses. Malabsorption of protein, carbohydrate, fat, and minerals is common, affecting between 20 and 40 percent of patients. Malabsorption of vitamins is less common, as are bacterial overgrowth and drug-induced abnormalities (reduced folate absorption secondary to sulfasalazine therapy). Increased requirements may occur in response to increased inflammatory activity, fever, intestinal fistulas, or periods of rapid growth, particularly during adolescence. Inflammation leads to negative energy and nitrogen balances as a result of decreased dietary intake and increased metabolic activity. Additional nutrient requirements also occur as a consequence of growth demands in children. With a peak weight gain of 7 kg per 6 month interval during puberty, and at an energy cost of approximately 4.4 calories per gram of tissue gained, an additional energy intake of 170 kcal per day may be needed during the adolescent growth spurt. Therefore, the stress imposed by inflammation and growth is an important factor in the development of chronic malnutrition in children with inflammatory bowel disease.

TREATMENT OF GROWTH RETARDATION

Medical Treatment

In the routine management of inflammatory bowel disease with or without growth failure, control of inflammatory activity is the first goal of medical treatment. Medications currently used in children with inflammatory bowel disease are listed in Table 4. Sulfasalazine (50 to 75 mg per kilogram per day, maximum of 3 to 4 g per day) is recommended for the treatment of mild acute attacks and maintenance of remission when the colon is involved. Some patients with small bowel Crohn's disease

TABLE 4 Commonly Used Drugs in Treatment of Inflammatory Bowel Disease

Drug	Daily Dose	Comment
Sulfasalazine	50 mg/kg	May increase to 75 mg/kg or standard adult dose
Steroids		
Prednisone	1–2 mg/kg	Single AM dose when possible
Prednisolone		Dose depends upon severity
		Not to exceed standard adult dose
Adrenocorticotropic hormone (ACTH)	1.6–2.0 units/kg	Administer as a continuous infusion
Azathioprine	2 mg/kg	Not to exceed standard adult
6-Mercaptopurine	1.5 mg/kg	dose
Metronidazole	20 mg/kg	Not to exceed 1 g

will also respond to sulfasalazine therapy, but less predictably so. In contrast, prednisone (1 to 2 mg per kilogram per day, maximum 60 to 80 mg per day) is more effective in treating moderate to severe disease activity.

Corticosteroids are effective in inducing remissions but do not prevent relapses and may increase overall morbidity when used in a maintenance fashion. Therefore, corticosteroids are generally recommended in courses. A single morning dose is preferable when the severity of the disease permits this form of therapy. Twice daily oral doses are sometimes necessary.

When intravenous therapy is required, methylprednisolone should be used (1 to 2 mg per kilogram per day) in two or three divided doses. Adrenocorticotropic hormone (ACTH) (1.6 to 2.0 units per kilogram per day) is recommended for treatment of newly diagnosed active disease or recurrent disease when oral steroids are not being used. If therapy has been initiated with intravenous steroids or ACTH, oral prednisone may be given when symptoms abate, first using the twice daily schedule and then switching to a daily morning dose. Therapy is maintained for 4 to 6 weeks with tapering to an alternate-day regimen by decreasing the dosage 5 mg every other day at 5- to 7-day intervals. If necessary, prolonged alternate-day therapy may be maintained. In most patients, this regimen allows for gradual decrease of medication without flare-up of disease. Low-dose, alternate-day steroid therapy is an acceptable alternative form of long-term treatment.

Pharmacologic doses of corticosteroids have been associated with urinary excretion of nitrogen and have been implicated in linear growth delay in chronic disease. Nevertheless, some patients with inflammatory bowel disease demonstrate accelerated linear growth despite high-dose steroid therapy, presumably because of suppression of inflammatory activity. An improvement in appetite, however, may account in part for the growth response owing to increased dietary protein and energy intake associated with corticosteroid use. This may be particularly true when alternate-day steroid therapy is used for a prolonged period.

Other medications may be valuable in bringing disease activity under control. Azathioprine and 6-mercaptopurine may allow reduction in the dosage of steroids required, prolong remission, obviate the need for surgery, and allow prolonged maintenance in patients who would not be candidates for other forms of therapy. Metronidazole is valuable for perianal disease, and vancomycin may be helpful in those patients whose disease flare-ups are associated with *Clostridium difficile* overgrowth.

Surgical Treatment

Surgical resection of disease has been considered as an alternative in the management of growth failure in patients with inflammatory bowel disease, but the results of this approach have not supported its routine use. In most studies, children with Crohn's ileocolitis have only limited response to removal of active disease, with only 14 to 28 percent of patients showing postoperative catch-up growth. Virtually all children who have had catch-up growth after surgery were prepubertal at the time of operation; in general, pubertal patients have shown no catch-up growth after surgery. These patients have either ceased to grow or have grown at the same rate as they did prior to surgery.

At the present time, surgical intervention should be reserved for those patients in whom there is a clear indication other than growth failure. In selected prepubertal children in whom medical and nutritional therapy have failed to alter growth arrest, surgical treatment may be beneficial.

NUTRITIONAL TREATMENT

Even in the absence of nutritional failure or growth retardation, the indications and benefits of nutritional therapy in inflammatory bowel disease have become apparent. The indications for nutritional therapy are listed in Table 5. With respect to disease activity, nutritional regimens have been advocated as primary modes of therapy in newly diagnosed cases of Crohn's disease, and there is adequate documentation that clinical, biochemical, and nutritional abnormalities are reversed by nutritional therapy alone. Even in patients who have been maintained on corticosteroid treatment, with adequate nutritional support it is often possible to reduce or discontinue steroids entirely.

In terms of growth failure, both chronic enteral and parenteral regimens have produced nutritional repletion in children and adolescents with this complication of inflammatory bowel disease. Improved linear and ponderal growth rates have been observed in adolescents with Crohn's disease who received continuous enteral feedings by the nasogastric route for 6 weeks, and a dramatic rehabilitation of nutritional status and stimu-

TABLE 5   Indications for Nutritional Therapy

Primary therapy for disease activity:
   Newly diagnosed inflammatory bowel disease
   Chronic disease unresponsive to medical management
   Short bowel syndrome
   Closure of fistulas
   Small bowel obstruction
   Ostomy care

Supportive therapy for disease activity:
   Inoperative diffuse disease
   Preoperative nutritional rehabilitation

Drug-nutrient interactions:
   Sulfasalazine/folic acid

Abnormalities of specific laboratory tests:
   Anemia (microcytic, macrocytic)
   Hypoproteinemia
   Fat malabsorption
   Lactose intolerance
   Serum mineral deficiencies (Fe, Ca, Mg, K^+)
   Serum vitamin deficiencies (folate, B_{12}, A, D)
   Prolonged prothrombin time (vitamin K)
   Depressed alkaline phosphatase (Zn)

Complications of inflammatory bowel disease:
   Malnutrition
   Growth failure

lation of growth have been achieved using total parenteral nutrition with or without enteral feedings.

In our own clinics, programs of long-term nutritional supplementation have been initiated for severely growth retarded adolescents with Crohn's disease. These patients have received a daily protein and energy intake of 3.2 g per kilogram and 95 kcal per kilogram per day, respectively. Results of supplementation in these patients are shown in Table 6. After 3 weeks of nutritional supplementation, a weight gain of 4 kg occurred, nitrogen balance improved fourfold, and total body potassium increased significantly. After 7 months of nutritional supplementation, average height and weight velocities were at least five times greater than those observed during the 10 months prior to supplementation and equaled or exceeded velocities of normal adolescents. These observations demonstrate that the abnormalities in the nutritional status of adolescents with Crohn's disease, malnutrition, and growth failure are not related to intrinsic defects in metabolic pathways and that with appropriate supplementation, nutritional rehabilitation and stimulation of growth occur. Moreover, neither the presence of chronic inflammation nor the use of corticosteroids interferes with the ability to rehabilitate these patients nutritionally.

TABLE 6 Effect of Nutritional Supplementation on Body Composition, Protein and Energy Metabolism, and Growth in Adolescents

Measurement	Dietary Interval (Data)	
	Presupplementation	Postsupplementation
Body composition:		
Weight (kg)	37	41
Nitrogen retention (mg/kg/day)	36	137
Total body potassium (g)	80	87
Whole body protein and energy metabolism:		
Amino acid incorporation (mg/kg/day)	269	447
Amino acid oxidation (mg/kg/day)	262	154
"Basal" oxygen consumption (ml/min/m²)	156	206
Growth velocity:		
Height (cm/6 mo)	0.6	3.0
Weight (kg/6 mo)	1.3	7.3

In clinical situations in which abnormal symptoms, such as severe diarrhea, abscesses, or fistulas, prevent enteral rehabilitation, parenteral nutritional therapy can reverse nutritional failure and stimulate growth.

Goals of Nutritional Therapy. In the nutritional management of children with growth failure and inflammatory bowel disease, the major aim is to replace the nutrient losses associated with the inflammatory process, to correct body deficits, and to provide sufficient nutrients to promote energy and nitrogen balance for normal metabolic function. In children, additional nutrients must be provided to restore normal growth and to produce catch-up growth. To accomplish these aims, appropriate assessment of nutritional status should be performed routinely as described above. The frequency and extent of nutritional assessment will vary for each individual and should be reviewed frequently.

The methods available for treatment of nutritional disorders in inflammatory bowel disease include the enteral and parenteral routes (Table 7). The easiest way to provide nutritional supplementation is to increase dietary intake by the enteral route using standard table foods. No specific diet has been shown to alter the course of ulcerative colitis or Crohn's disease in patients who are in remission. There is also no clear evidence that the consumption or avoidance of specific foods influences the severity of disease or the frequency of relapse or induces remission. Accordingly, patients are encouraged to eat a well-balanced adequate diet and to avoid food fads. In children and adolescents, it is preferable to allow the intake of favorite foods and beverages rather than force a limited energy intake. When disease is active, when specific foods exacerbate symptoms, or when laboratory tests suggest specific abnormalities such as lactose intolerance, the diet should be modified accordingly. In the presence of severe postprandial pain, a low-residue diet administered as frequent small meals is often recommended. In children with watery diarrhea due to hydroxy-fatty acid or bile acid excretion, a low-fat diet supplemented with medium-chain triglycerides or the use of cholestyramine may be helpful in controlling symptoms. Care must be taken, however, to ensure adequate energy intake when patients are provided with instructions for a low-fat diet.

Multivitamins with minerals should be administered routinely to replace deficits in the diet. Oral iron and folic acid therapy should be provided when laboratory findings are consistent with a deficiency state. Parenteral administration of vitamin B_{12} may be necessary in patients with extensive small bowel disease or ileal resection. Despite an association

TABLE 7 Nutritional Therapy for Inflammatory Bowel Disease

Well-balanced, high-protein and energy diet:
± Low residue
± Lactose-free
± Low-fat, medium chain triglyceride (MCT) and cholestyramine supplemented

Enteral supplementation (140% to 150% of Recommended Daily Allowances for height age):
Continuous or intermittent nasogastric tube feeding
Feeding gastrostomy—continuous, or intermittent

Total parenteral nutrition (140% to 150% of Recommended Daily Allowances for height age):
Peripheral
Central

Vitamins and Minerals:
Supplemental
  Multivitamins with minerals (daily)

Therapeutic:

Folate	
Iron	1 mg daily
Ferrous sulfate (20% Fe)	6 mg elemental Fe/kg/day,
Ferrous gluconate (11.5%)	divided in 3 oral doses
Iron dextran (IM) (Imferon)	Follow directions on package insert
Magnesium	200–400 mg elemental mg/day IV
Vitamin B_{12}	1,000 g at 3-month intervals (SC or IM)
Zinc sulfate (22% Zn)	50–100 mg elemental Zn/day
	divided in 3 oral doses

between serum zinc levels and linear growth delay, very few patients with growth failure have low serum zinc levels. Those who do are generally treated with oral zinc supplements.

When the patient is unable to increase dietary protein and energy intake with larger meals or palatable snacks, oral supplementation with a commercially available liquid formula should be attempted. Successful supplementation of dietary intake may be achieved with such formulas; however, many patients will experience early satiety when taking these formulas and will not increase their total nutrient intake significantly. Under these circumstances, nutritional supplementation can be accomplished by intragastric feedings or parenteral alimentation.

Nasogastric infusions used either continuously or intermittently have been effective in reversing metabolic imbalances and improving nutritional status, linear and ponderal growth rates, and the clinical well-being of patients with inflammatory bowel disease. With this method, a silicone rubber nasogastric tube of small diameter may be passed through the nose into the stomach and left in place for continuous slow drip or pump feedings. Alternatively, the nasogastric tube may be passed in the evening for an overnight liquid infusion and removed when the patient awakens. We prefer the latter method because it does not interfere with school attendance or the social development of the adolescent. If the patient does not tolerate this form of therapy, a gastrostomy may be performed for either continuous or intermittent tube feedings in the same manner as the nasogastric regimen. The gastrostomy tube is advantageous in that it is cosmetically acceptable and easily cared for. In our experience, the only complication associated with intragastric tube feedings has been reversible diarrhea secondary to too rapid administration of the nutritional supplement.

The amount of nutritional supplementation administered via the nasogastric or gastrostomy tube will vary, depending upon the nutritional requirements and tolerance level of the individual. In our adolescent patients, 1,500 ml of a commercial formula (Ensure or Osmolite) administered nightly for 8 to 10 hours was well tolerated. This volume of supplemental formula, in addition to usual meals and snacks, provided protein and energy intakes of 3 g per kilogram per day and 95 kcal per kilogram per day, respectively. We also recommend that commercially prepared formulas be used as adjuncts rather than as the sole source of long-term nutritional intake to avoid potential nutrient imbalances.

When patients with inflammatory bowel disease are unable to tolerate adequate amounts of enteral alimentation because of disease activity or diarrhea, parenteral alimentation may provide substantial benefits. Peripheral nutrition with standard solutions providing 10 percent glucose, 2.5 percent amino acids, vitamins, and minerals may be an acceptable primary or supplemental form of therapy for short periods. Under these circumstances, peripheral alimentation must be accompanied by an intravenous lipid preparation to provide adequate energy and essential fatty acid intake. Alternatively, central venous parenteral nutrition may provide long-term support; it appropriately improves nutritional status as demonstrated by linear and ponderal growth rates, lean body mass deposition, and postoperative recovery. Parenteral alimentation may also induce a clinical remission. Home parenteral alimentation is available for those patients who require long-term nutritional support for active disease, short bowel syndrome, or growth failure. In general, the nutritional recommendations have been similar to those used for enteral nutrition support. Patients may be monitored by their own hospital programs or by a commercial nutritional maintenance company. (See *Home Parenteral Nutrition.*)

SUGGESTED READING

Grybosky JD, Spiro HD. Prognosis in children with Crohn's disease. Gastroenterology 1978; 74:807–817.

Kirshner BS, Klich JR, Kalman SS, et al. Reversal of growth retardation in Crohn's disease with therapy emphasizing oral nutritional restitution. Gastroenterology 1981; 80:10–15.

Motil KJ, Grand RJ. Nutritional management of inflammatory bowel disease. Pediatr Clin North Am 1985: 32:447–469.

NUTRITION AND LIVER DISEASE

JAUNDICE

KHURSHEED N. JEEJEEBHOY, M.B., B.S., Ph.D., F.R.C.P.(C)

Patients with jaundice have a variety of nutritional difficulties. These are related partly to the disease causing the jaundice and partly to the lack of bile in the intestine.

NUTRITIONAL EFFECTS OF DISEASE IN JAUNDICED PATIENTS

There are three major pathophysiologic causes of jaundice: (1) increased hemolysis, (2) hepatocellular disease, and (3) obstruction to the biliary passages.

Hemolytic Jaundice. This does not pose any special nutritional problems, but because it causes anemia, it can be treated mistakenly by iron and vitamin supplementation. Iron supplementation should not be given to these patients because they are often overloaded with iron.

Hepatocellular Jaundice. Liver disease causes nausea, anorexia, and vomiting. The major objective for these patients is to maintain adequate nutrient intake in the face of these symptoms. In most cases the use of high-carbohydrate, low-fat diets is helpful, not because fat is harmful to these patients but rather because fat delays gastric emptying and enhances the sense of nausea and early satiety, which limit food intake. Thus, empirically, it is easier to feed these patients diets that do not adversely affect gastric emptying. In patients with severe vomiting, it may be necessary to resort to parenteral nutrition for short periods. A peripheral system of partial parenteral nutrition works well in such patients. There is no evidence for the use of unbalanced or altered diets except in patients with liver failure who may not be able to tolerate a high protein intake.

Obstructive Jaundice. The diseases causing obstructive jaundice—
i.e., stones in the biliary tract, strictures of the common bile duct, and
cancer of the bile duct and pancreas—are often associated with abdominal pain. Under these circumstances food intake is curtailed because eating
is associated with increased pain. In addition, chronic pain and use of
analgesics may reduce appetite. Bile duct obstruction may be associated
with sepsis, causing increased catabolism. Cancer results in weight loss
due to a variety of factors, among which are the metabolic effects of neoplasia. Thus patients with obstructive jaundice often lose weight and become malnourished.

EFFECT OF LACK OF BILE
ON DIGESTION AND ABSORPTION

Bile contains salts that are essential for the absorption of fats and
fat-soluble vitamins. These salts are composed of a nonpolar steroid core
and polar side chains, which are hydroxyl groups and an amino acid.
Thus bile salts are amphipathic, i.e., they have an affinity for both fats
and water. When present in excess of a specific concentration called the
critical micellar concentration (CMC), they form small particles called
micelles. The polar groups are deployed on the outside of these and mix
with the water, and the steroid is within the micelle. These particles dissolve the products of fat digestion, fatty acids, monoglycerides, and vitamins in their lipid center and disperse them in the aqueous intestinal
contents. Such dispersal markedly increases the area of contact between
the enterocyte and the lipid. It can be shown that a gram of fat that oc-
cupies the area of a postage stamp is dispersed in micelles over an area
of three football fields! Without this interaction with bile salts, fats and
fat-soluble vitamins do not disperse in the intestine and therefore do not
come into close contact with the enterocytes that absorb the nutrients.

It it clear that in the absence of bile, fat and fat-soluble vitamins are
poorly absorbed. In consequence these patients have fatty diarrhea, lose
weight, and develop deficiencies of vitamins A, D, and K, which can
cause night blindness, metabolic bone disease, and easy bruising, respectively.

NUTRITIONAL MANAGEMENT OF JAUNDICE

Patients should be encouraged to increase caloric and protein intake
to meet target energy requirements. They should be assessed to determine their energy requirements, and diet histories should be obtained

to determine whether intake is restricted. Even if there is no restriction in intake, it is safe to assume in the presence of obstructive jaundice that there is malabsorption of fat-soluble vitamins and of about 20 to 40 percent of fat intake. These patients should take water-soluble analogues of these vitamins as supplements and a high-carbohydrate diet to permit absorption of most of the calories eaten and to avoid diarrhea. If they also have severe pancreatic insufficiency, they may need nasogastric feeding with an elemental diet low in fat in which the macronutrients are in a monomeric form. Parenteral nutrition is rarely required for obstructive jaundice per se but may be required if patients have peritonitis and sepsis in conjunction with jaundice.

JAUNDICE AND PARENTERAL NUTRITION

Another aspect of the relationship between jaundice and nutrition is the occasional development of jaundice during intravenous feeding for reasons that remain obscure. The incidence of jaundice in patients on total parenteral nutrition (TPN) is variable but is more likely to occur in children, in patients with sepsis, in those with a short bowel, and in those receiving excessive calories. The jaundice is of the so-called obstructive type and the liver is only infrequently injured. However jaundice and hepatocellular injury may occur in patients on long-term TPN and may lead to cirrhosis. While it has been claimed that jaundice does not occur in enteral nutrition, a recent controlled trial suggested that the incidence is no lower in patients on enteral nutrition than in those on TPN. The treatment of this condition is debatable; however, reduction of caloric intake, resumption of oral feeding, treatment of sepsis, and even the empirical use of metronidazole may be useful. The single most effective measure is to resume a normal oral diet.

SUGGESTED READING

Bengoa JM, Honauer SB, Sitrin MD, et al. Pattern and prognosis of liver function test abnormalities during parenteral nutrition in inflammatory bowel disease. Hepatology 1985; 5:79–84.

Miller DJ, Keetan GH, Webber BL, et al. Jaundice in severe bacterial infection. Gastroenterology 1976; 71:94–97.

Schaffner F, Popper H. Classification and mechanisms of cholestasis. In: Wright R, Alberti; KGMM, Karran S, Millwar-Sadler GH, eds. Liver and biliary disease. Philadelphia: WB Saunders, 1979:296.

Tweedle DEF, Skidmore FD, Gleave EN, et al. Nutritional support for patients undergoing surgery for cancer of the head and neck. Res Clin Forums 1979; 1:59–65.

ACUTE HEPATITIS

JENNY HEATHCOTE, M.B., B.S., M.D., F.R.C.P., F.R.C.P. (C)

The term "hepatitis," meaning inflammation of the liver, is frequently used synonomously with viral hepatitis. In North America, inflammation of the liver is as commonly caused by alcohol abuse as it is by a viral infection, and therefore the nutritional management of both viral and alcoholic hepatitis will be considered in this chapter. Because the liver has a major metabolic function, nutritional management of patients with hepatitis can be fairly complex.

VIRAL HEPATITIS

A number of viruses may infect the liver. Some of these are liver specific, namely hepatitis A and B and the group of viruses termed collectively "non-A, non-B." Other viruses affect the liver within the context of a systemic infection, and in North America the most common of these are the Epstein-Barr virus and cytomegalovirus. Fortunately, the more severe herpes simplex virus hepatitis is rarely seen.

Acute viral hepatitis is generally a benign, short-lived illness. This is fortunate since there are no antiviral drugs known to be particularly effective against the hepatitis viruses. Rarely, viral hepatitis takes a fulminant course (0.1 percent of hepatitis virus infections). An increased prevalence of fulminant, particularly non-A, non-B, hepatitis in pregnant women from third-world countries may be related to their general malnutrition and the increased nutritional requirements demanded by the fetus. However, in all patients with acute viral hepatitis, the potential for inadequate nutritional intake is present. In acute viral hepatitis anorexia is probably the most common, and often the only, symptom. It is more likely that the nutritional status of the patient with acute viral hepatitis will depend on the severity of the disease. Loss of appetite may be so severe that the very thought or smell of food will lead to profound nausea. Vomiting is not uncommon but should it continue past a day or two it may herald particularly severe hepatitis. Protracted vomiting is one of the indications for hospital admission and careful observation and manage-

182

ment. However, the usual pattern of events is for appetite to gradually improve without the need for nutritional support.

There are a number of idiosyncratic reactions to drugs such as halothane and predictable toxic hepatic drug reactions such as overdose of acetaminophen that may also lead to the development of severe acute hepatic failure, indistinguishable clinically from fulminant viral hepatitis. Management of these conditions is the same as for viral hepatitis, plus the use of antidotes when applicable.

General Nutritional Support

In the 1950s, a study on servicemen with acute viral hepatitis showed that those fed (via tube feeding) a high-calorie diet with more than 150 g of protein and fat per day had a shorter course of illness compared to those given a regular diet. The reason for the apparent benefit from a high-calorie diet is uncertain. Recently, some evidence has emerged that glucagon and insulin may be "hepatotrophic" factors, hence it is possible that a diet high in calories may exert its benefit via the stimulation of these two hormones. There is no evidence to support the "old wives' tale" that fat should be avoided in acute hepatitis. A high-fat diet may precipitate nausea in anyone who is anorexic, but low-fat, calorie-sufficient diets are bulky and unappetizing. Therefore, there should be no fat restriction.

Clotting Factors and Glucose Metabolism

Patients with fulminant hepatitis will rapidly develop symptoms and signs of liver failure leading to a decreasing level of consciousness, coma, and frequently death. The mortality rate in such patients is approximately 80 percent even with the best medical care. Under these circumstances the role of the liver as the body's major synthesizer and metabolizer of essential nutrients becomes highlighted. Clinically, the two most evident manifestations of the liver's failure to synthesize adequately are easy bruising and hypoglycemia.

The liver alone manufactures all the clotting factors except for Factor VIII. Factors II, VII, IX, and X are dependent on normal liver function and an adequate supply of vitamin K. It is recommended that 10 mg of vitamin K be given subcutaneously (never intramuscularly, as this may give rise to further bruising) when a coagulopathy is present.

As vitamin K is fat soluble, its absorption may be impaired in the presence of jaundice due to a reduction in the concentration of bile acids in the duodenum. Hence, the vitamin should be administered parenterally, probably for 3 consecutive days. As might be expected, vitamin K replacement therapy frequently does not reverse the coagulation abnormalities. If bleeding occurs, blood coagulation factors will need to be replaced by intravenously administered fresh frozen plasma and blood.

Hypoglycemia is one of the few avoidable causes of death in fulminant viral hepatitis. Its exact etiology is unclear. Examination of the liver has revealed low glycogen levels, and therefore, defects in glycogen synthesis and gluconeogenesis have been suggested. It is also likely that hepatic metabolism of insulin and glucagon is impaired under such circumstances. Prolonged hypoglycemia may lead to irreversible brain damage, and hence its development should be anticipated and prevention attempted. How this may be achieved is uncertain. In view of the fluid and electrolyte abnormalities that occur in fulminant viral hepatitis, it is best to avoid intravenous feeding when possible and to use nasogastric tube feeding; this will also aid in maintaining adequate oral caloric intake. Hypoglycemia may be so severe that even continuous intravenous glucose administration may fail to reverse the condition.

Fluid and Electrolytes

Marked fluid and electrolyte disturbances always accompany fulminant viral hepatitis. Rapid fluid retention takes place initially due to abnormalities in the renal excretion of free water, which gives rise to a dilutional hyponatremia. However, total body sodium levels are generally elevated owing to progressive renal failure and secondary hyperaldosteronism. As the liver failure progresses, renal function deteriorates rapidly. The hepatorenal syndrome, the exact cause of which is unknown, is present in most cases of fatal fulminant viral hepatitis.

The most common electrolyte problem encountered early in the course of the fulminant disease is hypokalemia, which may require as much as 600 mEq of potassium daily. Hypocalcemia and hypomagnesemia may also be present. Once renal failure is evident and electrolytes as well as fluid cannot be adequately excreted, any combination of electrolyte abnormalities may be observed and each needs to be treated individually. Because of the rapidly changing picture, it is probably safest to try to maintain the fluid and electrolyte balance by enteral administration when possible since there is a slightly lower risk of fluid overload via the oral-enteral route.

Hepatic Encephalopathy and Protein Metabolism

The sine qua non of fulminant viral hepatitis is the presence of hepatic encephalopathy. Its exact etiology is unknown, but it is well established that protein loading worsens and protein restriction improves hepatic encephalopathy. There is a marked disturbance of protein metabolism in severe acute and chronic liver disease. Since the half life of albumin is 20 days, there may be little fall in serum albumin levels in rapidly fulminant viral hepatitis (apart from the spurious effect of hemodilution), but disruption of the normal amino acid pattern is observed. There is a relative lack of the branched–chain amino acids—leucine, isoleucine, and valine—but administration of these amino acids does not improve mental status in the long term. Hence, the only recourse is to restrict total protein intake, which has the additional benefit of reducing sodium intake. Reduced protein load can be further achieved by enhancing the evacuation of protein from the bowel obtained by the use of purgatives. The most commonly used is lactulose, a nonabsorbed disaccharide that not only acts as a purgative but also lowers the pH of the bowel lumen, thereby further enhancing nitrogen excretion by promoting the formation of NH_4 ions. Lactulose can be administered either orally or via enema if the patient is unconscious. Magnesium-containing purgatives should be avoided as they may precipitate hypermagnesemia in the face of renal failure.

Unfortunately, the depression of the nervous system in acute fulminant viral hepatitis is generally complicated by cerebral edema. Therefore, despite energetic treatment of hepatic encephalopathy, improvement of the level of consciousness may not occur. Fluid overload may well predispose to the development of cerebral edema and should be avoided.

Alcohol

As alcohol is preferentially metabolized by the liver, patients with acute viral hepatitis are advised to abstain from alcohol during the acute and recovery phases of their illness. There is no hard data to support this, and physicians really use this dictum to remind their patients of the harmful effects of too much alcohol upon the liver.

ALCOHOLIC HEPATITIS

A small percentage of alcoholics (defined as the consumption of 80 g or more of alcohol daily) develop alcoholic hepatitis. The factors that together with excess alcohol consumption promote liver damage are as yet undefined. Similarly, the exact route by which alcohol and/or its metabolites exert their damaging effect upon the liver remains unclear. Alcoholic hepatitis is a diagnosis that can be made only by examining liver tissue obtained at liver biopsy as there are no clinical features that will distinguish it from any other form of alcohol-induced liver disease (e.g., fatty liver or cirrhosis).

There is no good evidence of a link between diet and the development of alcoholic liver disease. In vivo experiments have shown that alcohol-induced liver injury may occur despite a more than adequate diet. However, there may indeed be an as yet undefined interaction between diet, alcohol, and other factors (e.g., genetic) that predispose an alcoholic to develop liver disease. The severity of alcoholic hepatitis is variable. There is an attendant mortality that varies from 0 to 50 percent depending on the series being reported.

Nutritional Deficiencies

Many nutritional deficiencies are observed in association with alcoholic hepatitis. These abnormalities are due partly to poor dietary intake and partly to the effects of alcohol upon the liver and other organs. To fully consider the nutritional requirements of the alcoholic with alcohol-induced hepatitis, it is essential to first establish the baseline nutritional deficiencies that may be present as a result of alcoholism per se.

Although small preprandial doses of alcohol have long been recommended to stimulate the appetite, it has been observed that excess alcohol consumption (i.e., more than 10 percent of ingested calories) actually suppresses the appetite. Inadequate food intake may also be the result of financial problems caused by heavy alcohol consumption.

Initially, reduced food intake in the alcoholic leads to a deficiency of vitamins whose body stores are normally small, such as folic acid, thiamine, and vitamin C. Long-term alcohol abuse gives rise to a much broader range of nutritional deficits, including riboflavin, nicotinic acid, pyridoxine, and pantothenic acid deficiencies. If the diet is chronically reduced, deficiency of fat-soluble vitamins A, D, and K, as well as protein deficiency, may occur. More recently, deficiencies of zinc, magnesium, and calcium have been described in chronic alcoholics. There is some evidence that zinc deficiency may lead to further hepatic deterioration, but further research is needed in this area.

These deficiencies probably result from a combination of decreased intake and reduced absorption. For instance, iron deficiency which is never purely nutritional, may also result from the toxic effects of alcohol on bone marrow or chronic blood loss secondary to alcoholic gastritis. Gastritis can also contribute to malnutrition by causing anorexia.

Malabsorption and Malnutrition

In vitro experiments have shown that alcohol may also have a direct toxic effect upon the small bowel mucosa, thereby affecting glucose, amino acid, fatty acid, folate, thiamine, and even vitamin B_{12} absorption.

Chronic alcohol abuse tends to give rise to pancreatic damage before it induces liver disease. Chronic pancreatitis causes maldigestion of protein, fat, and carbohydrate. Severe chronic pancreatitis in the alcoholic results in diabetes. In alcoholics with pancreatitis and liver disease, diabetes is extremely difficult to control as these patients have marked insulin resistance. Severe chronic pancreatitis also causes vitamin B_{12} deficiency by impairing secretion of the pancreatic enzymes needed to degrade the vitamin B_{12}–R factor complex.

Fat-soluble vitamin deficiencies occur only when there is marked cholestasis due either to a bile duct stricture secondary to pancreatitis or to severe alcoholic hepatitis. However, vitamin K deficiency, and rarely vitamin D deficiency, may on occasion be purely nutritional.

The metabolism of alcohol and its effect upon the liver seem to lead to increased requirements for certain nutrients, such as folic acid and vitamin B_6. It makes sense to provide supplements of those nutritional factors known to be reduced in the alcoholic as well as to advise withdrawal from alcohol. Those factors whose long-term deficiency may lead to irreversible damage (e.g., thiamine) should certainly be administered to all alcoholics.

Alcohol Withdrawal

Alcohol withdrawal is mandatory in the treatment of alcohol-related disease of any organ. There is no evidence to suggest that this should not be done "cold turkey." There is a direct correlation between long-term mortality from alcohol-related liver disease and maintenance of alcohol abstention. Nevertheless, despite cessation of alcohol intake, alcoholic hepatitis carries with it a significant mortality.

Treatment

Numerous treatment regimens have been tried, but none has had significant success. Among these have been various nutritional therapies, the latest of which has been the oral or intravenous administration of branched-chain amino acids (BCAA). Early reports on the use of this new nutritional supplement were encouraging, but the most recent randomized controlled trials have failed to show any difference in the mortality rates of those who received the therapy and those who received a calorically equivalent diet minus BCAA, despite the finding that administration of BCAA may lead to a return to normal of the blood amino acid profile. Thus, expensive protein formulas containing BCAA have been rendered redundant. Unless the patient's course is complicated by the development of hepatic encephalopathy, a high-protein diet from regular sources should be prescribed as most patients are malnourished. While high-protein diets are unpalatable to patients with gastritis, this problem is shortlived since gastric mucosa heals rapidly.

Complications

When complications of portal hypertension accompany alcoholic hepatitis with or without background cirrhosis, more complex dietary management is indicated. Portal hypertension may give rise to ascites, hepatic encephalopathy, and/or bleeding from esophageal and/or gastric varices.

In patients who manifest signs of hepatic encephalopathy, electrolyte imbalance, sepsis, or constipation should be treated first, and only if there is still no improvement should protein intake be reduced.

All patients with ascites resulting from liver disease have marked sodium retention, although the serum sodium may be normal or even reduced (secondary to hemodilution). An essential aspect of ascites management is salt restriction, which in turn necessitates a degree of protein restriction. Patients with moderate ascites and normal serum sodium need only be restricted to 1 to 2 g of NaCl per day, but patients with marked fluid retention and hyponatremia require sodium intake to be restricted to as little as 500 mg per day. Particularly in those with peripheral edema and hyponatremia, fluid restriction to a liter per day may be indicated. Occasionally this therapy may be complicated by hypovolemia, which is best treated with intravenous colloid replacement in the form of salt-poor albumin.

Diuretic therapy, which will not be discussed in detail here, is a necessary part of the therapeutic regimen for fluid retention in alcoholic hepatitis. The major diuretic used in the control of ascites is the aldosterone antagonist spironolactone, a potassium-sparing diuretic. Hence, the salt substitute KCl should not be used in these patients. Hyperkalemia is not a problem despite the chronic use of spironolactone unless renal failure supervenes or the patient has a type IV renal tubular acidosis (seen most frequently in diabetics). In fact, many patients with alcoholic hepatitis have hypokalemia on the basis of the more common forms of renal tubular acidosis as well as secondary to hyperaldosteronism. In the event that renal failure of any etiology supervenes, the usual dietary and fluid restrictions should be applied.

Our incomplete knowledge of the importance of nutritional support in viral and alcoholic hepatitis reflects the lack of expertise in this field demonstrated by practising physicians to date.

SUGGESTED READING

Chalmers TC, Eckhardt RD, Reynolds WE, et al. The treatment of acute infectious hepatitis: controlled studies of the effects of diet, rest, and physical reconditioning on the acute course of the disease and on the incidence of relapses and residual abnormalities. J Clin Invest 1955; 34:1163–1235.

Felig P, Brown WV, Levine RA, et al. Glucose homeostasis in viral hepatitis. N Engl J Med 1970; 283:1436–1440.

Mendenhall CL, Anderson S, Weesner RE, et al. Protein-calorie malnutrition associated with alcoholic hepatitis. Am J Med 1984; 76:211–222.

Mezei E. Liver disease and nutrition. Gastroenterology 1978; 74:770–783.

Mezei E. Alcoholic liver disease: roles of alcohol and malnutrition. Am J Clin Nutr 1980; 33:2709–2718.

Nefzger MD, Chalmers TC. The treatment of acute infectious hepatitis: ten year follow-up study of the effects of diet and rest. Am J Med 1963; 35:299–309.

Neveau S, Pelletier G, Poynard T, et al. A randomized clinical trial of supplementary parenteral nutrition in jaundiced, alcoholic cirrhotic patients. Hepatology 1986; 6:270–274.

Sherlock S. Nutrition and the alcoholic. Lancet 1984; 1:436–438.

HEPATIC ENCEPHALOPATHY

BRAD W. WARNER, M.D.
JOSEF E. FISCHER, M.D., F.A.C.S.

Nutritional management of the failing liver is basically supportive, as the liver possesses a great capacity for regeneration following injury. Of the numerous factors known to promote hepatic regeneration (triiodothyronine, adrenocorticosteroids, insulin), nutrition is the most easily manipulated by the physician. Metabolism of carbohydrate, protein, and fat is altered in liver failure, but abnormal metabolism of protein is the factor that most severely limits nutritional repletion. Provision of inadequate amounts of protein results in suboptimal support of hepatic protein synthesis, permitting continued protein catabolism, and therefore is of limited value. Alternatively, administration of large amounts of protein to the failing liver precipitates hepatic encephalopathy. Optimal nutritional management of liver failure and encephalopathy, therefore, should provide protein sufficient for support of hepatic regeneration while at the same time avoiding the development (or worsening) of encephalopathy.

ETIOLOGY

An understanding of the etiology of hepatic encephalopathy is essential in the treatment of this condition. No single agent has been found to be responsible for hepatic encephalopathy, and no single theory adequately explains its etiology. Most hypotheses, however, arise from the general concept that the failing liver is no longer able to inactivate or metabolize certain substances. The four main hypotheses are as follows:

The Ammonia Hypothesis. Unfortunately, no correlation exists between blood or brain ammonia levels and the degree of encephalopathy. There is little disagreement that ammonia is a component of a set of factors responsible for inducing encephalopathy, or at least that elevated levels are associated with encephalopathy, but it is not accepted as the sole causative agent.

The Synergistic Hypothesis. This hypothesis proposes that the combination of ammonia, mercaptans, methanethiols, and short-chain fatty acids causes hepatic encephalopathy. Owing to the difficulty in measurement of these combined factors in different laboratories, this hypothesis has not gained widespread acceptance. Furthermore, short-chain fatty acids have been administered to patients with a history of encephalopathy without causing encephalopathy.

The Amino Acid/Neurotransmitter Hypothesis. This hypothesis suggests that the plasma amino acid imbalance induced by the failing liver allows the accumulation of a greater proportion of aromatic amino acids (phenylalanine, tyrosine, and tryptophan) as well as methionine and histidine in the central nervous system. These amino acids are all aminergic neurotransmitter precursors, and when there exists an imbalance of aminergic products, encephalopathy ensues. Much support for this theory has evolved.

The GABA Hypothesis. The inhibitory neurotransmitter, gamma-aminobutyric acid (GABA), is normal in advanced hepatic coma and in animals following total hepatectomy. However, there has been a recent interest in GABA as a possible cause of hepatic encephalopathy, especially with the finding of increased GABA in plasma of animals and patients with hepatic coma. In its current form, the GABA hypothesis suggests (1) increased rates of entry, through an abnormal permeable intestine, of GABA formed by colonic bacteria; (2) decreased rates of extraction of GABA by the liver; (3) increased rates of GABA formation by extracerebral tissue, such as liver and kidney; (4) entry of GABA into the brain through an impaired blood-brain barrier; (5) up-regulation in the brain of components of GABA receptor complex, including the GABA-amplifying benzodiazepine and barbiturate binding sites and of the glycine receptor; and (6) down-regulation of receptor sites for putative excitatory neurotransmitters, such as glutamate and aspartate. It is likely that if GABA has any applicability at all to hepatic coma, it is largely in the area of acute hepatic necrosis, as no studies of acute-on-chronic hepatic encephalopathy have revealed increased amounts of GABA in any site in the brain. It does, however, remain a very active area of investigation with respect to hepatic encephalopathy.

CLASSIFICATION OF LIVER FAILURE

The development of liver failure can be conveniently divided into three general categories:

Acute. This usually involves a previously normal liver and is associated with a viral or toxic etiology. This type of liver failure is progressive and outcome is decided rapidly (within 2 to 3 weeks).

Chronic. This is most commonly associated with alcoholic cirrhosis. Typically, the liver shows signs of acute necrosis superimposed upon chronic damage.

"Acute-on-Chronic." This implies an acute insult (e.g., infection, shock, starvation) to a liver with preexistent disease. While most patients with acute liver failure benefit from nutritional support (and we have demonstrated that patients with chronic liver disease have improved survival with prolonged and aggressive nutritional repletion), patients with acute-on-chronic liver failure probably benefit the most from nutritional intervention, and it is toward this group of patients that the remainder of the discussion will be directed. Management of the patient with acute-on-chronic liver failure consists of treatment of the underlying cause of the acute event and correction of associated hepatic functional abnormalities. Furthermore, therapy directed toward specific treatment of associated encephalopathy is warranted.

Precipitating Factors

The development of encephalopathy in a patient with known liver disease should prompt a thorough search for the acute insult, as treatment of the initiating event alone may resolve the encephalopathy. Easily recognized and common initiators include constipation, dehydration, and overdiuresis. Other important initiators are discussed below.

THERAPY OF HEPATIC ENCEPHALOPATHY

The optimal management of hepatic encephalopathy should include the following therapeutic measures:

Identification and Treatment of Infection

Urinary tract infection and pneumonia are common in this population, and work-up should include urinalysis and culture as well as chest films. The possibility of intravenous catheter sepsis should be entertained in a patient who has been hospitalized with a long-term indwelling central or peripheral venous catheter. Spontaneous bacterial peritonitis is an entity increasingly recognized in cirrhotic patients with ascites and must be considered when acute deterioration occurs, as mortality in this patient population is very high (up to 90 percent). To exclude this possibility, paracentesis should be performed with removal of a small amount of ascitic fluid, which is gram-stained and sent for culture and sensitivity as well as a cell count. Prompt therapy is indicated and consists of parenteral antibiotics to which the cultured organism is sensitive (usually pneumococci or gram-negative rods).

Treatment of Gastrointestinal Bleeding

While patients with cirrhosis are at higher risk for the development of gastric and duodenal ulcers as well as gastritis, esophageal varices account for the majority of cases, depending, of course, on the patient population. Hemorrhage results in diminished liver perfusion and further compromises hepatic function. Additionally, the blood in the gastrointestinal (GI) tract is high in protein, and gut absorption of this protein contributes to encephalopathy.

Treatment of upper GI bleeding consists of insertion of a Foley catheter, at least two large-bore peripheral intravenous lines, and a large-diameter nasogastric (NG) tube. Iced saline lavage is performed through the NG tube and continued until clear. Blood pressure is restored with volume replacement in the form of crystalloid and packed red blood cells as dictated by hematocrit changes. Fiberoptic upper GI endoscopy is performed as soon as possible to define the source of bleeding and direct more specific therapy. Maintenance of adequate urine output (0.5 to 1.0 ml per kilogram per hour) is important to prevent the development of acute tubular necrosis. In patients who are hemodynamically unstable, insertion of a Swan-Ganz catheter and arterial catheter permits continuous hemodynamic monitoring while adding valuable diagnostic information.

If variceal bleeding is the etiology, the quicker the bleeding is stopped the better the outcome. Endoscopic sclerotherapy is attempted when available, and intravenous Pitressin is begun at 0.4 units per minute and slowly tapered once bleeding has been controlled. A Sengstaken-Blakemore tube may be used to control bleeding if the previously mentioned techniques fail; this tube provides only temporary hemostasis but is often life-saving. Finally, emergent portosystemic shunt procedures may be indicated in selected patients, but these have a high mortality. (Further discussion is beyond the scope of this chapter.)

Correction of Electrolyte Abnormalities

Hypokalemia and alkalosis often occur and should be aggressively treated with parenteral potassium-chloride supplementation. Enteral administration of potassium is not recommended, as absorption is likely to be impaired with the concomitant administration of enemas and cathartics, and potassium is irritating to the gut mucosa. Potassium chloride may be administered as "piggybacks" over 1 hour in dosages of 7.5 mEq in 50 ml D_5W peripherally or 20 mEq in 50 ml D_5W centrally. Serum electrolytes are checked every 4 hours to guide subsequent replacement.

Hyponatremia is also common and is usually dilutional. The best approach is fluid restriction (less than 1,000 ml per 24 hrs). The best guide to sodium requirements is the measurement of 24-hour urinary sodium excretion; no more sodium is given than the amount excreted in the urine each day, which is usually small, as urine sodium is usually less than 10 mEq per liter. One should also measure sodium losses from other sources if applicable (e.g., NG tube, drains).

Protein Restriction

This is very important in the patient capable of oral intake. The minimum intake is 40 g of protein per day. Oral intake of less than 20 g of protein per day is incompatible with long-term survival.

Catharsis

This removes protein load from the gut and is an important consideration for the patient with large amounts of blood in the GI tract. Cleansing tap water or soapsuds enemas are sufficient. Oral magnesium citrate (300 ml) or castor oil (30 ml) may also be tried. Alternatively, lactulose as an enema or cathartic may be substituted.

Lactulose

The exact mechanism of action is unknown, but lactulose reduces absorption of intraluminal ammonia by the creation of an acidic pH and an increase in intestinal transit time (cathartic effect) and may stimulate secretion of nitrogenous compounds from the gut into the intestinal lumen. The dosage is titrated to the clinical appearance of 2 to 3 soft stools per day. Lactulose is prepared as a syrup and 30 ml is given by mouth every hour until diarrhea ensues and then once or twice per day as a maintenance dose. Lactulose may also be given as an enema consisting of 300 ml of 50 percent lactulose in 700 ml tap water.

Intestinal Sterilization

Nonabsorbable antibiotics such as kanamycin or neomycin may be tried in an attempt to reduce the urea-splitting organisms within the bowel. These antibiotics must be used with caution in patients with preexisting renal insufficiency, as up to 1 percent of orally administered neomycin may be absorbed, which may worsen renal function or subject the patient to ototoxicity. The dosage most often administered is 1 to 2 g of neomycin given orally every 6 to 8 hours.

Colon Exclusion

This is a rarely used procedure, since operative morbidity and mortality in this patient population is substantial. When utilized, end ileostomy is performed rather than ileorectal anastomosis; the latter procedure allows for bacterial overgrowth of the terminal ileum, which decreases the effectiveness of the procedure.

Parenteral Nutrition

Parenteral nutrition is considered for patients who have an anticipated lack of oral intake for more than 72 hours. Usually, in a patient with grade zero or grade I encephalopathy, a standard balanced amino acid solution is slowly introduced with a goal of 50 to 60 g of amino acids to be administered daily. Up to 60 percent of these patients can be expected to tolerate this protein load and require no further specialized therapy. Any sign of worsening encephalopathy or lack of improvement of encephalopathy for 1 week warrants a switch to a more specialized amino acid solution containing high branched-chain amino acids (BCAA) (e.g., Hepatamine). Additionally, a plasma amino acid profile is drawn just prior to institution of therapy and then twice weekly. The need to switch to Hepatamine would be supported by a worsening of the plasma amino acid profile (increasing concentration of aromatic amino acids and decreasing amounts of BCAA).

Parenteral nutrition with Hepatamine (35 percent BCAA) is indicated as the first-line treatment in patients with grade II or greater encephalopathy, as many of these patients will not tolerate a standard amino acid formulation.

Potential benefits to the use of high BCAA-containing formulations include the abrogation of the peripheral energy deficit that exists in these patients, as the BCAA can be completely oxidized by skeletal muscle for energy and may supply up to 30 percent of energy requirements. Furthermore, the BCAA are capable of stimulating protein synthesis and inhibiting protein degradation within skeletal muscle. Hepatic protein synthesis is also stimulated by the BCAA when administered with an energy source. By curtailment of skeletal muscle proteolysis and stimulation of muscle and hepatic protein synthesis, fewer aromatic amino acids are unloaded into the circulation and thus provide less competition for amino acid transport at the blood-brain barrier. Finally, the infused BCAA compete for transport at the blood-brain barrier with aromatic and other "toxic" amino acids.

Generally, Hepatamine is administered in a 25 percent dextrose base, with approximately 41 g of amino acids given the first 24 hours and advanced at 20 g per day until a final goal of 80 to 100 g of amino acids per day is reached. Therapy is continued for as long as the patient remains encephalopathic (grade II or greater) and is unable to tolerate enteral intake.

Prospective, randomized trials that have demonstrated improved survival and reversal of encephalopathy have used dextrose as the sole substrate. Only two trials have shown no benefit to the use of high BCAA solutions, and both have used some type of fat as substrate. Therefore, we do not recommend the use of lipids as a principal energy source during Hepatamine infusion, but some lipid should be given both to prevent essential fatty acid deficiency and to serve as a source of energy for the viscera. Serum fatty acids should be monitored.

The management of the patient with acute hepatic encephalopathy mandates a careful search for its etiology and therapy directed toward removal of potentially toxic substances and nutritional support of the failing liver. Optimal therapeutic modalities for the patient with hepatic encephalopathy should result in lower morbidity and improved survival.

SUGGESTED READING

Fischer JE. Portal systemic encephalopathy. In: Wright R, Millward-Sadler GH, Alberti KGMM, and Karran S, eds. Liver and biliary disease, 2nd ed. London: WB Saunders, 1985: 1245.

James JH, Jeppsson B, Ziparo V, Fischer JE. Hyperammonemia, plasma amino acid imbalance, and blood-brain amino acid transport: a unified theory of portal-systemic encephalopathy. Lancet 1979; 2:772–775.

Nachbauer CA, Fischer JE. Nutritional support in hepatic failure. In: Fischer JE, ed. Surgical nutrition. Boston: Little, Brown, 1983: 551.

NUTRITION AND SURGERY

PREOPERATIVE NUTRITIONAL SUPPORT

GORDON P. BUZBY, M.D.

The goal of nutritional support is to provide appropriate nutrient intake under a given set of clinical circumstances. Over the past two decades the development of parenteral nutrient solutions and technologic improvements in delivery of enteral and parenteral feedings have made it possible to feed the great majority of patients. In the preoperative period, it is now possible to maintain or even improve nutritional status in all but the most severely stressed or septic patients. Few would deny that patients requiring surgery should be encouraged to eat an adequate diet when per os intake is both possible and not inconsistent with other aspects of the therapeutic plan. But when are invasive, potentially dangerous, and/or expensive interventions warranted in order to provide nutritional support prior to operation, especially when this necessitates a delay in surgery? Data are insufficient to define with precision when such interventions are definitely indicated or contraindicated. Clinicians must make their decisions based on a synthesis of hard and soft data, and of clinical experience and judgment being aware of economic realities and constantly vigilant in keeping abreast of new developments.

The goal of preoperative nutritional support is to maintain nutritional status in the well-nourished patient or to improve it in the malnourished patient in the days immediately preceding operation. Although improved nutrition per se is a legitimate objective, in most cases it does not justify the potential morbidity and expense of preoperative enteral or parenteral feeding unless it provides some other direct tangible benefit to the patient. If there is such a direct benefit, it will lie mostly in the reduction of the high operative morbidity and mortality associated with surgery performed in the face of untreated protein-calorie malnutrition. Thus preoperative nutritional support is indicated when it can be expected to reduce such operative morbidity and/or mortality.

PREREQUISITES FOR PREOPERATIVE NUTRITIONAL SUPPORT

Rational application of preoperative nutritional support is based on the following:

1. The patient is malnourished or likely to become substantially so prior to operation should nutritional support be withheld.
2. Malnutrition is associated (as a potentially causative factor) with an increased incidence of complications following the particular operation i.e., an incidence exceeding that experienced with well-nourished patients undergoing the same operation.
3. No delay in surgery is involved in providing preoperative nutritional support, or if a delay is required it will not be detrimental to the patient.
4. Treatment of the malnutrition prior to surgery (or maintenance of normal nutrition) can be achieved safely and is known (or strongly suspected) to reduce the operative complications otherwise experienced.

Patients for whom all these criteria are satisfied are definite candidates for preoperative nutritional support, while failure to meet one or more puts the value of such support in question. For an individual patient, determination of whether each criterion is met is frequently both an art and a science. However, most clinicians would agree that optimal assessment must include input from the patient's primary physician, surgeon, and nutritional support team. An approach to patient selection for preoperative nutritional support is presented below. It is consistent with the prerequisites mentioned above and has proven useful in our clinical experience. By no means is it the only reasonable approach to selection and modification to fit the peculiarities of other patient populations and local situations can be readily envisioned.

PATIENT SELECTION

"Is the patient malnourished?" This is the first question that should be asked at the time of patient presentation. In an emergency, even if malnutrition is severe, operation cannot be delayed to permit preoperative repletion. However, preoperative recognition of nutritional deficits may assist the surgeon in planning the operative procedure. For example, intraoperative placement of a jejunal feeding tube to permit postoperative enteral repletion may be indicated in a malnourished patient undergoing emergency partial gastrectomy for a bleeding gastric ulcer. In contrast, the surgeon may forego jejunostomy in a well-nourished patient who will better tolerate the several weeks of suboptimal oral intake that follow this procedure.

Although most would agree that baseline nutritional status should be assessed, there will be far less agreement on how this is best accomplished. From the abundance of proposed markers, the clinician must pick which measures to use routinely in the preoperative setting, and which one to follow when two or more measures give conflicting results. Some clinicians avoid this problem by shunning tests altogether and basing nutritional assessment on a careful history and physical examination, focusing on dietary and weight loss history and physical stigmata of malnutrition (muscle wasting, edema, etc.). This approach has been termed Subjective Global Assessment (SGA) by its proponents. When properly used by experienced individuals, SGA is sufficiently sensitive and specific for malnutrition to make it useful for preoperative assessment and identification of patients likely to suffer nutrition-related postoperative complications.

An alternative to subjective assessment is the use of selected objective nutritional markers which, either alone or in combination with other markers (sometimes in multivariate equations), are known to be associated with increased operative risk. The Prognostic Nutritional Index (PNI) is perhaps the best known of several multivariate models relating nutritional status to risk of operative complications in a quantitative way. Although the PNI has proven highly useful in both clinical and research settings, its dependence on skin tests makes its routine use for preoperative screening inconvenient since the skin test results are not available for 48 hours.

A simplified modification of the PNI has been used recently to screen for malnutrition in a large multi-institution clinical study funded by the

Veterans Administration (VA). This index is termed the Nutrition Risk Index (NRI) and is based on serum albumin (g per deciliter) and recent weight loss (% usual body weight (UBW) = current weight/weight 6 months ago). The NRI is given by the relationship:

$$NRI = 15.19 \times serum\ albumin + 0.417 \times \%UBW$$

An NRI greater than 100 indicates normal nutritional status; an NRI of 97.5 to 99.9 indicates mild malnutrition; and an NRI below 97.5 indicates moderate to severe malnutrition.

Both the SGA and the NRI have been shown to correlate well with other more sophisticated measures of nutritional status. In the VA study these two measures showed a remarkable degree of concordance. When both techniques were used independently to assess baseline nutritional status in 447 preoperative patients, in only seven cases did one technique indicate normal nutritional status where the other indicated severe malnutrition. Agreement between the two techniques in assessing the *severity* of malnutrition (moderate versus severe or mild versus moderate) was less pronounced. From a practical point of view, based on the VA experience, it would appear reasonable for the experienced, nutritionally astute clinician to utilize subjective assessment as a screening technique for preoperative malnutrition when the assessment is based on a rigorous, thorough, and objective examination. When SGA suggests malnutrition, more objective measures like the NRI or PNI become useful in gauging its severity.

After assessing baseline status, one must ask whether malnutrition will be associated with increased morbidity following the anticipated operation. Good data exist for a variety of diseases and operations relating excess postoperative complications to preexisting malnutrition as diagnosed by subjective (SGA) or objective (NRI, PNI, etc.) criteria. The strongest data exist for major abdominal operations involving the gastrointestinal (GI) tract from thoracic inlet to anus, including gynecologic and urologic procedures in which bowel is resected or anastomosed. Increases in complications and mortality ranging from twofold to tenfold are commonly reported in malnourished patients. The most substantial increases are seen in complications related to impaired wound healing (anastomotic leaks, wound disruption, etc.) and increased susceptibility to infection, both of which may be caused by malnutrition.

In contrast, the relationship between nutritional status and outcome following cardiac or vascular surgery is far less convincing. Although more complications occur in malnourished patients, they tend to relate to technical factors and/or extent of disease. Malnutrition may be a "marker" for more severe underlying disease and thereby be associated with increased morbidity. This relationship may not be causative, however, and correction of malnutrition may not influence the risk factors that are truly responsible for the excessively high morbidity (extensive atherosclerotic disease, poor myocardial function, etc.). Prompt, technically superior surgery and anesthetic support are probably the keys to a favorable outcome in these patients.

For operations involving a variety of other organ systems (head and neck, major orthopaedic procedures in the elderly, etc.) the relationship between malnutrition and poor outcome also exists. For these procedures, the nature of the association is probably somewhere between the cause and effect relationship seen in GI surgery and the fortuitous association through common etiology seen in cardiovascular surgery, but further high-quality studies are needed to clarify these relationships.

The third (and sometimes last) step in determining whether preoperative nutritional support is indicated is to determine the urgency of the surgical procedure. For some patients immediate operation will be mandatory (GI obstruction or perforation, active bleeding, intra-abdominal sepsis, etc.), and preoperative nutritional support cannot be considered. As previously noted, however, nutritional assessment should be done even before urgent operations to permit any appropriate intraoperative maneuvers that will facilitate postoperative support.

For other patients an interval of days, weeks, or even months may be necessary before operation to permit additional testing, preparation, and/or adjuvant therapy. All patients requiring a major operation and in whom an operative delay is required should be considered candidates for nutritional counseling, often with dietary supervision, and sometimes with aggressive nutritional support. Whether just one, two, or all three of these are required depends upon the patient's baseline nutritional status, the type and magnitude of the proposed operation, the functional status of the patient's GI tract, and the anticipated time interval between presentation and operation. Well-nourished patients who can eat should be counseled to consume an appropriate diet and instructed on how to optimize intake during preoperative testing, bowel preps, and other disruptions in normal eating patterns. Defined formula diets may prove useful when solid food or high-residue liquids are not permitted. Similarly, malnourished patients with functional GI tracts should receive aggressive counseling and dietary supervision to minimize further deterioration or improve nutritional status. Although admittedly somewhat arbitrary, a reasonable caloric goal for maintaining the well-nourished patient is 130 percent of resting energy expenditure (REE) plus 1.5 g per kilogram protein. To replete the malnourished patient a reasonable goal is 150 percent of REE plus 2.0 g per kilogram protein. When these goals can be achieved by counseling and supplements, involuntary enteral or parenteral feeding should not be considered.

Patients who cannot eat and who are not candidates for immediate operation are likely to be candidates for enteral or parenteral feeding. Sufficient data exist relating malnutrition to poor operative outcome that permitting nutritional deficits to develop under watchful supervision is clearly unacceptable. In this setting, the risks and expense of preoperative nutritional support are limited only to those factors associated directly with the feeding per se and do not include the risks of delaying operation or the expense of prolonged preoperative hospitalization since these would occur even in the absence of nutritional support. The question is whether significant nutritional deterioration will occur before surgery can be undertaken if nutritional support is withheld. It is not known how long a patient can be starved before his ability to tolerate surgery is compromised. Alterations in nutritionally sensitive circulating plasma proteins are known to occur within 5 days of starvation in previously well-nourished patients and within 3 days in previously malnourished patients. It therefore seems unwise to permit starvation to exceed 3 to 5 days depending upon baseline nutritional status. If the interval between admission and operation is likely to be longer, nutritional support should be instituted immediately. In the preoperative patient, enteral feeding via nasoduodenal tube is often possible and should be considered as a cost-effective alternative to parenteral feeding.

To this point we have considered patients in whom a delay between admission and operation is contraindicated (and in whom preoperative nutritional support is not an option) and patients for whom such a delay is mandatory (where preoperative support is also mandatory if the patient cannot eat and the delay is more than a few days). So far, the decisions have been relatively easy. We now consider the patient for whom immediate operation is possible but not mandatory and in whom preoperative nutritional support would necessitate delaying surgery specifically to provide this therapy. Now the decision becomes more difficult. For this patient the benefits of such therapy must outweigh the risks of nutritional support itself, the risks of delaying surgery, and the risks of an added period of preoperative hospitalization. Further, the benefits must be sufficiently great to justify the cost of this therapy. This includes not only the costs directly related to providing the nutrition, but also those related to the extended preoperative length of stay unless these are offset by equal or greater reductions in postoperative costs (through decreased postoperative complications). Clinicians must therefore be highly selective in their application of preoperative nutritional support in this clinical setting.

A methodical approach must be rigorously applied to ensure that all the prerequisites for rational preoperative nutritional support have been met. We have said already that a delay in operating will not prove detrimental to this patient, so that prerequisite 3 (see section on Prerequisites for Preoperative Nutritional Support) has been satisfied. We must now verify that the patient is malnourished and that malnutrition plays a role in causing complications after operations of the type anticipated for this patient. The practice of routinely providing preoperative enteral or parenteral feeding prior to certain high-risk procedures (e.g., esophagogastrectomy, pancreaticoduodenectomy, etc.) is not justified. Among candidates for essentially any operation, there will be a spectrum of nutritional deficits ranging from none to severe. Preoperative nutritional support will be of no benefit to a patient who does not have the disease that nutritional support is intended to treat (malnutrition) and is unlikely to develop it before the operation if that is performed expeditiously. Well-nourished patients who *can* go to surgery immediately *should* go immediately, and preoperative nutritional support is not indicated.

For patients who are malnourished prior to operations with high nutrition-related morbidity, the final question is, will preoperative nutritional support reduce postoperative complications? Although numerous clinical trials have evaluated this issue, few have provided reliable answers that are broadly applicable. Data from Cologne, West Germany, suggest a clear benefit in patients undergoing major resective procedures for upper GI malignancies. For other diseases and/or operations, data are less definitive, and one must base one's decision on a synthesis of suggestive but inconclusive data, clinical judgment, and common sense. Our current practice is to offer preoperative enteral or parenteral feeding to patients who cannot achieve reasonable oral intake (previously defined) if they are moderately to severely malnourished by subjective and objective criteria *and* they require a major operation involving the esophagus, stomach, gut, pancreas, or biliary system. We define a major operation as one that involves (1) opening the peritoneum and/or pleural space, (2) anastomosis and/or resection, and (3) a major complication rate (in excess of 10 percent). One could certainly argue with our definitions and limits so that the threshold for instituting preoperative nutritional support would be somewhat lower or higher, but we believe that this approach is conceptually valid and consistent with available data.

HOW MUCH AND FOR HOW LONG?

Once preoperative nutritional support is instituted, how much should be given and for how long? Once again, common sense must dictate this choice in the absence of definitive data. There appears to be no benefit to nonprotein caloric intakes in excess of 150 percent of resting energy expenditure, and indeed, caloric intakes above this level may be detrimental. Protein should probably be provided in quantities of 1.5 to 2.0 g per kilogram.

The duration of support must be individualized. Less than 4 days will probably not have a significant effect on any clinically relevant measure of nutritional status, and studies evaluating the efficacy of regimens of less than 4 days duration have uniformly shown no benefit. At the other extreme, the marginal benefit of continuing a regimen in excess of 14 days seems unlikely to justify the added expense and marginal increase in complications associated with such prolonged support. One exception to this may be the patient in whom support can be provided at home via the enteral route and in whom there is no risk whatever associated with a prolonged operative delay. Most clinicians would agree that 7 to 14 days is a reasonable duration for in-hospital preoperative nutritional support when the goal is to improve nutritional status. Obviously, more prolonged periods may be indicated when other considerations make a delay in operation clinically desirable.

On the other hand, the decision to embark on a course of preoperative nutritional support is never irreversible. Patient tolerance must be assessed continuously, and changes in clinical status that make further operative delay dangerous can develop quickly and with little warning. Development of a delay-related or feeding-related complication will quickly negate any benefit associated with improved nutritional status. Preoperative nutritional support provided poorly is worse than no support at all.

There is no "test" to determine when the goal of preoperative support has been achieved and operative risk has been decreased. Reversal of skin test anergy and improvement in circulating levels of serum transferrin have been associated with decreased operative risk and may be useful in selected patients. More often, the decision to proceed with operation is subjective and is based on observation of the patient's level of physical and mental activity, sense of well-being, and general appearance. Whether more objective endpoints can be defined requires further evaluation.

In this chapter an approach to preoperative nutritional support has been presented that has evolved over several years, through multiple clinical research studies, and that reflects experience gained from thousands of patients. The evolutionary process will undoubtedly continue as new and better data become available to tell us what to do and as technologic improvements permit us to do it better.

SUGGESTED READING

Buzby GP, Williford WO, Peterson OL, et al. A randomized clinical trial of total parenteral nutrition in malnourished surgical patients: the rationale and impact of previous clinical trials and pilot study on protocol design. Am J Clin Nutr (in press).

Dempsey DD, Buzby GP, Mullen JL. The link between nutritional status, and clinical outcome: can nutritional intervention modify it? Am J Clin Nutr (in press).

Health and Public Policy Committee, American College of Physicians. Perioperative parenteral nutrition. Ann Intern Med 1987; 107:252–253.

GASTROINTESTINAL FISTULA

MARK T. JAROCH, M.D.
EZRA STEIGER, M.D.

Gastrointestinal fistulas are potentially lethal complications of intra-abdominal surgery or intestinal disease. Enteric contents draining from an incision or a drain site herald the presence of a gastrointestinal fistula. The etiology includes Crohn's disease, malignancy, radiation enteritis, or postoperative complications and can frequently be identified by reviewing the patient's past medical and surgical history. Management of the fistula takes place over a period of weeks and consists of several phases including the initial stabilization, improvement of nutritional status, and surgical intervention if necessary.

STABILIZATION

This initial phase of management includes the treatment of sepsis, correction of fluid and electrolyte imbalances, localization of fistula site, and initiation of nutritional support. The treatment of sepsis associated with an enterocutaneous fistula consists of providing adequate drainage for both the fistula and any abscesses that may be present. Adequate drainage may be facilitated by placing a mushroom catheter in the skin at the fistula exit site or removing several skin clips if the fistula is draining through the wound. An abscess identified after adequate drainage of the fistula should be drained either percutaneously using computed tomography (CT) or operatively. The corrosive effect of enteric contents on the skin can be minimized by the placement of skin barriers and collection devices with the assistance of an enterostomal therapist.

Fever and leukocytosis are quite common until adequate drainage of the fistula is achieved. Broad-spectrum antibiotics are often started at this time. The fever generally does not resolve until the sepsis is adequately drained.

Empiric antibiotic therapy should consist of a penicillin derivative for gram-positive organisms and an aminoglycoside for gram-negative organisms. Anaerobic coverage should be included if this type of organism is suspected. A third-generation cephalosporin may be substituted for the aminoglycoside if concern over nephrotoxicity arises, especially in the elderly. Specific therapy can be initiated after review of the gram stain, culture results, and sensitivity tests. The duration of antibiotic therapy must be individually determined based on the response in resolution of fever, leukocytosis, and left shift of the differential. Persistent fever despite adequate antibiotic coverage and appropriate drug levels suggests the presence of undrained sepsis. CT examination of the abdomen may identify an intra-abdominal abscess. Particularly difficult to diagnose is an inter-loop abscess located between the loops of small bowel and the small bowel mesentery.

Finally, one must always be concerned with catheter sepsis associated with central venous catheters for total parenteral nutrition (TPN). Fever without an obvious source suggests catheter sepsis, which is initially managed by changing the catheter over a guide wire. Bacterial growth from the catheter tip or from blood drawn through the catheter requires insertion of a new catheter at a different site.

Fluid and electrolyte balance can often be deranged, particularly with a proximal small bowel fistula. The distinction between a high-output fistula (greater than 200 cc per day of output) and a low-output fistula is important since increased mortality is associated with the high-output fistula. We begin our fluid orders with a maintenance solution and the volume is based on the patient's height and weight. The fistula output is then replaced cc per cc with a solution having an electrolyte composition similar to that of the fistula output. This is facilitated by sending a specimen of fistula output for sodium, potassium, and chloride determination. Once the fistula output stabilizes, we design a single solution that will provide both maintenance and replacement fluids and electrolytes. Accurate stoma fluid replacement is generally needed only with a high-output fistula. H_2 receptor blockers (cimetidine or ranitidine) are used to decrease the volume of gastric secretions and thus minimize fistula output. Patients are kept NPO during the initial evaluation.

Diagnostic studies used in the evaluation of gastrointestinal fistulas include an upper gastrointestinal and small bowel series, barium enema, fistula injection studies, and CT. Not all these studies are needed with each patient, and they generally have specific indications. The upper gastrointestinal and small bowel series is useful in Crohn's disease to document recurrence, locate disease, and identify distal obstruction. The extent and severity of small bowel involvement in radiation enteritis can also be estimated with contrast studies. Identification of the fistula source with a fistulogram is helpful since a colonic fistula will generally close more rapidly than a more proximal small bowel fistula. The CT scan will help to identify any sites of undrained sepsis.

With certain exceptions, early surgical correction of the acute fistula during the stabilization phase is generally not advised because of an increased mortality rate. However, early operation is needed to provide adequate drainage for fistulas associated with undrained intra-abdominal septic foci. Patients with multiple fistulas may benefit from early operation to provide proximal diversion of the enteric stream to facilitate skin care, fistula closure, and control of sepsis.

Emotional support during these often catastrophic situations is needed, and assistance from the Social Service and Psychiatry Department is best initiated during the stabilization phase.

NUTRITIONAL MANAGEMENT

The second phase of fistula management consists of improvement of the patient's nutritional status. Most gastrointestinal fistulas in our experience are best managed by keeping the patient NPO, using cimetidine or ranitidine to decrease gastric secretions, and providing nutritional support with TPN.

The caloric requirements are determined by the Harris-Benedict equation and are increased by a factor of 1.5 to 1.7, depending on the degree of stress. Amino acids are added to provide 1.0 to 2.0 g of protein per kilogram of weight. The caloric and protein requirements are adjusted as the serial nutritional assessments are evaluated. Intravenous fat emulsions are given to prevent the development of essential fatty acid deficiency. We have demonstrated that the emulsions can be given to patients with pancreatic fistulas without an increase in the fistula fluid volume or enzyme output.

The volume of fluid and electrolyte composition in the TPN consists of maintenance fluids for the patient's size and a supplement to make up for fluid and electrolyte losses from the fistula. Trace elements are added to the TPN. We have noted increased requirements of zinc, chromium, and selenium if fistula output is large. Serum magnesium levels are measured weekly. Trace element levels should be monitored if TPN is to be given for longer than 4 to 6 weeks or sooner if clinically indicated.

Serial nutritional assessments are performed to both initially evaluate the patient and assess progress during treatment at 1 to 2 week intervals. The nutritional assessment includes the evaluation of delayed hypersensitivity skin testing (antigens include *Candida*, mumps, *tuberculin purified protein derivative (PPD)*, and *Trichophyton*), triceps skinfold thickness, midarm circumference, change in weight, total lymphocyte count, serum albumin, prealbumin, and transferrin values are obtained weekly. Lack of improvement in transferrin can occur in patients with malignancy, ongoing sepsis, or inadequate amounts of protein or carbohydrate in the TPN. Transferrin and prealbumin measurements are the best objective criteria of improvement of the patient's nutritional status. Recent surgery will significantly depress the serum transferrin and prealbumin levels for the first 3 to 5 postoperative days.

The duration of TPN depends on the underlying gastrointestinal pathology, type of fistula, and nutritional assessment. A patient with Crohn's disease, malnutrition, and an enterocutaneous or enteroenteral fistula (ileoileal or ileocolic) is generally given 7 to 10 days of TPN followed by surgery. Generally, fistulas secondary to Crohn's disease will become dormant on intensive medical therapy including TPN and steroids but will usually begin to drain when an oral diet is resumed. Knowledge of the natural history leads us to favor early operation in this setting.

An enterocutaneous fistula that develops after a laparotomy and lysis of adhesions or after a bowel resection will generally close while on TPN. Closure will occur provided that protein and calorie requirements are met in addition to following the surgical principles of draining any associated sepsis and making sure that no distal obstruction exists. In most patients, fistula output decreases within the first 5 to 10 days after starting TPN. Complete fistula closure takes 3 to 5 weeks. After radiographic or clinical evidence of closure is obtained, an additional 5 to 7 days of TPN is given to ensure closure. Oral intake is resumed after this period beginning with clear liquids and advancing to a regular diet. Reopening of the fistula can occur if the patient resumes oral intake immediately after fistula closure. We feel that keeping the patient NPO allows for more rapid fistula closure.

The actual value of TPN in the management of gastrointestinal fistulas is controversial. Prior to the introduction of TPN, the mortality rate from fistulas decreased with improved parasurgical care, respiratory support, and improved antibiotics. In our view, TPN is a method for providing early nutritional support, and it has allowed more fistulas to heal spontaneously while maintaining or improving the patient's nutritional status.

SURGICAL MANAGEMENT

If the fistula closes spontaneously, no further treatment is needed. Esophagocutaneous, gastrocutaneous, pancreaticocutaneous, biliary cutaneous, and enterocutaneous fistulas can all be closed with TPN as long as the sepsis is cleared, patients are kept NPO, and protein and caloric requirements are met with TPN. Some fistulas will never close due to distal obstruction, mucosalined tract, malignancy, and other factors; in these cases surgery should be considered. Prior to operation, adequate time should be given for resolution of the peritoneal inflammation associated with the fistula. Contrast studies of the gastrointestinal tract and fistula should be done preoperatively to define the anatomy.

Various surgical options are available and include resection of the fistula-bearing segment with end-to-end anastomosis, isolation of the fistula-bearing segment without resection and end-to-end anastomosis, and exclusion bypass. In those patients with proximal nonclosing fistulas who have dense inflammatory adhesions precluding a safe operation, home TPN may be used for 2 to 6 months until an operation is possible. Patients with multiple fistulas, intra-abdominal sepsis, and dense inflammatory adhesions may benefit from a proximal diverting jejunostomy and home TPN for 3 to 6 months. Diversion of enteric contents and home TPN allows the dense adhesions to become less vascular and more supple, ensuring a safer definitive procedure.

Gastrointestinal fistulas can be a life-threatening complication of gastrointestinal pathology or surgery. Current treatment consists of several phases. Initially the patient is stabilized, the sepsis is treated, fluid and electrolyte imbalance is corrected, and nutritional support is initiated. The second phase of nutritional support continues until the fistula closes or operation is undertaken. TPN is frequently used in this phase, and it has been associated with an improved rate of spontaneous fistula closure. It should be remembered that TPN is a useful adjunct in fistula management, but it never replaces sound surgical principles, especially when dealing with infection. Low-output distal fistulas may be managed with low-residue or elemental diets. Options for surgical management include removal or exclusion of the fistula-bearing segment or proximal diversion and home TPN.

SUGGESTED READING

Fazio VW, Coutsoftides T, Steiger E. Factors influencing the outcome of treatment of small bowel cutaneous fistula. World J Surg 1983; 7:481-488.

Soeters PB, Ebeid AM, Fischer JE. Review of 404 patients with gastrointestinal fistulas: impact of parenteral nutrition. Ann Surg 1979; 190:189-202.

Steiger E, Marein C, Misny P, et al. Total parenteral nutrition and fluid/electrolyte therapy in the home: nine years experience. Cleve Clin Q 1985; 52:317-327.

HEAD AND NECK SURGERY

MERVYN DEITEL, M.D., F.R.C.S.(C), F.A.C.S., F.I.C.S.

Diseases of the head and neck may be accompanied by nutritional deficiencies related to cancer, inability to ingest food orally, radiotherapy or chemotherapy, or the metabolic stress of staged operations. Malnutrition results in an increased incidence of infection, delayed wound healing, wound breakdown, pharyngocutaneous fistulas, flap necrosis, intolerance to oncologic therapy, and poor enteral absorption of nutrients. Nutritional depletion may prevent the optimal surgical procedure from being undertaken (e.g., one-stage gastric "pull-up" and transposition to the neck for pharyngocervical esophagectomy), because the patient cannot tolerate an extensive radical operation.

ETIOLOGY

Obstruction

Obstruction by hypopharyngeal, pyriform sinus, and postcricoid tumors will result in increasing dysphagia and weight loss. Many head and neck tumors grow large before metastasizing. They may be localized and resectable, and hence, nutritional repletion may be worthwhile. A large Zenker's diverticulum containing food may cause high dysphagia from pressure on the upper esophagus. Marasmus, brainstem strokes, and bulbar polio may be associated with cricopharyngeal achalasia with aspiration pneumonia.

Cancer

Cancer of the head and neck may produce pain because the tumor involves the mandible or soft tissue. Mastication may be impossible. Patients with other types of cancer may have physiologic or psychologic anorexia problems. There is commonly a lowered threshold for "bitter" (aversion to meat and vegetable proteins), possibly related to subnormal levels of vitamin A, niacin, copper, and nickel. Cheilosis and gangrenous stomatitis have been associated with magnesium deficiency.

Radiotherapy. Radiotherapy is commonly used in the treatment of carcinoma of the larynx, tongue, floor of mouth, oronasopharynx, tonsil, and hypopharynx. Sequelae are listed in Table 1. After therapy, hard, spicy, or hot foods produce pain. Patients should eat bland foods, and rinse with topical Xylocaine Viscous (lidocaine) before the first mouthfuls of food. For the dry mouth, moist foods and food lubricants such as gravy, butter, margarine, sauce, and milk can be used, which will also increase caloric intake. A synthetic saliva or a sialogogue such as trithioparamethoxphenylpropene (Sialor, Herdt & Charlton Inc., Montreal, Quebec), 25 mg t.i.d. or b.i.d. before meals, may overcome dry mouth. Some patients use more sugar because of the decline in taste acuity ("mouth blindness"), but others have a dislike for sweets. Taste acuity generally returns within 1 year. Zinc sulfate orally may improve disorders of taste in patients with low levels of zinc.

Decreased salivary gland secretion continues for up to 6 months after radiotherapy. Saliva is alkaline, and its absence lowers intraoral pH, leading to dental caries. Strict oral hygiene and frequent brushing of teeth are necessary.

Osteoradionecrosis of the mandible will interfere with mastication and swallowing. Trismus may occur with fixation of the temporomandibular joints.

Chemotherapy. Oral ulcerations with pain on food ingestion may occur. Anorexia, nausea, vomiting and diarrhea also will decrease oral intake.

TABLE 1   Radiotherapy–Induced Injuries

Mucositis, sore throat, pain on swallowing
Anorexia
Altered taste
Xerostomia
Dental caries
Esophageal edema and fibrosis, obstruction,
    regurgitation, pneumonia
Osteoradionecrosis
Trismus

Smoking and Alcohol

Heavy smoking and chronic alcohol intake have respiratory and metabolic nutritional sequelae. These patients frequently have poor oral hygiene with poor dentition, so that mastication is impossible. Leukoplakia in the mouth may lead to further carcinomas with compromise of the alimentary mechanism.

Postoperative Complications

A chylous fistula of the thoracic duct (close to its entrance to the subclavian vein) is a dreaded complication of radical neck dissection or resection of extensive tumor at the base of the neck. The lymph leak is sutured if noted at surgery, although this can enlarge the defect in the thin-walled lymphatics. Postoperatively, each time the patient eats, chyle fills the wound, and the patient may lose more than 2,000 ml of chyle daily. Initial aspiration or drainage is done, followed by local pressure dressings. The standard hospital diet has a high content of long-chain triglycerides, which are transported via chylomicrons into the lacteals and increase lymph flow, with resulting loss of protein-rich milky appearing lymphatic fluid. The chyle also contains a high concentration of fat-soluble vitamins and massive amounts of lymphocytes, with resulting malnutrition and immunologic deficiency. With persisting drainage and progressive malnutrition, surgical ligation of the thoracic duct above the right diaphragm has been necessary. However, abstinence from oral intake with a course of TPN of up to 3 weeks will prevent the accumulation of chyle. Intravenous fat emulsion can be included, as this does not enter the lymphatic circulation. Fat-free elemental diets may be tried, with the addition of medium-chain triglycerides (Portagen) which are absorbed directly into the portal circulation, bypassing the lymphatics and decreasing the pressure in the lymphatic system so that spontaneous closure can occur.

Pharyngoesophageal stenosis may require a liquid diet and dilatation. After extensive hypopharyngeal procedures which interrupt the swallowing mechanism or supraglottic laryngectomy, dysphagia and aspiration from cricopharyngeal achalasia may be relieved by myotomy (see p 217). Approximately 50 percent of the tongue can be removed without significant disability, but greater amounts may lead to problems with deglutition and cricopharyngeal achalasia. Dentures cannot be worn following a hemimandibulectomy "commando" operation, and the patient may require nasogastric feeding for a period followed by proper liquid and pureed diet.

A tracheostomy tube may anchor the larynx, preventing it from rising in juxtaposition to the base of the tongue in order to prevent aspiration as the patient swallows. Furthermore, air that could be used on expiration to clear the larynx is shunted through the tracheostomy tube.

Following parotidectomy, in up to 25 percent of patients Frey's syndrome of gustatory sweating and flushing occurs in overlying skin upon the sight of food. This syndrome is due to abnormal neural connections between parotid parasympathetic and skin sweat gland sympathetic fibers; it generally causes no problem when the patient is given explanation.

NUTRITIONAL ASSESSMENT

Nutritional status should be ascertained from percent weight loss, dietary history, anorexia, change in food preferences, visible changes particularly in the skin and skeletal muscle mass, serum albumin and transferrin, hypersensitivity skin-test anergy, and weekly anthropometric measurements. Dietary counseling is indicated, and patients in need of anabolic nutrition should be started on an aggressive feeding program before treatment if an extensive procedure is contemplated. Operations with a high level of metabolic stress include the "commando" procedure, laryngopharyngectomy, and cervical esophagectomy; operations usually associated with a low level of metabolic stress include hemiglossectomy, thyroidectomy, and parotidectomy.

NUTRITIONAL SUPPORT

Oral Feeding

The gastrointestinal tract is normal in most head and neck patients, and whenever possible, nutritional therapy should be carried out via the enteral route, which is cheaper and safer. If possible the oral route is used. Food may have to be very soft, pureed, or liquid. Between-meal supplements such as Ensure, Sustacal, Resource, Meritine, and Enrich (containing fiber) can be valuable. Head and neck patients who do not like sweet flavours will often prefer unflavored Isocal, Isosource, or Osmolite. These supplements contain 250 kcal and 9 to 14 g of protein per can. Commercial pudding supplements are well tolerated after chemotherapy but often must be thinned with liquids for easier swallowing.

After a radical antrectomy, a cavity may be left in the roof of the mouth that allows food and liquids to escape through the nose. A special occluding dental prosthesis or obturator may replace missing hard or soft palate and separate the nasal from the oral cavity.

Cricopharyngeal Dysphagia

If the cricopharyngeous muscle or sphincter has inadequate or in-coordinated relaxation during swallowing, cricopharyngeal achalasia will result with the potential for frequent expectoration, aspiration, pneumonia, and weight loss. This can follow brainstem disease (e.g., bulbar stroke or bulbar polio); major resection of the posterior tongue, hypopharynx, or supraglottis; amyotrophic lateral sclerosis; myopathy of thyrotoxicosis; or gastroesophageal reflux. Swallowed liquids are aspirated, as they spill readily into the laryngeal inlet. These patients can handle custards and pureed foods better. After supraglottic laryngectomy patients can be trained to inhale, swallow, and then exhale, which serves to clear food from the laryngeal aditus.

Extramucosal vertical myotomy in the posterior part of the cricopharyngeous muscle permits pharyngeal emptying, and patients may be fed orally 8 hours postoperatively. This procedure is recommended during extensive hypopharyngeal resection. However, the results of myotomy are poor in patients with myoneurogenic disorders or when the problem is a result of weakness of the pharyngeal constrictor muscles. In the latter instance, nutritional replenishment of the skeletal muscles is indicated.

Tude Feeding

A small bore (8 or 10 Fr) soft polyurethane or silicone rubber tube with a tungsten-weighted tip will reduce the risk of gastroesophageal reflux with aspiration and of irritation and erosion of an oropharyngeal wound. The Acutrol bag may be used to provide a buretrol for safe volume delivery. However, most patients prefer intermittent feeds, particularly outpatients, delivered over a fairly short period via a funnel or syringe.

The slightly wider bore tubes required to have a greater flow-rate are well tolerated in head and neck patients and allow a more viscous feeding without clogging. The patients can pass their own tube and some use nocturnal feedings.

In depleted hypoalbuminemic patients, malabsorption and diarrhea may ensue, because of impaired jejunal absorption due to decreased cell replication, decreased brush border enzymes, and decreased oncotic pressure in the intestinal villus. Bloating and cramps will occur if the patient is lactose intolerant and the diet is milk based. Constipation can result from lack of residue. The oropharyngeal lesion may be so large that the nasogastric tube cannot be inserted. The balloon on a cuffed tracheostomy tube may have to be deflated (after pharyngeal suctioning) in order to permit passage of the nasogastric tube. While being tube fed, the patient should be erect or the head of the bed should be elevated. For bolus feedings, the patient can be given 500 ml full strength after every 4 hours. However, adequate water must be included to avoid hypertonic dehydration. Nasogastric tubes can cause excess salivation, otitis media, and acute parotitis. One must watch for complications in patients who are aphonic and cannot express themselves.

Tube feedings can guarantee that the patient gets adequate intake. During radiotherapy, intensive outpatient nasogastric tube feeding has improved nutritional status significantly better than the best nutrition that could be taken orally. After laryngectomy or resection of a Zenker's diverticulum, nasogastric feeding can provide nutrition for 5 days during which the suture line is protected from irritation from swallowed food.

Ostomy Feeding

When the oral route is not available and for prolonged feeding, a gastrostomy may replenish and maintain the patient pre- and postoperatively, as, for example, when deglutitory function is permanently lost after a very extensive head and neck operation. Percutaneous gastrostomy by the Ponsky-Gauderer "pull" (string) method or Russell "push" (obturator peel-away sheath) method are being used widely, with the latter method preferred since oropharyngeal bacteria are not drawn through the abdominal wall. We have dilatated hypopharyngeal tumors, which enabled passage of the gastroscope for percutaneous gastrostomy.

A percutaneous pharyngostomy (pyriform sinusostomy) under local anesthesia may be done during or after radical maxillofacial surgery when extraoral alimentation is required for more than 7 days, or when there is inability to swallow due to neurologic disease. A cervical esophagostomy under local or general anesthesia may be performed through a supraclavicular approach or when the esophagus is already exposed during surgery. In this procedure, injury must be avoided to the recurrent laryngeal nerve. When a good tract has developed, the patient may insert his or her own feeding tube as needed. A feeding jejunostomy may be considered in the patient with gastroesophageal reflux. Isocal, Osmolite, and Enrich (containing fiber) are suitable liquid diets for tube feeding.

Total Parenteral Nutrition

When oral or enteral feeding is not feasible, (e.g., due to irritation by the nasogastric tube on an oropharyngeal wound, diarrhea, hypersalivation, or regurgitation), total parenteral nutrition may be used. For central TPN, a catheter should be inserted on the side *opposite* the tumor or known lymph node metastases or radical neck dissection. It is unsuitable (1) with bilateral radical neck dissection; (2) with deltopectoral and myocutaneous flaps; (3) in the early period after radiotherapy to the neck, when moist desquamation and superficial infection may occur; (4) in the late period after radiation therapy to the neck because of fibrosis; and (5) for burns about the neck.

Oral and salivary secretions from an adjacent pharyngeal stoma, fistula, or tracheostomy could contaminate the hyperalimentation site. A plastic sheet placed over the dressing and changed as necessary (e.g., twice daily) may be effective, although the transparent membrane dressings (OpSite, Tegaderm) may provide a barrier to contamination. Subcutaneous tunneling of the catheter inferiorly or a long silicone catheter in the deep brachial vein above the elbow may be used. We have implanted the subcutaneous infusion device (Chemo-Port—HDC Corporation) in the pectoral region, with smooth TPN delivery. No tape is applied to the skin of the neck or upper thorax that is to be included within a radiation portal so that skin bullae will not form. While peripheral TPN has some use in head and neck surgery, it is not as effective as central TPN in the long-term; furthermore, malnourished patients often have fragile peripheral veins.

SUGGESTED READING

Bucklin DL, Gilsdorf RB. Percutaneous needle pharyngostomy. JPEN 1985; 9:68–70.

Dudrick SJ, O'Donnell JJ, Weinmann-Winkler S, Jensen TG. Nutritional assessment: indications for nutritional support. In: Deitel M, ed. Nutrition in clinical surgery, Baltimore: Williams & Wilkins, 1985:24.

Gagic NM. Cricopharyngeal myotomy. Can J Surg 1983; 26:47–49.

Hearne BE, Dunaj JM, Daly JM, et al. Enteral nutrition support in head and neck cancer: tube vs. oral feeding during radiation therapy. J Am Diet Assoc 1985; 85:669–677.

Ramos W, Faintuch J. Nutritional management of thoracic duct fistulas. A comparative study of parenteral versus enteral nutrition. JPEN 1986; 10:519–521.

HEPATIC SURGERY

PAUL D. GREIG, M.D., F.R.C.S.(C)

As a result of the underlying disease, patients undergoing hepatic surgery are often malnourished and are at significant risk for developing further nutritional depletion in the postoperative period. These patients can be considered in the following three categories according to the nature of the liver disease and the surgical procedure:

1. Those with no intrinsic hepatocellular disease, e.g., the patient scheduled to undergo liver resection for primary or secondary liver tumor, or for drainage of an intrahepatic cyst or abscess, or the traumatized patient with liver injury.
2. Those with significant liver disease, e.g., the patient with hepatitis or cirrhosis, or obstructive jaundice scheduled to undergo major abdominal surgery.
3. Those needing liver transplantation, in which the patient has end stage liver disease preoperatively and requires nutritional and metabolic support of the transplanted liver postoperatively.

NORMAL LIVER FUNCTION

No Intrinsic Hepatocellular Disease

In patients scheduled to undergo a liver resection for tumor, or for drainage of an hepatic cyst or abscess, the uninvolved hepatic parenchyma is normal, as is hepatocellular function. The surgery is usually elective, and the patient is otherwise well with normal nutritional status. No specific preoperative nutritional intervention is needed.

Postoperatively, consideration should be given to metabolic support of the regenerating liver, particularily in those patients undergoing a major resection. Hepatic regeneration begins almost immediately following resection, and the rate of regeneration is age dependent, being more rapid in the younger patient. Of the many hormonal "hepatotrophic factors" that have been described, insulin appears to be the most important factor in portal blood, although glucagon and other gut hormones as well as nonportal factors are also important.

Nutritional factors are also important in liver regeneration. Preoperative starvation delays and reduces the rate of liver regeneration. Postoperative nutritional support is important to overall nutritional status, particularly with the increased requirements for nitrogen and energy following major surgery. Dietary protein has been shown to be an important regulator of hepatocyte proliferation. Certain amino acids, particularily lysine, methionine, tryptophan, isoleucine, valine, and threonine appear to be essential to this process. Whether intravenous solutions enriched with branched-chain amino acids (BCAAs) enhance liver regeneration remains unclear. However, overfeeding of amino acids or fat has an inhibitory influence on hepatic regeneration. During the early postoperative period, the replicating hepatocytes may have increased requirements for magnesium and phosphate, as well as for macronutrients.

INTRINSIC LIVER DISEASE

Obstructive Jaundice

The patient with obstructive jaundice is often anorexic and, with the reduced absorption of fat, may have considerable preoperative protein-calorie malnutrition. Specifically, with the malabsorption of fat-soluble vitamins, particularly vitamin K, a coagulopathy may occur with prolongation of prothrombin and partial thromboplastin times. There is an increased risk of renal failure associated with hyperbilirubinemia, therefore it is important to keep the patient well hydrated, particularly if nephrotoxic agents, such as aminoglycosides or intravenous radiographic contrast media for a CT scan, intravenous pyelogram, or angiogram are to be used.

In the preoperative intervention for obstructive jaundice, biliary tree decompression with percutaneous transhepatic cholangiography and internal drainge (PTCD) or endoscopic retrograde cholangiopancreatography (ERCP) with papillotomy and stent does not appear to reduce the postoperative morbidity or mortality. However, if there is to be a significant surgical delay, this may reduce anorexia and allow normal fat absorption, thereby resulting in improved oral intake preoperatively. Alternatively, enteral or parenteral feeding may be indicated. Fat-soluble vitamins, particularly vitamin K, should be given parenterally.

If total parenteral nutrition is used, both copper and manganese should be omitted as they are excreted in the bile. Postoperatively, with decompression the nutritional support of these patients is similar to that of any surgical patient.

Hepatitis and Cirrhosis

Patients with cirrhosis and/or hepatitis are often malnourished as a result of anorexia from their chronic disease, of abdominal fullness from ascites, of dietary protein restriction for encephalopathy, and of the malabsorption associated with portal hypertension. Patients are often anergic and have a significantly higher postoperative morbidity and mortality than those without liver disease.

Cirrhosis is associated with significant alterations in protein and energy metabolism. There is an increase in "whole body" protein breakdown, including the myofibrillar protein predominantly in skeletal muscle. There are also increases in amino acid turnover and in protein synthesis rates including albumin synthesis. Despite the presence of protein-calorie malnutrition, the resting energy expenditure of the patient with end stage liver disease is similar to normal values. Exogenous lipid clearance in cirrhosis may be slightly reduced; however, triglyceride synthesis is maintained and the reduced respiratory quotient (RQ) measured in cirrhotics after an overnight fast indicates a significant utilization of fat for calories. An imbalance of the ratio glucagon: insulin may result in glucose intolerance. Nonprotein calories should therefore be administered as a daily combination of glucose and lipid. A mixture of 50 percent carbohydrate and 50 percent fat is usually well tolerated.

Although the increased rate of amino acid turnover and protein synthesis in cirrhosis would suggest an increased protein requirement, it is often necessary to restrict the protein component of the diet as part of the treatment of hepatic encephalopathy. The pathogenesis of hepatic encephalopathy is complex and not completely understood, but includes the following:

1. The accumulation of toxins with coma-producing potential, such as ammonia, mercaptans, and fatty acids that may act alone or synergistically
2. An increase in the inhibitory neurotransmitter GABA
3. Impaired energy metabolism by the brain, and

4. An imbalance of circulating amino acids, thus resulting in the production of false neurotransmitters.

Patients with severe encephalopathy (stage III or IV) should receive no protein and should have the gastrointestinal tract cleared with enemas, in combination with oral lactulose or neomycin. With mild to moderate encephalopathy, a restriction of oral protein to 40 g per day, with lactulose or neomycin, is indicated. Vegetable protein may be associated with less encephalopathy than animal proteins. Intravenous amino acids appear to be less encephalopathic to patients with advanced liver disease than does oral protein, and 0.75 to 1.0 g per kilogram per day with sufficient nonprotein calories to meet total energy expenditure is usually well tolerated.

There is considerable theoretical and experimental rationale for the use of BCAAs in the metabolic and nutritional support of advanced liver disease. A consistant finding is an increase in circulating concentrations of aromatic amino acids (AAAs) and methionine, and a relative decrease in the BCAAs. This may be due to the increased protein degradation, particularly in skeletal muscle, with release of amino acids. The BCAAs that are released can be directly oxidized by skeletal muscle for fuel leading to the reduced plasma concentrations; however, with the hepatic dysfunction, there is a reduced clearance of AAAs. The increased ratio of AAA to BCAA is thought to result in increased brain uptake of AAAs. (The AAAs and BCAAs are neutral amino acids and compete for the same carrier across the blood brain barrier.) The increased intracerebral concentrations of tyrosine and tryptophan result in an increased production of the neurotransmitters dopamine and serotonin, respectively, and of false neurotransmitters such as octopamine. This may be important in the pathogenesis of hepatic encephalopathy.

It is postulated that the provision of BCAAs should ameliorate the condition in two ways. First, BCAAs, particularly leucine, act directly on skeletal muscle to decrease protein degradation, thereby reducing the AAA load to be cleared by the liver. Second, by increasing the plasma levels of BCAAs and reducing the AAA:BCAA ratio towards normal, there should be reduced synthesis of false neurotransmitters with improvement in encephalopathy.

BCAA-enriched formulations (40 to 50 percent of AAs as BCAAs), both oral and intravenous, have been reported to be superior to conventional amino acid solutions (20 to 25 percent AAs as BCAAs), or to placebo or neomycin alone, in reversing hepatic encephalopathy and/or improving overall nutritional status. However, this has not been a constant finding, with many studies unable to identify an advantage of BCAA-enriched solutions over conventional formulations.

Managing fluid and electrolyte levels in advanced liver disease can be difficult. With their advanced liver disease, cirrhotic patients display sodium and water retention, which is particularly pronounced in the presence of ascites and peripheral edema. The nutritional support should include sodium restriction to 20 to 40 mmol per day in compensated cirrhosis and zero sodium in the presence of severe ascites and edema. Calcium, magnesium, and phosphate requirements are usually unchanged in liver disease. Vitamin and trace element requirements are similarly unaffected by liver disease with the exceptions that the fat-soluble vitamin dosage may be increased and the chromium and manganese should be omitted.

LIVER TRANSPLANTATION

The nutritional requirements of the patient undergoing orthotopic liver transplantation (OLT) are unique. Preoperatively, the OLT candidate has end stage liver disease, with severe hepatocellular dysfunction (uncorrectable coagulopathy, hypoalbuminemia, ascites, and jaundice), whereas postoperatively, the transplanted liver requires the metabolic and nutritional support to recover from the "harvesting injury" associated with hypothermic anoxic preservation for up to 8 hours.

The liver transplant candidate often has advanced protein-calorie malnutrition with subnormal triceps skinfold thickness, low creatinine-height index, hypoalbuminemia, and anergy to skin testing. This places the patient at significant risk for postoperative morbidity and mortality.

A preoperative program aimed at improving nutritional status while a suitable organ donor is sought is important in reducing complications. Resolution of ascites with sodium and water restriction, and judicious use of spironolactone and furosemide should result in an improved appetite (with less abdominal "fullness") and increased activity. A dietary consultation to advise the patient on a diet that is tailored to the individual's protein tolerance, and adequate nonprotein calories with a daily vitamin supplement is important to optimize intake. Liquid nutritional supplements should not be used instead of food but may be used as snacks. BCAA-enriched supplements may be useful in improving nitrogen balance. This nutritional regimen should be combined with an exercise program aimed at increasing skeletal muscle power and endurance and cardio-respiratory reserve.

Occasionally, the preoperative liver transplant candidate requires hospitalization for the treatment of complications of the underlying liver disease (spontaneous bacterial peritonitis, bleeding esophageal varices, increasing encephalopathy, etc.). It is important that during the hospitalization, daily nutritional requirements are met to prevent further malnutrition. This may necessitate nasoduodenal tube feedings or parenteral nutrition, which should not be delayed.

The nutritional requirements of the liver transplant candidate are the same as those of patients with advanced liver disease as outlined in the previous section. The average resting energy expenditure is similar to that of normal subjects but is significantly elevated when expressed per gram of urinary creatinine. This is in keeping with the normal or increased rate of protein turnover measured in cirrhotic patients. The energy requirements increase with infection and may be provided as a daily combination of glucose and lipid. Hepatic encephalopathy usually limits the protein intake, although intravenous amino acids (0.75 to 1.0 g per kilogram per day) are better tolerated than oral protein loads. BCAA-enriched formulations of enteral or parenteral products may provide some benefit to overall nutritional status and may improve hepatic encephalopathy; however, the results of the various studies are conflicting, as outlined in the previous section. Fluid, electrolyte, vitamin, and trace element requirements have been described previously.

Postoperative nutritional and metabolic support must take into consideration the preexisting protein-calorie malnutrition, the metabolic response to major surgery, and the transplanted liver that is recovering from the hypothermic ischemia-reperfusion injury associated with organ preservation (the "harvesting injury"). The presence of malnutrition makes the early postoperative institution of nutritional support important in preventing further nutritional depletion. In the immediate postoperative period this usually requires parenteral nutrition. With the metabolic response to transplantation, there may be an estimated 10 percent increase in resting energy expenditure. Glucose intolerance may result from elevated circulating levels of catecholamines and glucagon and the corticosteroids used for immunosupression, and it may necessitate an insulin infusion to maintain euglycemia and to limit the amount of glucose that can be utilized. Lipid emulsions are usually well tolerated.

Postoperative nutritional support should also consider metabolic support of the transplanted liver. Much is known regarding the injury that occurs during hypothermic preservation and subsequent reperfusion in the experimental animal, and the nutritional support may be used as part of liver preservation. The mechanism of hepatocellular injury is complex and likely includes the production of oxygen-derived free radicals (OFRs) by xanthine oxidase. Two methods of neutralizing these toxic radicals are scavenging with glutathione and using the "membrane stabilizing" effects of vitamin E and selenium. Provision of cystine, glycine and glutamate, the three amino acid components of the glutathione molecule, may in theory increase glutathione levels and decrease the effect of OFRs. Provision of selenium and alpha-tocopherol may also reduce OFR injury. The clinical use of these agents in liver transplantation has yet to be reported.

With liver preservation there is a decrease in ATP with loss of adenosine and phosphate from the cell. Hypophosphatemia and hypomagnesemia are common immediately following liver transplantation, and replacement of magnesium and phosphate are essential to the postoperative nutritional support of the recovering liver. Cyclosporine A, an important immunosuppressive agent in liver transplantation, increases urinary magnesium losses, and a dietary supplement is often required.

SUGGESTED READING

Block RS, Allaben RD, Walt JA. Cholecystectomy in patients with cirrhosis. Arch Surg 1985; 120:669–672.

Bucher NLR, McGowan JA. Regulatory mechanisms in hepatic regeneration. In: Wright R, Millward-Sadler GH, Alberti KGMM, Karran S, eds. Liver and biliary disease. London, England: WB Saunders, 1985:251.

Crossley IR, Wardel EN, Williams R. Biochemical mechanisms of hepatic encephalopathy. Clin Sci 1983; 64:247–252.

Fischer JF, Bower RH. Nutritional support in liver disease. Surg Clin North Am 1981; 61:653–660.

Greig PD. Hepatic disorders. In: Askanazi J, Starker PM, Weissman C, eds. Fluid and electrolyte management in critical care. Stoneham, MA: Butterworth, 1986:267.

Hehir DJ, Jenkins RL, Bistrian BR, Blackburn GL. Nutrition in patients undergoing orthotopic liver transplant. J Parenter Enter Nutr 1985; 9:695–700.

Mullen KD, Denne SC, McCullough AJ, et al. Leucine metabolism in stable cirrhosis. Hepatology 1986; 6:622–630.

O'Keefe SJD, Abraham RR, Davis M, Williams R. Protein turnover in acute and chronic liver disease. Acta Chir Scand [Suppl] 1981; 507:91–101.

Shanbhogue RLK, Bistrian BR, Jenkins RL, et al. Resting energy expenditure in patients with end-stage liver disease and in normal population. J Parenter Enter Nutr 1987; 11:305–308.

NUTRITION AND RENAL DISEASE

CHRONIC RENAL FAILURE

EBEN I. FEINSTEIN, M.D.

Chronic renal failure (CRF) is a syndrome in which there is a decrease in the glomerular filtration rate (GFR), which is usually progressive and irreversible. The syndrome occurs in association with a variety of primary renal diseases, including chronic glomerulonephritis and interstitial nephritis; familial disorders, such as polycystic kidney disease; and congenital abnormalities such as vesicoureteral reflux. CRF also occurs in patients with systemic diseases, of which diabetes mellitus and hypertension are important examples. CRF may be identified at any level of decreased renal function. The disease is classified in several stages; early renal failure refers to a reduction in GFR from normal to 75 ml per minute, mild renal failure occurs with a GFR between 75 to 50 ml per minute, moderate renal failure occurs with a GFR between 50 and 20 ml per minute advanced renal failure refers to a GFR of 20 ml per minute or below. At levels of GFR below 5 ml per minute, dialysis or transplantation is required. A common feature with CRF is the progressive loss of renal function. The rate of decline of GFR varies; some patients require hemodialysis therapy within weeks to months after the onset of their illness. In other patients, such as those with polycytic kidney disease, the loss of renal function proceeds over many years.

As the GFR declines, alterations in the renal handling of water and solutes occur. A number of important adaptations take place, which maintain homeostasis of important electrolytes such as sodium and potassium. As a result, sodium retention and hyperkalemia do not usually occur until advanced CRF. In the case of other electrolytes and solutes, abnormalities in homeostasis are evident earlier in the course of renal failure. For example, elevated levels of blood urea nitrogen (BUN) and serum creatinine occur in early CRF, and metabolic acidosis is frequently evident in moderate CRF. At this stage, early renal osteodystrophy, along with deficiency of 1,25-vitamin D and secondary hyperparathyroidism, have been demonstrated. The uremic syndrome, including anemia, neurologic symptoms, hyperkalemia, and hyperphosphatemia, develops when the GFR falls to 20 ml per minute or lower. It is at this stage of CRF that dietary intervention becomes a key element in management.

In view of the importance of measuring renal function in the management of patients with CRF, a few remarks about the usual clinical indicators of GFR are appropriate here. The BUN, serum creatinine, and creatinine clearance are the most commonly used tests of renal function. The serum creatinine is a more reliable measure of GFR than the BUN because the latter may be elevated by increased protein intake, by any condition that increases endogenous protein breakdown, and by decreased urine flow rate. In interpreting the serum creatinine, one should remember that it rises above the normal range only after the GFR has declined to about 50 percent of normal. In fact, advanced renal failure may be present with only a minimally abnormal serum creatinine concentration. A better method for measuring GFR is the creatinine clearance. However, this test requires a carefully collected urine specimen. Furthermore, as renal function declines, creatinine clearance may overestimate the true GFR by as much as 50 percent. The best clinical methods available for measuring GFR require the use of radionuclides. Since these techniques are not in widespread use, the clinician continues to rely upon the BUN and serum creatinine.

GOALS OF NUTRITIONAL THERAPY

In the following discussion, various components of dietary management are considered. In the case of protein intake and certain electrolytes, the dietary alteration is guided by the BUN or the level of the respective electrolyte. For most patients, dietary alteration is necessary when CRF reaches an advanced stage. However, dietary intervention earlier in the course of the disease may become more widespread if reductions in the rate of progression of the renal failure can be effected by changes in the diet.

Protein Requirements

Modification of dietary protein intake is a crucial element in the management of CRF. Many uremic toxins are derived from protein metabolism. Reduction of the dietary protein content can diminish the accumulation of those toxic substances and can retard the development of uremic symptoms. A protein-restricted diet is usually prescribed when the creatinine clearance falls below 20 ml per minute. For patients with this level of renal function, I prescribe a diet containing 0.55 to 0.6 g per kilogram per day of protein, half of which is derived from foods with high biologic value protein. This term refers to protein sources, such as eggs and lean meats, which contain a relatively elevated proportion of the essential amino acids. This restricted protein diet is effective in maintaining the BUN below 80 mg per deciliter in most patients until they reach end-stage renal disease. With the initiation of dialysis therapy, the protein content of the diet should be increased to at least 1.0 g per kilogram per day. This change in dietary protein intake reflects the need to insure adequate protein nutriture and to counter the catabolic effects of dialysis therapy (see below).

In recent years, there has been renewed interest in the use of very low protein diets, containing about 0.28 g per kilogram per day of protein, supplemented by essential amino acids or keto acids. A number of investigators have reported that such regimens not only control uremic toxicity, but may also retard the rate of decline of renal function in moderate and advanced CRF. The amino acid supplements are required in order to provide necessary additional essential amino acids (up to 20 g daily) and to prevent protein malnutrition. The keto acids are analogues of amino acids in which a keto group is substituted for the alpha amino nitrogen. When keto acids are ingested by patients eating a low protein diet, a transamination reaction replaces the keto group with an amino group. As a result, the patient receives amino acids without exogenous nitrogen and produces fewer nitrogen-containing metabolic products. Keto-acid preparations are not currently available for clinical use in the United States. However, extensive, controlled clinical trials of protein-restricted diets are currently in progress and within the next 5 years should yield conclusive information as to their value in dietary management. The efficacy of these diets in slowing the progression of renal failure will be of special interest. However, until sufficient data are available I advocate the use of a very low-protein diet only for patients who are well motivated, reliable, and able to afford the extra cost of amino acid supplements.

Sodium

The ability to maintain sodium balance is remarkably well preserved in patients with CRF. Even in advanced CRF, severe restriction in salt intake may not be required. As renal function progressively declines, natriuretic forces effect a corresponding reduction in tubular reabsorption of sodium. Despite this adaptive response, the range of sodium intake within which the kidney can maintain sodium balance is narrower than normal. As a result, instead of a range of zero to several hundred mEq per day of urinary sodium excretion, patients with CRF may be limited to a minimum of 20 to 40 mEq (0.5 to 1 g) and a maximum of 150 mEq (3.5 g) daily. Under such conditions, sodium restriction below the minimum quantity excreted daily is not advisable since it may lead to volume depletion and hypotension. This sequence of events is often seen in the uremic patient who develops anorexia or nausea and stops eating for several days. Infusion of saline may be needed in order to restore extracellular fluid volume.

To determine the optimum sodium intake for an individual patient with CRF requires the measurement of body weight, blood pressure, and examination for peripheral edema. To attain salt balance, I place the patient on a 2 g per day intake. If weight and blood pressure remain stable after 1 week, the salt intake is increased to 6 g per day. Again, if weight and blood pressure do not change at this level of intake, salt intake is increased by 2 g per day. Most patients gain weight or develop edema at 8 to 10 g of salt intake. The prescribed salt intake is set at 2 g below the maximum level. I must emphasize that this approach can be used only in patients without coexistent salt-retaining disorders, such as the nephrotic syndrome or congestive heart failure. In such circumstances, sodium restriction is indicated and diuretic therapy is often needed.

In patients treated with hemodialysis, reduced salt intake is almost always required. The signs of excessive salt intake are easily recognized from interdialytic weight gain, blood pressure, and peripheral edema. For many patients, salt restriction is the most difficult dietary hurdle to overcome. Given the many restrictions of the hemodialysis diet, patients find that salt is the only thing that makes food palatable. Dietary adherence is further hampered by the popularity of so many high salt-containing foods and by the ubiquity of salt in processed food products. In my experience, most patients do eventually learn to reduce their salt intake in order to avoid the discomfort of peripheral or pulmonary edema.

Water

Maintenance of water balance is usually not a problem until patients reach end-stage renal disease. Excretion of free water, although reduced, is sufficient to allow the patient to drink up to 3 L per day. Since it is a common misconception that the volume of urine is an indicator of kidney function, some patients with advanced renal failure increase their water intake in order to increase urine output. Such patients require careful counseling in order to prevent hyponatremia due to excessive water ingestion.

For patients receiving maintenance hemodialysis therapy, who often have urine volumes of less than 500 ml per day, restriction of daily fluid intake to between 1,000 and 1,500 ml is needed. Some patients find limiting water intake very difficult. They complain of the difficulty of adhering to the limits for fluid intake when they must swallow six or more medications three to four times daily. Furthermore, in some patients with hypertension, increased renin activity may stimulate thirst. Several drugs, including clonidine (a frequently used antihypertensive agent) and aluminum hydroxide, cause dryness of the mouth, which also stimulates water ingestion.

Potassium

Most patients do not require potassium restriction until they reach advanced renal failure with oliguria. However, the reduced dietary protein intake of these patients entails a lowering of potassium intake since many protein-rich foods also have a high potassium content. For patients receiving hemodialysis therapy careful counseling is needed to prevent hyperkalemia. These patients should be advised of foods that have a high potassium content, such as citrus fruits, tomatoes, potatoes, nuts, beans, and chocolate. When a patient receiving hemodialysis therapy demonstrates hyperkalemia, a careful review of recent food intake is imperative. I have frequently been impressed with how easy it is for patients to forget which foods have a high potassium content. In order to provide variety in the diet and to encourage compliance, I suggest that fruits with a lower potassium content such as grapes, blueberries, apples, and pineapples can be substituted for the citrus fruits. Potatoes should be prepared by boiling rather than baking or frying. For those patients who find they cannot satisfactorily reduce their potassium intake, Kayexalate (a cation exchange resin that increases intestinal potassium excretion), is helpful in preventing hyperkalemia.

When hyperkalemia occurs before advanced renal failure has developed, the syndrome of hyporeninemic hypoaldosteronism may be present. This syndrome is usally seen with diabetic nephropathy or one of the interstitial nephropathies. Renal tubular acidosis is an associated finding. Administration of the mineralocorticoid—Florinef—is effective in some patients, but sodium retention and edema may result. Treatment with Kayexalate may also be required.

Phosphate

Retention of phosphate occurs early in the course of CRF, but hyperphosphatemia is not seen until CRF reaches an advanced stage. There is evidence in experimental animals and in some clinical studies that reduction of phosphorus intake in early CRF may slow the rate of progression of the disease. However, in current practice, the aim of the reduction of dietary phosphate is to control hyperphosphatemia. There are three ways of reducing phosphorus intake from the diet. First, reduction of protein intake necessarily entails a restriction of dietary phosphate. Second, avoidance of dairy products is important since they are a major source of phosphorus. Third, the use of intestinal phosphate binders is usually necessary. Phosphate binders, such as salts of aluminum, calcium, or magnesium, act by preventing absorption of phosphate from the gut. Aluminum carbonate or hydroxide are the most commonly used binders in patients with CRF. They are available as capsules, tablets, or liquid suspensions; the choice of which form to prescribe depends on patient preference. I usually recommend the capsules because they do not have the displeasing taste of the liquid or tablets. However, the capsules are large, and some patients are reluctant to swallow 4 to 6 capsules after each meal. Varying the capsule form with the liquid suspension may improve compliance. Therapy should begin with 1 or 2 capsules after each meal. A dose at bedtime is useful since swallowed salivary juices, which contain phosphate, are also absorbed from the gut. The serum phosphate concentration should be used as a guide to the dose of intestinal binder. As many as 20 capsules a day may be required. If high doses fail to maintain the serum phosphate below 5 mg per deciliter, the patient is either likely to be eating too much dietary phosphate or to have severe hyperparathyroidism. In the latter group of patients, control of serum phosphate is very difficult because of the release of large amounts of phosphate, from bone under the influence of parathyroid hormone.

With the recent concern over aluminum intoxication in patients with CRF, interest in nonaluminum-containing binders has increased. Magnesium salts should be avoided in renal failure due to the danger of hypermagnesemia. However, calcium carbonate is an effective phosphate binder and has gained in popularity. When large amounts of an aluminum binder are required, I begin by substituting calcium carbonate (1,300 mg) for one dose of aluminum binder. Frequent (bi-weekly or monthly) measurements of serum calcium and phosphate are required so that hypercalcemia or an elevated Ca-P product is detected early. Many patients require at least 6 g of calcium carbonate for effective control of serum phosphate.

Calcium

In addition to their use as phosphate binders, calcium supplements are sometimes needed to correct hypocalcemia. For patients with CRF who are eating a low protein diet, I prescribe up to 1 g of elemental calcium. Calcium carbonate (40 percent of which is elemental calcium) is cheap and readily available in several over-the-counter preparations such as Tums and Titralac. For patients who dislike the taste of the tablets, the syrup Neo-calglucon can be used. Its disadvantages are its high cost and cloying sweet taste. Most of the patients who require hemodialysis do not need calcium supplements to correct hypocalcemia since 1,25-dihydroxycholecalciferol is available in oral and intravenous forms. This vitamin D metabolite, used in doses of 0.25 μg to 1.0 μg, effectively raises serum calcium by enhancing intestinal calcium absorption. Since phosphate absorption is also increased by the drug, careful monitoring of serum calcium and phosphate is mandatory. If hypercalcemia or an elevated calcium-phosphorus product develops, the dose of vitamin D should be reduced. Many patients require an increased dose of aluminum phosphate binders early in the course of vitamin D therapy in order to prevent worsening of hyperphosphatemia. After prolonged treatment, the serum phosphage may decline, perhaps as a result of the healing of the osteodystrophy and the improvement in secondary hyperparathyroidism.

Hyperlipidemia

An elevated concentration of serum triglycerides is found in the majority of patients with CRF. This is largely due to defective clearance of these lipids from the circulation. With a low protein diet, the carbohydrate content is increased, and this may exacerbate the hypertriglyceridemia. The problem is even more pronounced in patients treated with CAPD who are absorbing considerable quantities of glucose from the peritoneum. Dietary management of this problem entails a reduction, where possible, of the amount of carbohydrate ingested. This requires an increased intake of fat in order to provide adequate calories. At least half of the fat should be in the form of polyunsaturated fats. In addition to diet, the importance of regular exercise in controlling hyperlipidemia should be stressed. I have seen impressive lowering of serum triglycerides within 4 to 8 weeks of starting a program of bicycle exercising for 20 minutes, thrice weekly.

NUTRITIONAL EFFECTS OF DIALYSIS THERAPY

Both hemodialysis (HD) and peritoneal dialysis (PD) have important effects on nutrition (Table 1). Hemodialysis is associated with increased protein catabolism. Negative nitrogen balance has been demonstrated on the days of dialysis therapy despite ingestion of an increased quantity of protein. Amino acids, but not protein, are lost by diffusion into the dialysate. I prescribe a daily intake of at least 1 g per kilogram of dietary protein for patients treated with hemodialysis. Patients treated with chronic ambulatory peritoneal dialysis (CAPD) lose proteins and amino acids. Accordingly, their protein intake should be even greater, 1.2 to 1.5 g per kilogram of body weight.

Calorie intake for patients receiving dialysis therapy should be 30 to 35 kcal per kilogram per day. The hemodialysis bath should contain a glucose concentration of 200 mg per deciliter to prevent loss of glucose into the dialysate. Patients treated with CAPD may receive substantial calories from absorption of dialysate gluscose. This calorie load must be taken into account when prescribing dietary calories.

A considerable number of patients experience serious malnutrition while receiving hemodialysis. Many of these patients have coexisting conditions, such as diabetes mellitus or severe congestive cardiac failure, that contribute to their poor nutritional status. In some cases, deteriora-

TABLE 1 Nutritional Effects of Hemodialysis (HD) and Peritoneal Dialysis (PD) Therapy

Protein:
   HD—increased protein catabolism, no loss of protein into dialysate
   PD—loss of 9 g/day (CAPD patients)

Amino acids:
   HD—loss of 4–8 g of amino acids
   PD—loss of 2–4 g of free amino acids

Dextrose:
   HD—use of glucose-free dialysis leads to loss of 50 g of dextrose during the treatment
   PD—gain of 800 kcal/day (varies depending on dextrose concentration of solutions)

Vitamins:
   HD and PD—water-soluble vitamins are lost during both treatments

tion in nutritional status develops during an intercurrent illness, such as peritonitis or pneumonia. Recovery to the preexisting nutritional status may be slow and difficult. I frequently use protein and calorie supplements in such circumstances (Table 2).

The hemodialysis treatment also provides a ready avenue for administering nutrients. Amino acids, dextrose, and lipid emulsions can be given by infusion into the dialysis tubing. One regimen consists of 40 g of amino acids and 250 ml of a 20 percent lipid emulsion (500 kcal) infused over a 4 hour period. Hypertonic dextrose may also be used as a source of intradialytic calories. Patients who receive a large dextrose

TABLE 2 Enteral Nutrition in Acute Renal Failure

	Product (Manufacturer)	Caloric Sources	Caloric Density
Calorie supplementation	Controlyte (Doyle)	Fat, carbohydrate	40 kcal/tbs
	Polycose (Ross)	Carbohydrate	2 kcal/ml
Amino acid and calorie-supplementation	Amin-aid (McGaw)	1.94 g% (all essential)	2.0 kcal/ml
	Travasorb Renal (Travenol)	2.3 g% (60% essential)	1.4 kcal/ml

load should ingest a carbohydrate-rich food such as soda pop at the end of dialysis in order to prevent hypoglycemia.

DIETARY COMPLIANCE

The success of dietary therapy depends in large part on the compliance of the patient. It is not surprising, considering the many restrictions which the diet entails, that adherence is difficult to achieve. To be successful, dietary management requires a team effort involving the physician, nursing staff, the patient and the family, and above all, a skilled dietitian. Most dialysis units have dietitians on staff who are knowledgeable concerning renal disease and can devote most of their time to the counseling of patients with renal failure. The dietitian must instruct the patient about the metabolic disturbances that make dietary intervention necessary. It is crucial to develop a diet program that adapts the dietary requirements to indivdual preferences. In many areas of this country, such an approach requires a knowledge of the cuisine of various ethnic groups that have recently immigrated here. Recently, I have had to become familiar with the food preferences of patients from Central America, Mexico, and Southeast Asia in order to provide them with appropriate dietary management. Frequent reinforcement of the need to limit the intake of certain foods is mandatory. Like many nephrologists, I review the results of serum biochemistry determinations with the patients and point out how the food in their diet affects these results. In conclusion, using an understanding, compassionate, team approach to nutritional therapy most patients with CRF can achieve an acceptable level of dietary compliance.

SUGGESTED READING

Brenner BM, Meyer TW, Hostetter TH. Dietary protein intake and the progressive nature of kidney disease: the role of hemodynamically mediated glomerular injury in the pathogenesis of progressive glomerular sclerosis in aging, renal ablation, and nitrinsic renal disease. N Engl J Med 1982; 307:652–659.

Kopple JD. Nutritional management. In: Massry SG, Glassock RJ, eds. Textbook of nephrology. Baltimore: Williams & Wilkins, 1983:8.3–8.12.

ACUTE RENAL FAILURE

EBEN I. FEINSTEIN, M.D.

Acute renal failure (ARF) is a syndrome in which there is a precipitous decline in glomerular filtration rate. ARF occurs in a variety of clinical settings. This chapter is concerned mainly with acute tubular necrosis (ATN), a form of ARF that occurs following a toxic or ischemic insult to the kidney. ATN is a potentially reversible disease; if the patient is supported during the period of uremia, full recovery of renal function can be expected. Dialysis (either peritoneal dialysis or hemodialysis) and nutritional therapy are the mainstays of ARF management. The goal of nutritional therapy in acute renal failure is the maintenance of optimal nutritional status with minimal exacerbation of uremic toxicity. By preventing the depletion of body proteins, it is hoped that recovery of renal function may be accelerated and that patient survival improved.

The use of intensive dialysis therapy, beginning early in the course of the disease, has greatly improved patient management, yet, the overall mortality of ARF remains about 50 percent. In postoperative or posttrauma patients, mortality is as high as 60 to 70 percent.

An important factor causing increased morbidity and mortality with ARF is an elevated rate of protein catabolism. This is greatly influenced by the disease(s) that underlies or is associated with the renal failure. Thus, patients who have sustained traumatic or thermal injuries or who have undergone surgery are more likely to have a high rate of protein breakdown than are patients who have renal failure due to a nephrotoxic agent, such as an aminoglycoside antibiotic. Protein breakdown can be assessed clinically by the rate of rise of blood urea nitrogen (BUN); an increment of 30 mg per deciliter per day or more indicates increased (or hyper) catabolism. However, a better measure is the urea nitrogen appearance rate (UNA).

The UNA is a close approximation of the daily urea production. Since urea distributes throughout the body water, a rise in BUN reflects an increment in urea in the total body water (approximately 60 percent of body weight). Urea is excreted mainly in the urine and is also removed in dialysate. Using data that is easily obtainable, the following equations can be used to calculate the UNA during a specific time interval (usually 24 hours):

1. UNA = change in body urea space + urinary urea nitrogen + dialysate urea
2. Change in body urea space = (change in BUN, g per liter) (initial body weight) (0.6) + (change in body weight) (0.6) (final BUN, per liter)

(Note: BUN must be converted from mg per deciliter to g per liter.)

The last expression in the second equation refers to the contribution to the urea space of an increase in body water from fluid retention that may occur in ARF. To obviate the need to measure dialysate urea, UNA can be determined during periods in which the patient is not undergoing dialysis therapy. A UNA of 10 g per day or more in a patient with acute uremia indicates a markedly elevated rate of protein breakdown. The UNA correlates well with the nitrogen output; thus, nitrogen balance can be estimated from the difference between nitrogen intake and UNA.

In general, hypercatabolic patients present the greatest challenge for nutritional therapy. However not all patients with elevated UNA have the very high mortality rates to which I have alluded. In particular, patients with ARF due to nontraumatic rhabdomyolysis have rates of UNA comparable to those seen in surgical patients, yet mortality in the former group is distinctly less than in the latter. This difference in mortality suggests that visceral injury, which is usually absent in rhabdomyolysis, may be an important risk factor for death in ARF.

Several issues must be addressed in any discussion of parenteral nutrition with ARF. First, what type of amino acid mixture should be administered—essential amino acids (EAA) or a mixed formula of essential and nonessential amino acids (ENAA). Second, how should the calorie requirement be provided. Third, how should the fluid balance be maintained in the face of the large volumes of nutritional solutions that are needed.

REVIEW OF CLINICAL EXPERIENCE

The use of EAA and glucose in the nutritional management of ARF was based on clinical experience in patients with chronic renal failure who showed a decreased rate of rise of BUN when they ingested a markedly protein-restricted diet (about 20 g of protein daily). The protein in such diets was mainly from foods with high biologic value, i.e., they contained an increased proportion of essential amino acids. Some advocates of this dietary regimen postulated that the low protein intake promoted utilization of urea nitrogen for protein synthesis. According to this hypothesis, urea nitrogen is metabolized to carbon dioxide and ammonia. The latter can then be used for the synthesis of nonessential amino acids. This concept of reutilization of urea nitrogen was extended to the therapy of patients with ARF. Indeed, the intravenous infusion of small quantities (13 to 30 g per day) of EAA and glucose does result in a diminished rise in BUN. The correction of hyperkalemia, hyperphosphatemia, and hypermagnesemia are also important effects of this therapy. The prospective trial of Abel et al, which compared patients receiving parenteral nutrition with EAA and hypertonic glucose to a control group receiving only glucose, showed improved recovery of renal function with EAA therapy, but showed no beneficial effect on overall hospital mortality. In other studies, this EAA regimen did not improve nutritional status. Negative nitrogen balance was observed in many patients receiving small amounts of EAA. The serum concentrations of albumin and transferrin remained below normal as did the plasma concentration of many amino acids. Furthermore, careful studies of the reutilization of urea nitrogen for protein synthesis showed that the amount incorporated into albumin was nutritionally insignificant.

Proponents of therapy with essential and nonessential amino acids and glucose have argued that, since all of the amino acids are necessary for protein synthesis, treatment with a mixed amino acid formula would enhance protein synthesis better than EAA alone. Experiments by Toback et al substantiated the beneficial effects of ENAA in the rat with experimental ARF. My colleagues and I compared therapy in three groups of patients with ATN and with moderate to marked catabolism who received either infusions of EAA (average 14 g per day), ENAA (average 33 g per day), or no amino acids. All patients received equal amounts of calories derived mainly from hypertonic dextrose. The UNA was elevated in the three groups and was highest in patients receiving ENAA. Negative nitrogen balance occurred in the majority of patients. There was no difference in recovery of renal function or survival among the three treatment groups. In further studies, we assessed the effects of larger quantities of ENAA with the goal of correcting negative nitrogen balance in patients with severe protein catabolism. The administration of ENAA (average 84 g per day) led to improved nitrogen balance in some patients, but neither the overall nitrogen balance nor the survival rate for the ENAA group was significantly better than that of the control group who were treated with small amounts of EAA.

What conclusions can we draw from these clinical trials? First, the efficacy of parenteral nutrition using EAA or ENAA and glucose in countering the effects of protein catabolism is limited, especially with high rates of catabolism. Second, no regimen tested has consistently produced an improvement in recovery of renal function or survival. Despite these negative conclusions, in my opinion, nutritional therapy remains an important element in the treatment of ARF. I hope that future improvements in therapy would occur in two areas, i.e., control of the catabolic response with pharmacologic agents and development of newer amino acid formulations to improve nitrogen balance and to promote protein synthesis.

The importance of adequate caloric intake should be stressed. Sufficient calorie intake is important for attaining nitrogen balance. The calorie requirement of the patient may be estimated using the Harris-Benedict equation or may be measured using indirect calorimetry. Observations in critically ill patients with ARF suggest that calorie intake has an important impact on patient outcome. In this regard, it is possible that insufficient calorie intake may have contributed to the high mortality rate in the studies described previously. Most of the patients whom we studied received about 35 kcal per day, but some may have required as much as 45 kcal per day.

In the past, there was a reluctance to treat ARF with large amounts of amino acids and hypertonic dextrose because of the danger of fluid overload. This concern is well founded; many patients require 1,500 ml to 2,000 ml of parenteral nutrition solutions in addition to various other intravenous solutions, such as blood, albumin, and antibiotics. In most patients frequent dialysis therapy can maintain fluid balance. However, in some patients hemodynamic instability and hypotension hamper the ability of hemodialysis therapy to remove fluid volume equal to the daily fluid intake. The development of newer techniques for extracorporeal ultrafiltration has all but eliminated this obstacle. Hemodialysis using bicarbonate-buffered dialysate causes less dialysis-associated hypotension and is now the preferred method of hemodialysis in critically ill patients.

Other recently developed methods of slow and continuous fluid removal are being used more commonly. Two of these techniques, slow continuous ultrafiltration and continuous arteriovenous hemodialysis, utilize cellulose membranes; continuous arteriovenous hemofiltration (CAVH) requires a more permeable membrane, such as the polysulfone membrane. These techniques, which are less complicated than hemodialysis, allow ultrafiltration to proceed around the clock, minimize fluctuations in extracellular fluid volume and blood pressure, and allow the administration of needed nutrient solutions with a lessened risk of producing volume overload.

Management of Nutritional Therapy

Before prescribing the nutritional regimen for a patient with ARF, I first determine the level of catabolic stress from the rate of rise of BUN and UNA. Next, I consider whether the patient has any other medical condition, such as diabetes mellitus or liver failure, which have an important impact on nutritional therapy. I then decide on the mode of nutrient administration.

For patients with mild degrees of catabolism (UNA less than 5 g per day), who can be fed orally, I prescribe a diet containing 0.6 g per kilogram of protein. At least half of the protein is derived from sources with a high biologic value, such as eggs and lean meats. The dietary salt intake is usually 2 g per day. The fluid intake depends upon the urine volume and insensible fluid losses (usually estimated to be at least 400 ml per day). The daily potassium intake should be about 2 g (or 40 mEq). Careful monitoring of the serum potassium concentration is mandatory. Nondietary sources of potassium that should not be overlooked include blood transfusions and potassium salts of certain drugs, such as penicillin.

When anorexia or nausea limits the patient's ability to receive all of the required nutrition from the diet, I prescribe dietary supplements. If inadequate calorie intake is a problem (as it is in many patients), I use a supplement such as Controlyte (Doyle) or Polycose (Ross), which contain no protein or electrolytes (see Table 2 in the chapter on *Chronic Renal Failure*). In addition, if protein intake is inadequate, a supplement containing amino acids, with a high calorie density, such as Amin-aid (Kendall-McGaw) is useful. Many enteral supplements have a high osmolality, which can cause diarrhea. Dilution of the supplements to one-half or one-quarter of their full strength may be necessary to prevent this complication, though this has the drawback of increasing the daily fluid intake.

Peripheral intravenous nutrition may also be useful as a supplement to enteral nutrition. I use a 10 percent or 20 percent lipid emulsion in conjunction with an essential and nonessential amino acid preparation (8.5 percent or 10 percent) in order to give up to 1,200 kcals and 40 g of amino acids daily.

TOTAL PARENTERAL NUTRITION

For patients who are catabolic (UNA of greater than 10 g per day) or who cannot be fed enterally, total parenteral nutrition (TPN) via a subclavian vein catheter is required.

The TPN regimen should contain amino acids, hypertonic dextrose, vitamins, and (frequently) minerals (Table 1). For the hypercatabolic patient, I use a preparation containing essential and nonessential amino acids at an initial quantity of 0.5 g per kilogram of amino acids daily. The amount is increased over 2 to 3 days to a maximium of 1.0 g per kilogram per day. Because of the importance of keeping the volume of fluid infused to a minimum, I use a 10 percent solution. For the same reason, I use 70 percent dextrose-water as the major source of calories. This provides about 2.4 kcal per milliliter and is the most concentrated calorie source available. Most patients treated with D70/W will need insulin therapy. I have found that infusing insulin through a separate infusion pump is preferable to adding it to the TPN solution since, in this way, the insulin infusion rate may be adjusted independently of the TPN infusion rate. As much as 10 units per hour of insulin may be required to maintain the serum glucose at 200 mg per deciliter or less.

Lipid emulsions may also be given to patients with ARF and may provide up to 30 percent of the daily calorie requirement. A 20 percent concentration provides 2 kcal per milliliter. The serum triglyceride concentration should be measured during therapy since the clearance of triglycerides is impaired in uremia.

During the first few days of TPN therapy, serum electrolytes and glucose must be measured at least twice daily. The serum phosphate, potassium, and magnesium decline in most patients. Infusion of electrolytes is needed then to prevent serious complications from low serum concentrations of these electrolytes. If these concentrations are in low normal range at the start of therapy, I add them to the initial TPN infusions.

TABLE 1   Total Parenteral Nutrition in Acute Renal Failure

Nutrient	Amount (Daily)
Amino acids:	
Essential or	13–26 g/day
Essential and nonessential	1 g/kg body weight
Calories:	
Hypertonic dextrose (50 or 70%) and	35–50 kcal/kg body weight
Lipid emulsion (20%)	Lipid may provide up to 30% of total calories
Vitamins:[*]	
Thiamin	2–5 mg
Riboflavin	1–2.5 mg
Niacin	10–40 mg
Pantothenic acid	2.5–10 mg[†]
Pyridoxine	1.5–10 mg[†]
Folic acid	0.4–1.0 mg
Cobalamin	3 μg
Ascorbic acid	50–100 mg
Electrolytes:[‡]	
Sodium	35–70 mEq
Potassium	30 mEq
Chloride	35–70 mEq
Calcium	10 mEq
Magnesium	5–mEq
Phosphorus	3–8 mmol

[*] Vitamin intake may vary depending upon the preparation used

[†] The higher quantity is preferable for patients with acute renal failure

[‡] Daily quantities will vary with the individual patients. The quantities given are a representative range.

SUGGESTED READING

Abel RM, Beck CH, Abbott WM, et al. Improved survival from acute renal failure after treatment with intravenous essential L-amino acids and glucose. Results of a prospective double-blind study. N Engl J Med 1973; 288:695–699.

Feinstein EI, Blumenkrantz M, Healy M et al. Clinical and metabolic responses to parenteral nutrition in acute renal failure a controlled double blind study. Medicine 1981; 60:124–137.

Wesson DE, Mitch WE, Willmore DW. Nutritional considerations in the treatment of acute renal failure. In: Brenner B, Lazarus JM, eds. Acute renal failure. Philadelphia: WB Saunders, 1983:618.

NUTRITION AND CARDIOVASCULAR DISEASE

CONGESTIVE HEART FAILURE

STEVEN B. HEYMSFIELD, M.D.
GEORGE W. CHRISTY, M.D.
ELBRIDGE BILLS, B.Sc.
YVONNE PAYNE, B.Sc., R.D.

Diet therapy is of fundamental importance in the medical management of congestive heart failure (CHF). The specific aspects of CHF diet therapy are based upon the physiologic interrelations among food ingestion, body composition, and the cardiovascular system. These basic considerations are briefly summarized in the following section. The remainder of the chapter provides a description of the practical aspects of nutritional management of the CHF patient.

METABOLIC AND CARDIOVASCULAR INTERRELATIONS

Cellular function requires the continuous generation of energy from organic fuels. The circulatory system delivers these fuels plus an appropriate supply of oxygen to cellular loci where oxidative reactions release useful energy. The waste products of this process include carbon dioxide, water, and urea (protein oxidation). These compounds are removed from the cellular environment by the circulatory system and excreted by the lungs and kidneys. Several key points related to this process are worthy of mention.

Cardiac output parallels changes in whole body oxygen consumption and carbon dioxide production. The fasting-resting oxygen uptake and carbon dioxide release are determined largely by the body cell mass.

Ordinarily about 4 ml of oxygen and 3.8 ml of carbon dioxide flow into and out of each kilogram of active cell mass per minute. Stress, injury, and fever all increase the rate of resting cellular gas exchange whereas starvation and depletion of cell mass lower the rate.

Meal ingestion is accompanied by an increase in cellular oxidation referred to as the thermic effect of food (TEF). The TEF usually lasts 4 to 6 hours; the magnitude and duration of this response are related primarily to meal total energy content and proportion of protein, fat, and carbohydrate. Large meals, especially those with a high protein content, are accompanied by a large and prolonged TEF. The meal-induced increase in oxygen consumption and the associated increase in splanchnic blood flow cause a fall in peripheral vascular resistance and an increase in heart rate and cardiac output.

The cardiovascular load of meal ingestion is relatively small; even a large meal is only 1.1 to 1.3 METS* whereas taking a bed bath is 2.6 METS.

Fuel administered continuously either by gastrointestinal catheter or intravenous line produces an increase in cellular oxidation. The magnitude of this response is directly related to the formula (energy) infusion rate. Minimal effects on gas exchange are observed at a maintenance infusion; oxygen consumption and carbon dioxide production increase progressively thereafter with advancing formula infusion rates.

Rather than the fluctuating response of regular meal ingestion, the metabolic effects of formula infusion are continuous and sustained. There are in addition corresponding increases in heart rate, cardiac output, and minute ventilation rate.

The metabolic effects of continuous formula infusion are determined by the quantity and quality of fuels provided in the solution. First, the proportion of formula protein, carbohydrate, and fat determines the in vivo uptake of oxygen and release of carbon dioxide at any given infusion rate. The most important consideration in this regard is the proportion of formula nonprotein calories supplied as carbohydrate and fat. Generally a high carbohydrate solution (CHO = 80 percent of total calories) is associated with a lower oxygen uptake and a higher carbon dioxide output relative to a high fat formula (fat = 50 to 60 percent of total calories).

Hence in vivo gas exchange is directly related to both the infusion

---

*1 MET=resting oxygen uptake.

rate and the composition of formula supplied. Correspondingly, the requirement for cardiac output and the stimulation of ventilation are related to the feeding process. For example, an infusion rate of a high carbohydrate formula aimed at promoting rapid weight gain would increase cardiac output and minute ventilation to a greater extent than a maintenance infusion of a high-fat solution.

The second effect relative to formula composition is a function of formula protein; the amount and quality of protein (i.e., biologic value) has a direct effect on the urea production rate. A small amount of high-quality protein minimizes the rate of urea production. The blood urea nitrogen is determined by both the rate of urea production and the rate of urea excretion by the kidney. As many patients with CHF are azotemic, the dietary control of urea production often becomes a relevant issue in clinical practice.

In addition to metabolic demands the cardiac workload is also determined by fluid status. Central blood volume plays a major role in venous return to the heart, preload, and cardiac output. Blood volume and its parent fluid space, the extracellular compartment, are closely regulated by the interplay of a number of dietary and physiologic factors. The most important consideration is the cation sodium, which in health has a serum concentration of about 140 mEq per liter; assuming a constant serum value each mEq of Na retained translates to 7 ml of extracellular fluid. As the daily intake of Na varies between 500 mg (22 mEq) and 10,000 mg (435 mEq), regulatory mechanisms at the renal level adjust urinary excretion so as to maintain the serum Na concentration and extracellular fluid volume constant.

With the onset of CHF, neuroendocrine and renal adjustments reduce urinary Na excretion and expand the extracellular fluid and plasma space. This compensatory mechanism preserves the stroke volume of the malfunctioning myocardium. Failure of this mechanism ultimately leads to excessive fluid accumulation, edema, and worsening CHF.

NUTRITIONAL MANAGEMENT

The central principle in the nutritional management of the CHF patient is to supply adequate nutrition without creating excessive demands on the cardiovascular and respiratory systems.

Outpatient Therapy

A useful approach is to consider management of the severe CHF patient; subjects with lesser degrees of heart failure can then be treated according to appropriately adjusted guidelines.

One or a combination of three nutritional components are usually managed in the severe CHF patient, undernutrition ("cardiac cachexia"), obesity, and fluid status. The patient suffering from severe CHF usually has the following conditions that favor undernutrition: reduced intake due to dyspnea and the potential anorexigenic effects of digitalis preparations; early satiety due to gastric compression by an enlarged liver and ascites; malabsorption secondary to hypoxia and edema of the bowel; hypermetabolism due to increased cardiac mass and other unspecified factors; and nutrient depletion secondary to repeated phlebotomy and drug therapy.

Atrophy of lean tissues and loss of associated cellular function have both positive and negative effects. A reduced cell mass and infrequent food ingestion lower the total 24-hour and peak resting oxygen requirement; cardiac demands are reduced accordingly. On the other hand the supply of nutrients for processes such as wound healing or the inflammatory response is limited. Hence the general approach is to guide the patient towards a dietary protocol that minimizes cardiac demands and yet supplies nutrients for essential cellular functions.

Our initial evaluation includes a food intake and drug history, anthropometric assessment (weight and simple upper arm measurements), and serum studies (albumin and transferrin/iron if anemic). Specific abnormalities such as iron deficiency are treated accordingly. Otherwise the following general guidelines are adapted.

Energy intake as fat, carbohydrate, and protein is recommended in the proportions 0.35/0.50/0.15. A maintenance energy intake is usually suggested. Several guidelines for establishing a maintenance energy intake are provided in Table 1. When undernutrition is severe and the patient's clinical condition sufficiently stable, slow repletion of the depleted subject is recommended. Soft, easily chewed, and digested sources of these nutrients are reviewed with the patient. Due to the metabolic effects of large meals and the early satiety mentioned above, the food is preferrably ingested in four to six evenly spaced servings. Very hot or cold food or beverage should be avoided in order to minimize the risk of a vagal response with associated physiologic derangements.

The abnormally expanded extracellular fluid and plasma volumes are treated by combining a reduced dietary Na intake with diuretic-induced Na excretion. This dual approach has the advantage of allowing the

TABLE 1   Estimating the Cardiac Patient's Daily Caloric Needs*

Energy balance = energy intake − thermal energy losses

Energy intake: compute energy intake based on stool- and urine-corrected fuel values†
    carbohydrate = 4 kcal/g
    protein = 4 kcal/g
    fat = 9 kcal/g

Thermal energy losses = BMR‡ IF ‡ PA‡

> **BMR:**
> Estimate (in kcal/day) from Harris-Benedict equations:
>   men = 66 + 13.7W + 5H − 6.8A
>   women = 655 + 9.6W + 1.8H − 4.7A§
> Measure in resting state following an overnight fast; measured value
>   will include IF.
> Both estimated and measured BMR can be used to calculate sleeping BMR
>   as 0.9 BMR.
>
> **IF:**
> Estimate as follows:
>   stable severe CHF# = BMR × 0.1–0.2 (in kcal/day)
>   minor surgery = 50–75 kcal/day
>   major surgery = 100–150 kcal/day
>   sepsis = 200–500 kcal/day
>   fever = 0.07 BMR × degree fever above 98.6 ° F (in kcal/day)
>
> IF is included in BMR when thermal losses are measured by indirect
>   calorimetry.
>
> **TEF:**
> Estimate as 5%–8% of ingested calories per day.
> Measure area under metabolic rate curve for 4–8 hr following
>   representative meal. Extrapolate to three meals a day.
>
> **PA:**
> Estimate as follows:
>   bedrest = 1.2 BMR
>   light activity = 1.3 BMR
>   moderate activity = 1.5 BMR
>   strenuous activity = 2.0 BMR
> Measure during representative activities. Then compute daily PA (in kcal)
>   from activity diary plus energy cost of each activity.

---

* Suggestions assume that no malabsorption is present. With malabsorption intake needs
to be adjusted upward based upon quantitative fecal analyses.
† The gross energy content of carbohydrate, fat, and protein are 4.1, 9.4, and 5.65 kcal/g
respectively. The corrected values are based upon average stool and urinary losses in
healthy adults.
‡ BMR = basal metabolic rate. IF = injury or disease factor. TEF = thermal effect of
food. PA = physical activity
§ W = weight (in kg). H = height (in cm). A = age (in yr).
# CHF = congestive heart failure.

TABLE 2 Sodium Conversion Factors and Basic Principles of 2 g/day Sodium Diet*

A	Na (mEq)	Na (g)	NaCl (g)
		B	
Na (mEq)	—	0.023	0.0585
Na (g)	43.5	—	2.54
NaCl (g)	17.1	0.393	—

Basic principles of 2 g/day Na diet

Do not use salt in cooking.
Do not use salt at the table.
Do not eat high salt foods; these tend to be preseasoned, instant, and convenience foods.
Avoid medications high in Na; consult your pharmacist for a list.

* Given A, convert to B by multiplying the appropriate coefficient in the table times A.

patient to ingest palatable foods while minimizing the adverse effects of high-dose diuretic therapy (K and other mineral depletion). Moreover, a reduced Na intake potentiates K retention, thereby reducing the severity of diuretic-induced hypokalemia.

The healthy adult ingests an average of 4 to 8 g of Na per day (for various Na conversions see Table 2). Palatable meals consisting of 2.0 to 2.5 g per day of Na can be prepared without purchasing specially prepared foods (see Table 2). Two additional suggestions are to use salt substitutes and imaginative methods of seasoning to improve food palatability. Hence a low but not severely restricted Na intake is generally recommended, and the remaining adjustments in fluid status are regulated by diuretic therapy.

As most diuretics promote K excretion, serum K must be monitored accordingly. Once again the serum level of this cation is clinically titrated by balancing K input and output. Conversion factors for K and food sources of dietary K are presented in Table 3.

Drug nutrient interactions (Table 4) are reviewed and appropriate adjustments are made in the diet. In addition, we recommend the patient moderate the intake of beverages containing caffein (increases whole body oxygen consumption and heart rate; potentially arrhythmogenic); limit alcohol ingestion (myocardial depressant; arrhythmogenic) and discontinue smoking (stimulates whole body oxygen uptake; also carcinogenic and atherogenic).

TABLE 3 Potassium Conversion Factors and Common Sources in Food

_A_	B^*	
	K (mEq)	K (g)
K (mEq)	—	0.0391
K (g)	25.6	—
Common food sources of K[†]		
Bananas		
Cantaloupe		
Milk		
Oranges		
Potatoes		
Raisins		
Spinach		
Tomatoes		

[*] Given A, convert to B by multiplying the appropriate coefficient in the table times A.
[†] 8–13 mEq/serving.

Upon follow-up, some patients will suffer persistent anorexia and weight loss. If malabsorption is suspected an appropriate gastrointestinal evaluation is undertaken. Hypermetabolism is considered if fever and/or infection are present. In the absence of an obvious cause of hypermetabolism it is unusual for the resting metabolic rate to exceed a level 15 to 20 percent above normal. Malabsorption and hypermetabolism are rarely the sole mechanism for weight loss in the CHF patient; usually these mild epiphenomena of CHF combine with anorexia to cause negative energy and protein balance.

The primary therapy of malabsorption is directed at the underlying cause. The dietary management of malabsorption usually includes several simple measures: reduce fat intake; reduce proportion of fat intake as long-chain triglycerides and increase proportion as medium-chain triglycerides; and consider use of water-miscible vitamin preparations.

Hypermetabolism is likewise managed medically with the primary cause receiving initial attention. When hypermetabolism is persistent, the patient's energy intake is adjusted upward accordingly.

Once satisfied that no correctable causes of weight loss are present (e.g., digitalis-related anorexia), we usually provide the subject with dietary supplements. Typically these liquid formulas are relatively high

TABLE 4 Drug-nutrient Interactions Related to the Therapy of Cardiovascular Diseases

Drug	Nutrient Interaction/Systemic Effect
Alphamethyldopa (Aldomet)	Diarrhea
Digitalis preparations	Intoxication caused by these compounds results in nausea, vomiting, anorexia, diarrhea, and fatigue.
Ethacrinic acid (Edecrin)	Gastrointestinal symptoms; hypokalemia; hyponatremia; hypercalciuria; hyperuricemia; hyperglycemia; azotemia
Furosemide (Lasix)	Hypokalemia; hyponatremia; hypercalciuria; hyperuricemia; hyperglycemia; azotemia
Guanethidine (Ismelin)	Diarrhea
Hydralazine (Apresoline)	Gastrointestinal symptoms recognized; vitamin B_6 and pyridoxine antagonist. Na and H_2O retention if given without diuretic.
Minoxidil (Loniten)	Fluid retention if given without diuretic
Methylxanthines	Includes caffeinated beverages and such drugs as theophylline. Stimulate respiration, have cardiotonic effects, have arrhythmogenic potential, and promote diuresis.
Nitroprusside	Accumulation of thiocyanate with prolonged infusion is associated with nausea and weakness.
Prazosin (Minipress)	Fluid retention if given without diuretic
Propranolol (Inderal)	Diarrhea
Quinidine	Diarrhea
Reserpine	Increases gastric emptying
Spironolactone	Hyperkalemia; hyperglycemia; hyperuricemia; azotemia; and hyponatremia
Thiazides	Hypokalemia; hyponatremia; magnesium depletion; hyperglycemia; azotemia; hyperuricemia

in calories (1.0 to 2.0 kcal per ml) and consist of easily digested and absorbed nutrients (Table 5). A critical consideration is long-term palatability with a minimum of taste fatigue.

In patients with refractory undernutrition, home enteral feeding should be considered. Some basic principles of enteral feeding are reviewed in a later section. The reader should review other appropriate chapters in the book for additional details.

Although the focus up to this point has been on undernutrition and

TABLE 5 Elemental and Polymeric Enteral Formulas

Product/Manufacturer	Caloric Density (kcal/ml)	kcal/N	H₂O %	Osmolality (mOsm/kg)	Vol for 100% RDA (ml)	K (mEq/L)	Na (mEq/L)
Elemental							
Travasorb-HN (Travenol)	1.00	140:1	86	450	2000	30	40
Vital High Nitrogen (Ross)	1.00	150:1	84	460	1500	34.1	20.3
Vivonex TEN (Norwich-Eaton)	1.00	163:1	83	630	2000	20	20
Criticare-HN (Mead Johnson)	1.06	173:1	83	650	1887	33.8	27.6
Polymeric							
Entrition/Entripack (Biosearch)	1.00	178:1	83	300	2000	30.7	30.5
Sustacal[†] (Mead Johnson)	1.01	104:1	84	625	1080	53.3	40.8
Osmolite (Ross)	1.06	178:1	84	300	1887	25.9	23.9
Osmolite-HN (Ross)	1.06	150:1	84	310	1321	40	40.5
Isocal[†] (Mead Johnson)	1.06	192:1	84	300	1887	33.7	23
Susta II[†] (Mead Johnson)	1.06	147:1	84	450	1420	36.2	30.7
Compleat-Modified (Sandoz)	1.07	156:1	84	405	1495	35.8	55.7
Enrich[†] (Ross)	1.10	173:1	83	480	1391	40	36.8
Precision Isotein HN[+] (Sandoz)	1.20	112:1	85	300	1750	21.7	29.5
Sustacal HC[†] (Mead Johnson)	1.50	160:1	78	650	1800	37.8	36.8
Ensure Plus[†] (Ross)	1.50	171:1	77	600	1600	59.5	49.6
Pulmocare[†] (Ross)	1.50	150:1	77.4	490	1000	48.8	56.9
Traumacal[†] (Mead Johnson)	1.50	115:1	78	490	2000	35.7	51.5
Isocal HCN[†] (Mead Johnson)	2.00	170:1	71	690	1500	35.8	34.7

[*] % of total kcal.
[†] Palatability permits use as long-term supplement.
RDA = recommended dietary allowance
CHO = carbohydrate
LCT = long-chain triglyceride
MCT = medium-chain triglyceride

TABLE 5 Elemental and Polymeric Enteral Formulas (Continued)

Phos (mg/L)	Protein (%*, g/L)	CHO (%*, g/L)	Fat LCT (%*, g/L)	Fat MCT (%*, g/L)	Comments
500	18/45	70/175	12/13.3	—	Hydrolized lactalbumin
667	16.7/41.7	73.9/185	5.2/5.9	4.2/4.86	70% protein as short-chain peptides
500	15.3/38.3	82.2/206	2.5/2.8	—	High branched-chain amino acids
528	14/38	83/222	3/3.4	—	70% free amino acids; 30% short-chain peptides
500	14/35	54.5/136	31.5/35	—	Ready to feed isotonic formula
930	24/61.3	55/140	21/23.1	—	High protein
549	14/37.2	54.6/145	15.7/19.25	15.7/19.25	Isotonic; unpalatable for oral use
761	16.7/44.4	53.3/141	15/18.4	15/18.4	Isotonic
528	13/34.2	50/133	29.6/35.5	7.4/9	Isotonic; unpalatable for oral use
707	17/45.1	53/140.5	30/35.3	—	Added soy polysaccharide
1320	16/42.8	54/140	30/36.8	—	Blenderized; contains dietary fiber
719	14.5/39.7	55/162	30.5/37.2	—	Added soy polysaccharide
576	23/67.8	52/156	18.8/25	6.3/8.3	High protein isotonic formula powder
845	16/60.9	50/190	34/57.5	—	High caloric density formula
634	14.7/54.9	53.3/200	32/53.3	—	High caloric density formula
1020	16.7/62.6	28.1/105.4	55.2/92	—	High fat, low carbohydrate formula
748	22/82.4	38/142	28/48	12/20.6	High caloric density formula
668	15/74.8	45/225	28/63.6	12/27.3	High caloric density formula

fluid balance, a major concern is the obese patient with severe CHF. With excess accumulation of adipose tissue the following physiologic adjustments occur: increased lean body mass; rise in whole body oxygen consumption and heat production; increased absolute energy and oxygen cost of a given physical activity; elevated cardiac output; and enlarged heart mass. These are all interrelated metabolic and cardiovascular effects of obesity. A logical conclusion is that weight loss lowers the metabolic demands on the failing myocardium. Thus weight reduction is a cornerstone in the management of obese patients with CHF.

We recommend regular visits to a dietitian for appropriate counseling. Often a simple review of foods eaten and beverages ingested will reveal easily trimmed sources of dietary energy. Our approach is to then encourage consistent but slow weight loss through modest caloric restriction with the application of a diabetic exchange program. Many medical centers now have weight reduction programs in which the patient can enroll.

Inpatient Management

Severe CHF is often found in intensive care unit patients. A stepwise approach is used in managing these individuals: ad libitum food intake followed by nonvolitional enteral and parenteral feeding.

Patients able to ingest solid foods are managed in a manner similar to that described for outpatients. Soft and easily digested foods are served in multiple small portions. Extremes in temperature are avoided. Sodium intake is limited to 2.0 to 2.5 g per day; use of a salt substitute or other seasonings should be considered. Ingestion of caffeinated beverages is minimized, although complete abstinence is unnecessary. The latter may invoke withdrawal symptoms or other psychogenic reactions that override the hoped-for benefit of prohibiting caffeine intake.

When food intake is subnormal and the patient is losing nonfluid body weight, the next step to consider is enteral feeding. Candidates for this therapy include those undergoing prolonged preoperative or postoperative intensive care unit stays and patients with nonsurgical decompensated CHF. The formula diet can be infused through narrow-bone nasogastric tubes, a percutaneous gastrostomy catheter, a conventional gastrostomy or jejunostomy, or a needle catheter jejunostomy.

A wide range of enteral formulas is available for managing the CHF patient. As mentioned, certain basic principles should be considered. First, H_2O balance usually requires 1.0 ml of fluid per kilocalorie of diet supplied. With extreme fluid restriction, high caloric density formulas can be purchased or prepared that provide less than 0.5 ml H_2O per kilocalorie (see Table 5). The formula Na should be low and consistent with the guidelines mentioned earlier. Almost all current liquid diets are low in or free of lactose. Unless obvious malabsorption is present the conventional intact-nutrient polymeric solution is recommended. Diarrhea or clinically evident malabsorption suggests the need for a predigested nutrient source or "elemental formula." For the patient with electrolyte or other metabolic abnormalities, a modular formula can be created either de novo by the dietitian or from currently available modular systems Table 6). Severe azotemia may require the infusion of a formula containing less protein. A balanced formula in which carbohydrate and fat are in the approximate proportions mentioned earlier is preferred. An excessive proportion of carbohydrate favors glucose oxidation, high carbon dioxide production, and an increase in ventilation. On the other hand, excessive formula fat increases the need for pancreatic activity, micelle formation, and intestinal fat absorption. The relevant features of some commonly used enteral formulas are presented in Table 5.

Administration should be slow initially and adjusted to patient tolerance. Full-strength formula can be provided to most patients, although intolerance suggests the need for dilution. Residual gastric volume should be checked regularly. Aspiration is a serious complication of tube feeding that can be avoided by elevating the head of the bed and by using long feeding tubes. Catheters come in a variety of lengths and lumen diameters; weighted tips aid in passage. Fluoroscopic placement is occasionally necessary.

Formula administration is accompanied by an increase in splanchnic blood flow and a rise in thermogenesis as mentioned earlier. A slow infusion at or near a maintenance energy input minimizes the cardiopulmonary demands related to feeding.

Complications of tube feeding, in addition to aspiration, are worthy of mention. Diarrhea is a common side effect of tube feeding, especially in the critically ill patient. Obvious causes of this problem are first ruled out: these include an excessive infusion rate of a hyperosmolar solution, concomitant antibiotic administration, formula bacterial contamination, and lactose intolerance. Removal of the underlying cause and antidiarrheal therapy are the preferred method of treatment. We occasionally find that changing the formula alleviates the diarrhea; the mechanism of this effect is uncertain. Serum electrolytes should be monitored regularly and adjustments made in formula composition when appropriate. Hyperglycemia, especially in patients on corticosteroids, is relatively frequent. Reducing the proportion of formula carbohydrate and slowing the formula

TABLE 6 Modular Formula Components

Product/Manufacturer	Source	Caloric Density (kcal/g)	Protein %*	CHO %	Fat %	NA (mEq/g)	K (mEq/g)	Ca (mEq/g)	Phos (mg/g)
						PROTEIN			
ProPac (Biosearch)	Whey protein; 19.5 g/packet	4.0	77	—	8	0.10	0.13	6.0	3.1
Pro Mix R.D. (Navaco)	Whey protein; 18.7 g/packet	3.85	80	5	4	0.11	0.22	3.94	3.4
Nutrisource Protein (Sandoz)	Lactalbumin, egg albumin; 19.8 g/packet	4.04	76	9	7	0.12	0.15	3.54	3.03
Nutrisource Amino Acids (Sandoz)	Amino acids; 15.4 g/packet	3.90	97	—	—	—	—	—	—
Nutrisource BCAA (Sandoz)	Amino acids with 6.6 g of 15.4 g/packet as branched-chain amino acids	3.90	97	—	—	—	—	—	—
Casec (Mead Johnson)	Calcium caseinate; powder	3.70	88	—	2	0.07	0.003	16	8.0

TABLE 6 Modular Formula Components (Continued)

| Product/Manufacturer | FAT | | | CARBOHYDRATE | | | |
	Source	Caloric Density (kcal/ml)	Product/Manufacturer	Source	Caloric Density	Osmolality (mOsm/kg)
Microlipid (Biosearch)	Safflower oil emulsion	4.5	Moducal (Mead Johnson)	Maltodextrin powder	3.8 kcal/g	—
MCT Oil (Mead Johnson)	Medium-chain triglycerides; fractionated coconut oil	7.7	Sumacal (Biosearch)	Maltodextrin powder	3.8 kcal/g	—
Nutrisource LCF (Sandoz)	Soybean oil emulsion	2.2	Polycose (Ross)	Glucose polymer of hydrolyzed corn starch	2 kcal/ml	850
Nutrisource MCT (Sandoz)	Deionized corn syrup solids; medium-chain triglycerides	2.0	ProMix (Navaco)	Glucose polymer of hydrolyzed corn starch	2.5 kcal/ml	315
			Nutrisource Carbohydrate (Sandoz)	Deionized corn syrup solids	3.2 kcal/ml	2000

* % of total kcal
CHO = carbohydrate

infusion rate are widely accepted initial measures. Insulin therapy is indicated in refractory cases.

Patients who do not tolerate tube feeding require parenteral support. Usually peripheral intravenous infusions are inappropriate in this patient group as the large fluid load needed for weight maintenance is prohibitive. Central intravenous feeding is the preferred approach. All of the metabolic, fluid, and electrolyte principles mentioned earlier for enteral feeding also apply to parenteral formula infusion. Occasionally patients will require a minimal fluid input; this can be accomplished by appropriate use of parenteral lipids and/or a concentrated "cardiac failure" parenteral formula (Table 7).

The practitioner can thus control the patient's Na intake, fluid input, and metabolic load during both enteral and parenteral feeding. This approach, coupled with appropriate pharmacologic therapy, is capable of maintaining nutritional status without adversely affecting cardiac function in most patients.

TABLE 7   2172 mOsm/Liter Central Vein Cardiac Formula

	Ml	kcal	CHO* (g)	Protein (g)
Freamine 8.5%	360	98	—	28
Dextrose 70%	500	1190	350	—
Total	860	1288	350	28

MVI-12, vitamin K, and trace elements added daily.
Electrolytes adjusted to patient's requirements; does not contain essential fatty acids; fat emulsion can be added.

* CHO = carbohydrate

To conclude this discussion, the general approach we profess throughout this brief review is one of moderation. Even with this conservative management, substantial gains in patient well-being can be accomplished through the application of the basic principles and clinical practices described herein.

SUGGESTED READING

Heymsfield SB, Smith JL, Redd S, Whitworth HB. Critical illness: cardiac failure. In: Mullen JL, Crosby LO, Rombeau JL, eds. Symposium on surgical nutrition. Surg Clin North Am 1981; 61:636–653.

Pittman JG, Cohen P. The pathogenesis of cardiac cachexia. N Engl J Med 1964; 271:403–409.

Wenger NK. Guidelines for dietary management after myocardial infarction. Geriatrics 1979; 34:75–83.

HYPERTENSION

ROBERT M. A. RICHARDSON, M.D., F.R.C.P.(C)

Hypertension may affect up to 20 percent of North Americans and is a major risk factor in the development of stroke, heart failure, renal failure, and atherosclerosis. It would therefore logically follow that detection and treatment of hypertension would have significant benefits for both individuals and society. While it is true that drug treatment of moderate to severe hypertension (diastolic BP >105 mm Hg) has been shown to reduce the risk of stroke, heart failure, and renal damage, it has not yet been conclusively proven that therapy of mild hypertension (diastolic pressure of 90 to 105 mm Hg) has similar benefits. In fact, no study has conclusively proven that mortality from coronary artery disease has been reduced by antihypertensive therapy. The question of which hypertensive patients would benefit from therapy is a difficult but important question that has not been answered satisfactorily: rather, consensus has been reached based on available information and common sense. This chapter will discuss the question of who to treat in some detail because it is so important and then will consider nutritional and drug therapy of essential hypertension. Consideration of secondary hypertension is beyond the scope of this chapter.

WHO TO TREAT

Although hypertension is usually defined as an arterial pressure of greater than 150/90, it does not necessarily follow that all patients with higher blood pressures will benefit from treatment. While it is clear that patients with diastolic blood pressure greater than 105 should be treated, those with diastolic pressures of 90 to 105 present a more difficult problem. The actual level of diastolic pressure that should be used as an indication for treatment is uncertain, but a Canadian Consensus Conference of hypertension specialists has recommended a value of 100 mm Hg in uncomplicated hypertensives. The Third Joint National Committee on Detection, Evaluation, and Treatment of High Blood Pressure (1984) in the United States has suggested a value of 95 mm Hg.

In assessing an individual patient, it is important to recognize that the stress of seeing a physician can raise blood pressure, so it is helpful to repeat blood pressure measurements after 5 to 10 minutes of quiet resting. Measurement of blood pressure should be repeated at least twice over a few weeks or months to document that hypertension is persistent, because there is a tendency for elevated pressures to fall with time in some individuals. Only patients whose pressures are consistently elevated need to be treated. Remember to use a large cuff in the obese individual.

Other factors to consider in deciding whether to initiate treatment are the patient's age, the presence of other risk factors for atherosclerosis, and hypertensive end organ damage. Elderly patients (over 65 years) are particularly difficult to make rational decisions about because there are very little data available on the benefits of antihypertensive therapy in this age group, and blood pressure, especially systolic, tends to increase with advancing age. In general, one should probably be more conservative in treating the elderly hypertensive, because drug side effects are usually more severe and benefits of treatment less clear than in younger individuals. Patients with other risk factors for atherosclerosis such as diabetes mellitus, hyperlipidemia, and smoking probably should be treated more aggressively, although the evidence that this is beneficial is not strong. It has also been suggested that patients with evidence of end organ damage such as heart failure, left ventricular hypertrophy, or renal insufficiency should also be treated more aggressively.

NUTRITIONAL TREATMENT

Salt

It has been recognized for decades that dietary sodium chloride has a major influence on blood pressure. There is no doubt that a proportion of hypertensive patients show a reduction in pressure on a restricted salt diet and that salt ingestion antagonizes the antihypertensive effect of many drugs used in the treatment of hypertension. Significant reductions in blood pressure are not usually seen until dietary sodium is reduced to a "no added salt" diet, equivalent to less than 90 mmol per day. This is considerably less than the average daily North American sodium intake of 150 to 300 mmol. There are few long-term studies showing significant benefit of dietary salt restriction; in part this is because compliance with salt restriction is erratic and difficult to achieve, and probably in part because not all hypertensives are salt sensitive. Therefore, although adherence to a "no added salt" diet should be recommended, it alone will not control hypertension in most patients.

Weight Reduction

Some obese hypertensives have improved blood pressure levels following weight reduction, although the mechanism of this response is unclear. Since long-term maintenance of weight reduction is notoriously poor, it may be recommended but is unlikely to be successful in the majority of patients.

Calcium

It has recently been proposed that altered calcium homeostasis is a major factor in the pathogenesis of hypertension. There is some evidence that diets low in calcium predispose to hypertension, but this is very controversial. On balance, it appears that dietary calcium supplementation as an effective treatment for hypertension is unproven.

DRUG TREATMENT

This discussion involves the treatment of stable essential hypertension, which is what the vast majority of hypertensives have. The treatment of severe hypertension or hypertensive emergencies is beyond the scope of this chapter.

A widely accepted approach to the drug treatment of hypertension is stepped care, which starts with a drug from one category and adds additional drugs from subsequent categories in a stepwise fashion (Table 1). The same approach will be used here with consideration of some general principles of treatment first.

1. Use medication that can be given once a day or twice at most. Medication that must be taken three or four times a day is unlikely to be taken reliably.
2. If pressure is resistant to low doses of a single medication, side effects can be minimized by using low doses of two or more drugs that

TABLE 1 Stepped Care Approach

Step 1.		Thiazide diuretic or β-blocker
Step 2.	(a).	If on a diuretic: β-blocker or central adrenergic inhibitor
	(b).	If on a β-blocker: Thiazide diuretic
Step 3.		Vasodilator

compliment each other rather than by using large doses of one drug.
3. Different combinations of medications must be tried until one is found that suits the patient best. Flexibility is necessary, for the regimen prescribed may be life-long therapy; if the patient is not comfortable with the drugs, he or she is unlikely to take them.

Classification of Antihypertensive Drugs

Table 2 lists most of the commonly used antihypertensive medications. It is clearly impossible for the average nonspecialist practitioner to be familiar with all of them, but it is useful to know the major categories and one or two drugs within each category. Side effects, indications, and contraindications tend to be similar to each group and are listed in Table 3.

Patients with mild hypertension may be started on either a diuretic or a β-blocker. In general, older patients and those with heart failure, obstructive pulmonary disease, asthma, or diabetes should be started on a diuretic. Younger patients, particularly those who are clearly anxious with resting tachycardia, may be started on a β-blocker. If after 4 to 6 weeks blood pressure remains above 150/90, one can try substituting a β-blocker for a diuretic or vice versa since some patients respond to one but not the other. Alternatively, if the patient is already on a diuretic, a β-blocker such as atenolol or nadolol could be added, or one could add aldomet or clonidine. If the step 1 drug was a β-blocker, then a diuretic should be added at step 2.

Should a step 3 drug be required, several classes of drugs are available. Hydralazine or prazosin can be used in most patients. Calcium

TABLE 2   Classification of Commonly Used Antihypertensive Drugs

Diuretics	Adrenergic Inhibitors	Vasodilators
Thiazides	β-blockers	Direct
Chlorthalidone	Propanolol	Hydralazine
Furosemide	Atenolol	Minoxidil
	Metoprolol	
	Timolol	Indirect (α-blocker)
	Oxprenolol	Prazosin
	Pindolol	
	Nadolol	Calcium Antagonists
		Nifedipine
		Diltiazem
	Combined α- and β-blocker	
	Labetalol	
	Central	Converting Enzyme Inhibitors
	Methyldopa	Captopril
	Clonidine	Enalapril

antagonists are equally effective but must be given three or four times daily, at least in present formulations, which makes them somewhat impractical. Captopril and enalapril are also very effective and are relatively free of side effects. They tend to be more expensive, however. In general the converting enzyme inhibitors and minoxidil are reserved for more severe or resistant hypertension, although recently the converting enzyme inhibitors have been recommended as step 1 therapy.

In practice, therefore, I would usually initiate therapy with hydrochlorothiazide 25 mg once daily; add a one-a-day β-blocker such as atenolol 50 mg or nadolol 40 mg, either of which could be doubled if necessary; and then add either hydralazine 25 mg twice a day or prazosin 1.0 mg twice a day, which could be gradually increased to 100 mg twice a day or 10 mg twice a day, respectively, if necessary. If pressure was still poorly controlled and there was no evidence of noncompliance, I would replace the vasodilator with either captopril starting at 12.5 mg twice a day and increasing to a maximum of 50 mg twice a day, or minoxidil (in men only) starting at 2.5 mg twice a day increasing to 20 mg twice a day. Clearly, many other options are available, but this type of regimen has gained broad acceptance.

TABLE 3 Antihypertensive Drugs—Side Effects and Contraindications

Drug Class	Example	Side Effects	Relative/Absolute Contraindications
Diuretics	Hydrochlorothiazide	Hypokalemia, hyperuricemia, hyperlipidemia	Gout
Adrenergic inhibitors β-blockers	Atenolol, nadolol	Fatigue, bradycardia, cold extremities	Heart failure, heart block, COPD, asthma, insulin-induced hypoglycemia
Central	Methyldopa	Sedation, depression, postural hypotension	History of depression
Vasodilators direct	Hydralazine	Headache, tachycardia, edema (prevented by concurrent use of diuretics and β-blockers)	Angina
	Minoxidil	Hypertrichosis	Use in women limited by hypertrichosis
Calcium antagonists	Nifedipine	Headache, edema	—
	Diltiazem	Headache, edema	Heart block
Angiotension converting enzyme inhibitor	Captopril	Altered taste, rash, hypotension (especially with concurrent use of diuretics)	Can cause acute renal failure with bilateral renal artery stenosis

Diuretics and Hypokalemia

A major area of controversy in the drug treatment of hypertension is the frequent occurrence of hypokalemia associated with thiazide diuretics. Although hypokalemia is rarely severe enough to cause symptoms such as weakness, there is definitely an increased incidence of asymptomatic arrhythmias associated with thiazide use, and there is some evidence that in men with preexisting coronary artery disease there is an increased risk of sudden death. The evidence that diuretic use causes an increase in ventricular premature beats is strong. The frequency of ventricular premature beats correlates with the presence (but not necessarily the severity) of hypokalemia, and prevention of hypokalemia with concommitant use of potassium-sparing diuretics prevents or reverses the tendency to ventricular premature beats. The clinical significance of this asymptomatic arrhythmia is unknown, and in the vast majority of patients the ventricular premature beats seem to be of no import. However, in the Multiple Risk Factor Intervention Trial (and in two other similar studies) a subgroup of male patients treated with thiazides who had previously documented electrocardiographic abnormalities had an increased incidence of coronary death. The explanation is not certain, but it has been suggested that reductions in serum potassium may have predisposed those with underlying heart disease to fatal arrhythmias. The other concern about hypokalemia is that the stress of myocardial infarction (should that occur) can cause a release of catecholamines that shifts potassium into cells and may cause significant hypokalemia. The incidence of serious ventricular arrhythmias after myocardial infarction is much higher in the presence of hypokalemia.

Based on these concerns, it would seem appropriate to use β-blockers rather than diuretics as initial therapy in patients with known or suspected coronary artery disease. In patients without coronary disease, thiazides may be used as initial therapy, but high doses (50 to 200 mg per day of hydrochlorothiazide or equivalent) should be avoided, since the risk of hypokalemia rises dramatically with increased dose, but the antihypertensive effect does not rise proportionately. If serum potassium levels fall below 3.0 mmol per liter, a potassium-sparing diuretic should be added to restore levels to normal. In patients who are asymptomatic and who have no known coronary artery disease, levels of 3.0 to 3.5 mmol per liter probably do not have to be treated.

To conclude this discussion, close and regular follow-up of patients with encouragement, positive feedback, and open discussion of side effects is extremely important in encouraging compliance and effectuating treatment. Patients who remain hypertensive while on three medications should probably be referred to practitioners with a special expertise in the evaluation and treatment of hypertension.

SUGGESTED READING

Kaplan NM. Clinical hypertension. 4th ed. Baltimore: Williams & Wilkins, 1986.
Kaplan NM. Should mild hypertension be treated? N Engl J Med 1982; 307:306-309.

NUTRITION AND CNS DISEASE

THE UNCONSCIOUS PATIENT

TOM JAKSIC, M.D., Ph.D.
GEORGE L. BLACKBURN, M.D., Ph.D.

The management of head-injured patients in the intensive care unit setting continues to pose a major challenge. Approximately 50 percent of traumatic deaths are secondary to intracranial injury. Current data suggest that the judicious use of nutritional support is a valuable therapeutic adjunct in this subset of unconscious patients. Central nervous system (CNS) insult, either accidental or operative, elicits a profound catabolic response that is quantitatively similar to that found in severe thermal trauma. In addition, it imposes restrictions upon the use of enteral nutrition due to risk of aspiration and places a premium upon the avoidance of CO_2 retention. Thus, in order to promote wound healing, potentiate an appropriate response to sepsis, and combat increased intracranial pressure, the use of specifically designed parenteral and enteral nutritional therapy is indicated. A reasoned approach to appropriate alimentation includes (1) careful patient assessment, (2) determination of nutrient requirements, and (3) choice of the optimal route for nutrient provision.

PATIENT ASSESSMENT

Generally, nutritional support should be offered to all unconscious patients in one or more of the following situations: no oral intake is anticipated for more than 5 days, further surgery is likely, or there is pre-existing malnutrition. Of particular clinical utility in the assessment of previously poor nutritional status is a history of unintentional weight loss of greater than 10 percent of body weight in the months prior to admission. Lowered serum levels of albumin and transferrin, as well as anergy to common skin test antigens, are concomitants of the stress response found in the majority of patients.

Prompt institution of nutritional support is mandated especially in unconscious individuals with head injury, in whom nitrogen losses often exceed 30 g per day. The severity of brain trauma has been correlated with the extent of circulating catecholamine elevation and the degree of catabolic stress. It is feasible to initiate parenteral nutritional support within hours of injury if relative hemodynamic stability has been achieved. Rapp and colleagues have reported a salutary effect upon patient survival, nitrogen balance, serum albumin, and total lymphocyte count with the expeditious institution of parenteral nutrition in head-injured patients. It also has been suggested that early parenteral nutrition promotes functional recovery in patients with cerebral edema.

NUTRITIONAL REQUIREMENTS

Once a decision has been made to commence nutritional support, a determination of individual nutrient requirements is necessary. This assessment should include estimates of total energy allotment and protein needs, as well as electrolyte and micronutrient replacement.

Energy Requirements

Measurements of resting energy expenditure following head injury consistently show a substantial increment over calculated values (Table 1). As in other types of trauma, the degree of hypermetabolism varies

TABLE 1 Measured Resting Energy Expenditure in Head Injury

Study	Percent of Calculated Basal Metabolic Rate
Haider et al (1975)	170
Long et al (1979)	161
Clifton et al (1984)	138 (nonsedated) 89 (sedated)

with the extent of stress (which in neurosurgical terms may be predicted by the Glasgow Coma Scale). One caveat, however, as demonstrated by the work of Clifton and co-workers, is that patients who are sedated, in phenobarbitol coma, or have been given neuromuscular relaxants tend to have a reduced level of energy expenditure. The energy requirements of a seriously head-injured patient may be assessed approximately by calculating the Harris-Benedict equation (Table 2) and multiplying by a stress factor of 1.5. Whenever possible, the actual energy needs of the patient should be measured; this is particularly true if a protracted period of feeding is planned or difficulty is encountered in weaning a patient from mechanical ventilation. With the advent of commercially available portable indirect calorimeters (metabolic carts), the precise measurement of resting energy expenditure is now quite easy. This obviates the problems of underfeeding and malnutrition as well as overfeeding and the attendant increased risks of cholestasis and CO_2 retention. CO_2 elevations are of particular concern in those patients with CNS trauma in whom vasoconstriction is sought to decrease intracranial pressure.

Our own work with surgical intensive care unit patients has shown that a relatively poor (though statistically significant) correlation coefficient of 0.48 ($p < 0.05$) exists between measured values and those obtained using the Harris-Benedict equation. Hence calculated values are only a rough guide to feeding and should be reevaluated in light of clinical response.

The optimal ratio of carbohydrate to lipid calories is discussed below within the context of specific routes of nutrient administration.

TABLE 2 The Harris-Benedict Equation for the Estimation of Basal Metabolic Rate*

Female:
  $$BMR = 655 + (9.6 \times W) + (1.7 \times H) - (4.7 \times A)^{\dagger}$$

Male:
  $$BMR = 66 + (13.7 \times W) + (5.0 \times H) - (6.8 \times A)$$

* For patient with severe head injury a factor of 1.5 $\times$ BMR may be used as a rough estimate of caloric requirements.
† BMR = Basal metabolic rate in kilocalories; W = weight in kilograms, H = height in centimeters, A = age in years.

Protein Requirements

The high excretion of urinary nitrogen in neurosurgical patients may be mediated by an increased level of circulating catecholamines and augmented further by the use of therapeutic steroids. Protein needs in head injury are thus in the range of 1.5 to 2.2 g per kilogram. An enteral feeding study in neurosurgical patients examining these two levels showed some improved nitrogen balance with the latter protein apportionment. The approach we use is to begin feeding at 1.5 g per kilogram and then sequentially increase the protein intake until nitrogen balance is attained. Twenty-four hour urinary nitrogen and creatinine collections constitute a routine part of the nutritional management of our intensive care unit patients.

Protein intake may have to be reduced if renal failure or hepatic dysfunction is present. We have set our upper limit of blood urea nitrogen as 100 before a decrease in protein nutriture is instituted. Often a clinical compromise between acceptable dialysis frequency and adequate nutrition must be sought. If hepatic encephalopathy is suspected and dietary nitrogen has been reduced to a minimum, a change to a branched-chain-enriched formula may be considered. In stressed patients a reduction in protein intake below 1 g per kilogram is not recommended.

In an effort to sustain oncotic pressure and minimize cerebral edema, serum albumin levels are maintained over 2.2 g per deciliter. Prompt repletion by the intravenous infusion of albumin is performed if serum levels fall below this value. Since the oncotic effects of albumin are not linear, little is gained by artificially increasing serum albumin further. The direct addition of albumin to a parenteral nutrition formula is a convenient means of administration and poses no incompatibility problems. Albumin supplementation of 12.5 to 37.5 g per day may be undertaken in this manner.

Electrolyte Replacement

Electrolyte requirements (Na^+, K^+, Cl^-, HCO_3^-, Ca^{++}) must be evaluated frequently in the critically head-injured patient. In addition to routine electrolyte monitoring, careful attention to phosphate and magnesium levels is needed as hypophosphatemia may lead to thrombocytopenia and respiratory muscle dysfunction, while magnesium deficiency can cause cardiac arrhythmias. The evolution of central diabetes insipidus may complicate management further. If this occurs, an assessment of urinary electrolytes is useful in deciding upon the appropriate replacement solution.

Frequently, neurologically compromised patients incur respiratory alkalosis either spontaneously or iatrogenically. Alkalosis tends to promote hypokalemia as well as a decrease in ionized calcium (the binding affinity of calcium to albumin is increased by alkalosis). Patients with respiratory alkalosis should not receive acetate salts in an effort to prevent the evolution of additional metabolic alkalosis. Alkalemia in excess of pH 7.50 incurs a risk of refractory cardiac arrhythmia. If a metabolic component is present due to diuresis or nasogastric suction, Cl^- administration may correct the alkalosis. H_2 antagonists also are useful in reducing high gastric losses and hence the evolution of metabolic alkalosis.

Micronutrient Replacement

There is no compelling evidence that a surfeit of any micronutrient above the recommended dietary allowances suggested by the National Academy of Sciences is of benefit in CNS trauma. Daily parenteral administration of MVI-12 (William H. Rorer, Inc.), with 2 mg of iron and a trace element mix, avoids any deficiency state. If diarrhea is present, 10 mg of zinc are added for every liter of stool output to compensate for the amount lost (zinc has an enterohepatic circulation). Serum zinc levels are of dubious value in assessing whole-body zinc status in stressed states, as hepatic sequestration of zinc takes place. Intravenously fed patients also are given 10 mg of vitamin K weekly by subcutaneous injection.

Commercially sold enteral formulas generally contain adequate micronutrient and vitamin supplementation, provided that a certain minimum volume is administered. There are exceptions, however, and a careful inspection of each preparation is recommended prior to use.

Monitoring of Nutrition Support

Twenty-four hour urine collection for electrolytes, urea nitrogen, and creatinine will provide valuable metabolic data for calculating micronutrient and electrolyte balance and monitoring recovery from acute injury.

ROUTE OF NUTRIENT PROVISION

After nutrient requirements have been established, the route of administration must be selected. Options include central intravenous hyperalimentation, enteral nutrition, and peripheral intravenous nutrition. Each has its specific role and attendant complications.

Central Intravenous Hyperalimentation

Because comatose patients have decreased gastric emptying and prolonged ileus, they are at risk for aspiration. Central intravenous nutrition offers a practical means of feeding, especially during the acute phase of illness. Subclavian insertion is preferred due to the ease of catheter management, and once the patient is conscious, enhanced relative comfort. A jugular approach may, however, also be utilized. In experienced hands (more than 50 insertions), central vein cannulation carries a minimal morbidity. Pneumothorax occurs in about 1 in 200 insertions, and serious arterial injury is rare. The latter may be minimized by carefully finding the vein using a 19-gauge needle before formal cannulation is attempted. Line contamination and infection are more frequent complications. For any fever spike the following procedures are performed: peripheral blood cultures, blood cultures through the central line, and a line change over a wire to obtain a tip culture. Table 3 outlines our approach to line sepsis as well as our criteria for its diagnosis. The incidence of central venous thrombosis may be reduced from 5.4 to 1.2 percent by the addition of 6,000 units of heparin to the parenteral nutrition solution. This protective level of heparinization will not alter the partial thromboplastin time (PTT).

One intravenous bag of hyperalimentation fluid containing amino acids, glucose, and lipid emulsion with appropriate additives (three-in-one solution) is ordered daily by the hyperalimentation physician and mixed by the pharmacy. We administer varying amounts of volume, calories (as glucose and lipid), amino acids, electrolytes, and micronutrients, depending upon the specific needs of the patient.

Lipid usually is limited to less than 30 percent of calories in stressed patients. Although controversial, there is evidence to support the theory that reticuloendothelial blockade may be engendered by higher rates of lipid infusion. In the case of CO_2 retention, lipid administration may be increased to 50 percent of calories. It should be noted that linoleic acid (an essential polyunsaturated fatty acid–PUFA) need comprise only 2 to 3 percent of total calories in order to obviate any risk of essential fatty acid deficiency in humans, and the requirement for linolenic acid appears to be even lower. Current commercially available lipid emulsions

TABLE 3 A Clinical Approach to Catheter Sepsis

| *Culture Results** | | | | |
CTC	CBC	PBC	*Diagnosis*	*Therapy*
−	−	−	No infection	None
−	−	+	Sepsis	None or change catheter
+	−	−	Contamination	Change catheter
−	+	−	Probable catheter tip infection	Change catheter
−	+	+	Sepsis	Change catheter or remove catheter
+	+	−	Catheter tip infection	Change catheter or remove catheter
+	−	+	Catheter tip sepsis	Remove catheter
+	+	+	Catheter tip sepsis	Remove catheter

* CTC = catheter tip culture: CBC = catheter blood culture; PBC = peripheral blood culture.

are more than 50 percent linoleic acid and also contain sufficient quantities of linolenic acid. The immunoreactive PUFA may be beneficial in shock lung patients.

Certain medications may be added directly to the parenteral solution by the pharmacy. Those of particular interest in head injury include steroids and cimetidine or ranitidine. If required, insulin is also administered in this fashion; however, it must be recognized that about one-half the dose will adhere to the bag and tubing. Although violating the nutrition line is discouraged, many lifesaving medications such as lidocaine, isoproterenol, aminophylline, dopamine, dobutamine, and furosemide can be infused into the hyperalimentation catheter without risk of incompatibility. If it is known that antibiotics or other medications are required on a regular basis, a multilumen catheter is strongly recommended.

ENTERAL NUTRITION

Foremost among the concerns regarding enteral nutrition in the unconscious patient is the risk of aspiration. In an autopsy study of 720 neurologic patients, Olivares and co-workers found that 43 of 134 or 32 percent of gastric tube-fed patients had aspirated while only 28 of 515 or 5 percent of patients without gastric tubes had done so. Though a reason for caution, these findings do not mean that enteral feeding should be abandoned in the comatose patient. Rather, than enteral route is a more physiologic and cost-effective means of nutrition, and in our experience, may be used safely. Once the patient is hemodynamically stable, is without significantly increased intracranial pressure, has bowel sounds, and is not in immediate need of operative intervention, a thin feeding tube with a wire stylet may be inserted through the nose. Several cases of intracerebral malposition have been documented when basilar skull fractures have been present and obviously care is advised. A far more frequent problem is the insertion of the feeding tube into the right lung in intubated patients. This can be avoided by inflating the endotracheal cuff and guiding the feeding tube posteriorly into the oropharynx. It is our practice to place all feeding tubes in unconscious patients in a postpyloric position. Under fluoroscopic guidance we often are able to advance the feeding tube to the ligament of Treitz.

With the head of the patient's bed at 30 degrees, feeding should commence at a slow rate (i.e., 20 cc per hour) by means of a continous infusion pump and be advanced gradually as tolerance is established. If enternal nutrition has not been given for several weeks, a low fat and low osmolarity formula is recommended. Dilution of formulas to half or quarter strength is usually not necessary. Diarrhea is the most common complication of tube feeding and must be investigated by sending stool for routine pathogens and *Clostridium difficile* toxin. A diminution of feeding rate and the administration of an antidiarrheal agent such as tincture of opium (DTO) at 1 to 2 drops per 250 cc of feeding often can eliminate diarrhea if no microbial etiology exists. The transition from parenteral to tube feeding usually can be accomplished in a graded manner over 2 to 3 days.

Peripheral Parenteral Nutrition (PPN)

PPN is used primarily as supplemental therapy if insufficient enteral calories are being administered and a central line is not available. The most commonly used peripheral regimen is a 3 percent amino acid, 3 percent glucose, and 3 percent lipid formula with appropriate additives. An advantage of the peripheral approach is that it circumvents the risk associated with central venous catheterization. Unfortunately, peripheral

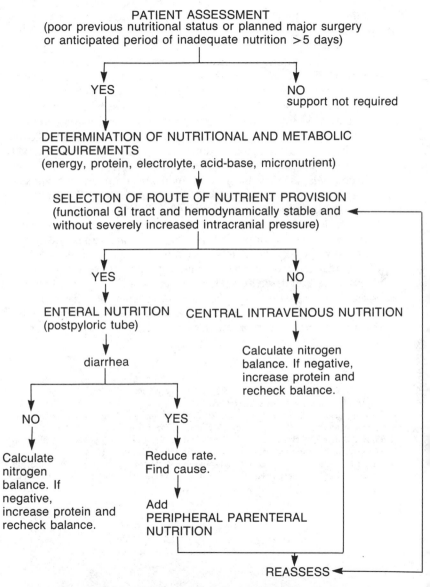

Figure 1 Metabolic support of the head-injured patient.

vein tolerance is limited to approximately 600 mOsm per liter. Thus the peripheral provision of all the nutrients necessary for the patient with a serious neurologic injury may result in fluid overload. After a period of time, the exhaustion of venous access sites also becomes a limiting factor. In an effort to preserve veins we administer 1,000 units heparin and 10 mg of hydrocortisone per liter of peripheral alimentation solution.

The presence of sepsis may enhance insulin resistance and lead to higher rates of VCO_2 (carbon dioxide production), and modification of the nutrition plan will be necessary to avoid overfeeding. The risks of feeding do not justify stopping therapy; rather, consultation and detailed critical care management are required.

To conclude, the early institution of nutritional support in hypercatabolic head-injured patients can be of significant benefit. Care must be taken in assessing nutritional requirements, tailoring a specific metabolic and nutritional strategy to meet individual needs, and then choosing the most suitable route of nutrient provision. An algorithm illustrating this process is provided in Figure 1. The role of adequate nutritional therapy is to potentiate wound healing, augment the immune response, and limit excessive lean tissue loss. Thus, the late sequelae of overwhelming sepsis and multiple system organ failure due to malnutrition may be avoided. Attention must be paid to metabolic balance studies that monitor oxygen consumption and carbon dioxide and urea nitrogen production.

SUGGESTED READING

Clifton GL, Robertson CS, Grossman RG, et al. The metabolic response to severe head injury. J Neurosurg 1984; 60:687–696.

Olivares L, Segovia A, Revuelta R. Tube feeding and lethal aspiration in neurological patients: a review of 720 autopsy cases. Stroke 1974; 5:654–657.

Rapp RP, Young B, Twyman D, et al. The favorable effect of early parenteral feeding on survival in head-injured patients. J Neurosurg 1983; 58:906–912.

Twyman D, Young B, Ott L, et al. High-protein enteral feedings: a means of achieving positive nitrogen balance in head injured patients. J Parenter Enter Nutr 1985; 9;679–684.

CHRONIC NEUROLOGIC DISEASE

ROGER G. P. REES, B.M.Sc., M.R.C.P.
DAVID B. A. SILK, M.D., F.R.C.P.

Chronic neuromuscular disability is becoming an increasingly important indication for nutritional support, which often needs to be long term. Patients with chronic neuromuscular disease can often be fed enterally as gut function is usually normal or minimally impaired. The decision to institute nutritional support in these patients should, however, be rationally based on sound ethical principles, taking into account wherever possible the natural history of the disease. Ideally, in our opinion, only those with reversible or stationary underlying disease should be treated. This section is based on the experience and policies of our unit in this special area of nutritional support, dealing largely with conscious patients.

PATIENT CLASSIFICATION

Patients with chronic neuromuscular disease who are nutritionally "at risk" comprise a heterogeneous group that may include those with any of the conditions broadly categorized in Table 1. These illnesses may lead either temporarily or permanently to a patient being unable to meet overall nutritional requirements through impairment of the intake, chewing, and/or swallowing of food.

Many patients falling within the diagnostic categories listed in Table 1 have multiple clinical problems associated with their underlying disease and may end up being managed in specialized units. In our experience, it is common for many of these patients to be referred for specific advice about nutritional management at some stage during assessment. In practice, many are initially managed in general medical wards. This is particularly true for those patients recovering from cardiovascular accidents and polyneuritis, as well as those with progressive bulbar palsy. Ideally, therefore, advice about nutritional management should be sought before the patient is referred to extended-care facilities.

279

TABLE 1 Diagnostic Categories of Nutritionally "At Risk"
Patients with Chronic Neuromuscular Disease

Cerebrovascular disease (stroke)

Traumatic brain damage and postneurosurgical patients
(gunshot wounds, tumors, subarachnoid hemorrhage)

Inoperable brain tumors

Cerebral palsy

Congenital hydrocephalus

Postmeningitis/encephalitis

Motor neuron and muscle disease

Polyneuritis (Guillain-Barré syndrome)

Spinal cord diseases

Demyelinating diseases

Extrapyramidal syndromes

INDICATIONS FOR NUTRITIONAL SUPPORT

While it may not yet be possible to specifically identify clinically
significant malnutrition with definable guidelines for management, there
is a scientific and clinical consensus that the sequelae of prolonged net
loss of nutrients are increased morbidity and mortality. While patients
can be grouped as "low" or "high" risk according to nutritional indices
and complex "weighting" systems, we do not recommend that the decision to institute nutritional support rests on the results of any formal series of objective assessments. In the context of chronic neurologic disease,
the clinician is usually already armed with the knowledge of the natural
history of the underlying disease (one of the most important aids in deciding whether nutritional support is necessary). The need for nutritional
support should be identified at this early stage, as the likelihood of malnutrition developing on account of reduced nutrient intake will be evident. Account should also be taken of the knowledge that bedridden
patients with head injuries sustain excessively high urinary losses of nitrogen. The same is also the case in paralyzed patients with polyneuritis
(Guillain-Barré syndrome). Hence, any loss of intake stemming from apathy, depression, weakness, or difficulty in chewing or swallowing quickly increases vulnerability to the vicious cycle of increasing negative
nitrogen balance with infection and decubitus ulcers.

There should be little difficulty in deciding which patients with potentially reversible or treatable disease should receive nutritional support. Occasionally colleagues (including nurses and dietitians) and patients' relatives may request or expect special attempts to be made to feed an individual when there has been complete agreement that the ultimate prognosis is hopeless. In these situations, we have followed the policy that if the patient has, in the opinion of their medical attendants, a terminal illness for which no further active treatment can be offered (for example, brain tumors unresponsive to treatment), then nutritional support is contraindicated. In contrast, although the prognosis for a given patient may be bad but specific treatment has been offered for the purpose of ameliorating symptoms or prolonging life, (e.g., in malignant disease or progressive bulbar palsy), then efficient feeding may well provide a useful adjunct to management. We have been referred such cases where nutritional support has improved the quality of remaining life by preventing hunger and pressure areas and allowing the patient to return home.

Despite these guidelines, there often remains uncertainty as to whether special attempts should be made to sustain nutritional status, and indeed for how long it is reasonable to provide nutritional support. In these difficult cases our policy is to provide nutritional support for defined periods, allowing ourselves the special task of reviewing the patient's progress at regular intervals with our medical colleagues.

ROUTES OF ADMINISTRATION AND FEEDING TECHNIQUES

Once the decision has been made to provide nutritional support, the aim is to maintain or promote positive nutrient balance with a minimum of risk and side effects. In the absence of any gross limitation of small bowel function, the majority of patients with chronic neurologic disease can be fed via the enteral rather than the parenteral route. The most practical way to do this will depend upon the clinical circumstances.

For some patients it may suffice for their oral intake to be supplemented by one of the commercially available palatable oral supplements or "sip" feeds. These offer a choice of flavors and may be energy dense (1.5 kcal per milliliter) and protein enriched. There have, however, been no properly controlled clinical studies of the clinical effectiveness of these supplements, particularly in relationship to actual documented intake.

In our opinion, therefore, when the patient is obviously malnourished (often with bed sores) tube feeding should be instituted so that intake can be guaranteed. Table 2 lists the available routes for tube feeding.

Nasogastric vs. Nasoenteral Route

Our standard technique for providing short-term enteral nutrition (up to 4 to 6 weeks) comprises 24-hour infusion of a formulated enteric diet usually assisted by a peristaltic pump via a pernasal fine-bore feeding tube positioned in the stomach. In our judgment the main disadvantage of nasoduodenal or nasojejunal feeding is that the pylorus is bypassed. Gastric emptying is mediated by the action of the pylorus, through the mechanism underlying the "duodenal braking effect," whereby the rate of gastric emptying is governed by the entry of gastric contents into the duodenum. The importance of the duodenal brake is often ignored in enteral nutrition, and the point that needs emphasizing is that the osmotic load of nutrients presented to the duodenum does not depend on the product of diet osmolality and rate of diet infusion, but on the product of gastric effluent osmolality and the rate of gastric emptying. The cramping, distension, and diarrhea that may occur during nasoenteric feeding are probably related, at least in part, to the rapid secretion of fluid and

---

TABLE 2   Routes of Administration for Tube Feeding

Short-term enteral feeding:
Nasogastric
Nasoduodenal
Nasojejunal

Long-term enteral feeding:
Cervical pharyngostomy
Cervical esophagostomy
Gastrostomy
   Stamm
   Witzel
   Janeway
   Percutaneous endoscopic gastrostomy (PEG)

Jejunostomy:
Witzel
Roux-en-Y
Needle catheter jejunostomy

electrolytes in response to the high osmotic load of nutrients infused directly into the upper small bowel. The duodenal braking effect of the pylorus should lower the osmotic load of nutrients in the upper small bowel and, in our opinion, will reduce the symptoms if enteral feeds are infused intragastrically. The use of the nasogastric rather than the nasoenteral route reduces the necessity of slowing the infusion rate to counteract the development of gastrointestinal side effects. The question that arises, however, is how often is it safe to use the nasogastric route in patients with neurologic disease?

While there are no control data to suggest that the positioning of fine-bore tubes in the duodenum or jejunum reduces unwanted tube removal, there is evidence that postpyloric feeding does reduce the likelihood of regurgitation and aspiration. Particularly at risk, in this regard, are aged, debilitated, demented, and stuporous patients; those with poor gag reflexes and motor neuron deglutition disorders; and neurosurgical patients in the immediate postoperative phase.

A case is often made, therefore, for feeding this subgroup of patients nasoenterally rather than nasogastrically. Despite the fact that at least 30 percent of our enterally fed patients have underlying neurologic or neurosurgical disease, our documented incidence of aspiration (9 of 781 patients enterally fed over 8,536 days) is lower than that of others. Since we believe that greater nutrition intake can be achieved via the nasogastric than the nasoenteral route, we usually resort to nasoenteral feeding in only the most difficult cases.

Routes for Long-Term Enteral Feeding

It is possible that as physicians our group had a propensity for advocating long-term enteral feeding via the nasogastric route rather than via a surgically created gastrostomy or jejunostomy. However, because of the limitations and drawbacks of fine-bore nasogastric feeding tubes used via the nasal route, the anticipated need for prolonged periods of enteral nutrition has stimulated the search for safe and secure enterostomy feeding. Details of the historical development and surgical fashioning of available ostomies are given in specialized texts (see Suggested Reading). It must be borne in mind that all of these require some form of formal surgical procedure which is an added risk to frail high-risk patients.

Of the gastrostomies, the Stamm and Witzel are technically the simplest but are prone to intra-abdominal leakage of gastric contents, especially the former. The Janeway procedure has been designed to overcome this complication through the construction of a gastric tube brought out to the anterior abdominal wall and appearing on the surface as a mucosal ring. An interesting recent refinement of this has been the development of the Sriram "continent gastrostomy," whereby the feeding tube can be removed between feeds without any spillage of gastric contents onto the skin.

We have been favorably impressed with the results of percutaneous endoscopic gastrostomy (PEG) feeding, which requires only local anesthesia plus mild intravenous sedation or analgesia. We are supported in this view by a large experience (see Suggested Reading) and would recommend this technique for patients with neurologic disability who are able to withstand endoscopy and are anatomically suitable (we declined one patient with gross abdominal obesity). It is likely that the PEG technique will become more widely used now that newly designed polyurethane PEG feeding tubes have become available (Corpak, Wheeling, IL, U.S.A.).

Although jejunostomy feeding avoids the risk of regurgitation and aspiration, our experience with this route, when using a Foley catheter as the feeding tube, has been complicated by the emergence of bile from the stoma. This has arisen through inadvertent overinflation of the catheter balloon, thereby preventing the free passage of luminal secretions from above. Needle catheter jejunostomy has an obvious advantage in this respect, although we have had limited experience with it. Of some practical importance in choosing the site for tube placement is that while duodenal and jejunostomy feeding require a steady and continuous infusion rate to control osmotic load (mOsm per minute) delivered to the small bowel, intermittent feeding may be used for intragastric or higher segment feeding, thereby providing greater freedom for the patient.

DIET AND METABOLIC CONSIDERATIONS

There is no indication for other than a whole protein polymeric diet for the great majority of patients, who will have normal or near normal gastrointestinal function. This is irrespective of the route of administration (diets are described in the tables found on pp 29, 57, 252–253, and

256). We have also documented that starter regimes, whereby 3 to 4 days are taken to infuse a full-strength diet, afford no advantage in minimizing gastrointestinal side effects when feeding nasogastrically. Consequently, we routinely prescribe full-strength diets from the outset when using this route. Diarrhea is most commonly associated with concomitant antibiotic therapy, which should be discontinued if possible.

Attention should always be given to the fluid, energy, protein, electrolyte, mineral, and vitamin requirements of the patient for repletion or balance. Fine adjustments may be necessary when nutritional support is total and prolonged, and it should be remembered that the patient's thirst and appetite no longer act to regulate intake during continuous enteral feeding.

There is now inceasing awareness of two aspects of nutritional metabolism that have implications for enteral diet formulation. The first is the increased requirement for nitrogen in many patients, quite apart from energy requirements that may be less than normal. Hence, in many neurologic patients with increased nitrogen losses, energy demands may be met before achieving nitrogen balance or repletion, and the importance of using high nitrogen formulations is now being realized. For example, controlled data from our wards has shown that overall positive nitrogen balance did not occur until a high nitrogen and energy (9.4 g per liter and 1.5 kcal per milliliter) enteral diet was employed, supplying a protein-energy content of 15.7 percent. The second aspect is that formulas containing high proportions of carbohydrate produce relatively more CO_2 per kcal than those containing more fat. This may be of clinical significance in patients who are receiving high diet infusion rates and who require ventilation or have respiratory insufficiency. In these patients, a specifically formulated diet containing relatively high proportions of fat and low proportions of carbohydrate would be indicated.

SUGGESTED READING

Keohane PP, Attrill H, Love M, Frost P, and Silk DBA. Relation between osmolality of diet and gastrointestinal side-effects in enteral nutrition. Br Med J 1984; 288:678–680.

Kirkby DF, Craig RM, Tsang T-K, and Plotnick BH. Percutaneous endoscopic gastrostomies. A prospective evaluation and review of the literature. JPEN 1986; 10:155–159.

Rombeau JL, Barot LR, Low DW, and Twomey PL. Feeding by tube enterostomy. In: Rombeau JL, Caldwell MD, eds. Enteral and tube feeding. Philadelphia: WB Saunders, 1984: 275.

NUTRITION AND HEMATOLOGIC DISEASE

IRON DEFICIENCY ANEMIA

SELWYN J. BAKER, M.B., B.S., M.D.(Melb), F.R.A.C.P., F.R.C.P.C.
ELIZABETH JACOB, M.B., B.S.(Madras), F.R.C.Path., F.R.C.P.C.

Iron is an integral component of hemoglobin, myoglobin, and the iron-containing enzymes essential for intermediary metabolism. Because of the limited supply of iron in most diets and because of the relatively poor absorption of food iron, iron deficiency is one of the most common human diseases.

PATHOGENESIS

The fetus gets a supply of iron from the mother, but postnatally, all iron must usually be obtained from dietary sources. There is normally a small continual loss of iron from the body via the skin, the urinary tract, and the gastrointestinal tract amounting to about 14 μg of iron per kilogram of body weight per day, or in a 65 kg adult male, about 0.9 mg per day. In women of childbearing age, additional losses are incurred through menstruation. Losses vary widely, but averaged over the month, median losses are about 0.5 mg of iron per day, with about 5 percent losing in excess of 2.0 mg per day. If iron balance is to be maintained, these physiologic losses must be made up by dietary iron. In addition, any increased iron needs, such as occur during growth in childhood and adolescence and during pregnancy, must be met. In pathologic states, where there is increased blood loss from any site, iron requirements will also be increased.

When absorption of dietary iron does not keep up with iron losses or demands, a state of negative iron balance develops. If this persists, iron deficiency results. Initially there will be a reduction of iron stores, which will be reflected by a fall in serum ferritin concentration. If the negative iron balance continues, when storage iron is exhausted, iron bound to transferrin will be utilized, resulting in a fall in serum iron concentration, a rise in circulating transferrin (TIBC), and a reduction in the percentage saturation of transferrin. When there is insufficient iron available for heme production, free erythrocyte protoporphyrin increases and the circulating hemoglobin concentration begins to fall, finally resulting in detectable anemia.

DIAGNOSIS

The diagnosis of iron deficiency anemia is most often made by the finding of an anemia with a hypochromic microcytic blood picture, associated with a low mean corpuscular hemoglobin concentration. A similar blood picture can, however, be caused by other conditions. The diagnosis should therefore be confirmed by one or more of the above measurements of iron status, such as serum ferritin, serum iron and TIBC, or erythrocyte protoporphyrin.

DIETARY MANAGEMENT

Theoretically, it is possible to increase iron absorption by increasing the consumption of foods rich in iron and particularly heme iron, which is far more readily absorbed than nonheme iron; increasing the consumption of foods that facilitate dietary iron absorption such as fish, meat, and ascorbic acid; and/or decreasing the consumption of foods known to inhibit iron absorption such as tea and eggs. Furthermore, dietary iron can be increased by fortification of foodstuffs with iron (e.g., infant formulas and bread).

The extra amounts of iron that can be made available by these maneuvers are relatively small. In adults, such increments in absorption are valuable in the long-term prevention of iron deficiency but are of little value in the therapeutic situation of an individual with overt iron deficiency. These patients require therapeutic supplemental iron in considerably larger amounts than can be achieved by dietary manipulation. However, in infants with iron deficiency, the use of iron-fortified formula is an acceptable way of managing less severe forms of the condition.

ORAL IRON THERAPY

Available Preparations

In some individuals, oral iron therapy produces gastrointestinal side effects. To reduce the prevalence of these side effects, many different formulations have been developed, resulting in a bewildering array of oral iron preparations on the market. Broadly speaking, these may be divided into two types: simple iron salts, either in liquid or tablet form, and various types of slow-release preparations. All soluble ferrous iron salts are equally well absorbed and all result in the same prevalence of side effects when given in amounts providing equivalent quantities of available iron. The slow-release preparations have been developed to reduce the concentration of free iron in the lumen of the intestine at any one time while still providing adequate amounts of iron for absorption as the preparation passes through the upper small intestine. Although some of the available slow-release preparations may produce somewhat fewer side effects than simple ferrous sulfate, they are so much more expensive that, in most cases, their use is not justified.

Preparation of Choice

Because of its low cost, the preparation of choice for oral therapy is ferrous sulfate, although all other soluble ferrous salts are equally effective. The method of formulation of the pill plays an important role in the bioavailability of the iron; in the extreme case, the pills may pass through the gastrointestinal tract unchanged. It is therefore important that manufacturing of the pills be done with strict quality control, and that the manufacturer carry out tests to confirm that the iron in the pills is readily available. In a given individual if there is any doubt, the bioavailability of the iron can be checked easily by measuring the rise in serum iron concentration 3 hours after giving the pill(s) and comparing it on a subsequent occasion, in the same individual, with the rise in serum iron after the administration of an equivalent amount of freshly prepared ferrous ascorbate. The rise in serum iron concentration after giving the pills should be at least equal to 70 percent of that obtained after giving the ferrous ascorbate.

Timing of Administration

Since the presence of food in the gastrointestinal tract reduces the amount of iron absorbed from a therapeutic dose, the pills should ideally be given between meals. However, in some people, this may produce gastrointestinal side effects, which can be prevented or at least mitigated by giving the pills with food thereby reducing the concentration of free iron in the upper intestine. In order to minimize the risk of side effects, it may be preferable to advise that the pills be taken with meals, even though the net effect will be a reduction in the amount of iron absorbed.

Dosage

In adults with iron deficiency anemia, a dose of 150 to 300 mg of elemental iron per day, in three divided doses, will usually produce a good hematologic response. Smaller doses will result in the absorption of smaller amounts of iron and a slower hematologic response. In infants and children the dose is 3 to 5 mg of iron per kilogram body weight per day in divided doses. Either tablets or an elixir may be used.

Side Effects

The side effects of oral iron therapy are mainly gastrointestinal and may be broadly divided into those affecting the upper gastrointestinal tract and those affecting colonic function. The former consist of varying combinations of upper abdominal pain, nausea, and vomiting; the latter are manifested by diarrhea or constipation. The prevalence of these side effects, particularly the upper gastrointestinal ones, is related to the concentration of iron in the lumen of the gastrointestinal tract. All soluble iron compounds produce a similar prevalence of side effects when given in equivalent amounts. Frequently, side effects are most troublesome in the first few days of therapy and tend to decrease in severity as therapy is continued. As mentioned, the amount of free iron in the lumen, and hence the prevalence of side effects, may be reduced by giving the tablets with food, but it should be noted that this also decreases the amount of iron available for absorption. It is our practice to prescribe iron to be taken when the stomach is empty, and only if side effects persist, to suggest that it be taken with meals. A small percentage of patients have persistent side effects that cannot be overcome by giving the tablets with meals. In these patients one of the slow-release preparations of iron may be tried.

Iron elixirs stain the teeth, but this is not permanent and can be removed readily by brushing. All oral iron preparations tend to turn the stool a slate grey-black color, which if an observer is not aware that the subject is taking iron, may at times be mistaken for melena.

PARENTERAL IRON THERAPY

Indications

The only indications for parenteral iron therapy are (1) inability to take oral iron due to severe uncontrollable side effects; (2) malabsorption of iron due to irreversible gastrointestinal disease; and (3) in rare cases, lack of compliance in taking oral iron. It is important to stress that the rate of hemoglobin regeneration is no more rapid with parenteral iron therapy than with optimal oral iron therapy; therefore, the need for a rapid hematologic response is *not* an indication for parenteral iron therapy.

Available Preparations

The only parenteral iron preparations currently available in North America are iron-dextran complexes (such as "Imferon"), which may be given either intramuscularly or intravenously, and iron-sorbitol complexes (such as "Jectofer"), which can only be given intramuscularly.

Method of Administration

Intramuscular iron should be given by deep intramuscular injection into one of the larger muscles such as those in the gluteal region. In order to minimize the risk of skin discoloration, injections should be given by the Z technique in which the skin and subcutaneous tissue are displaced laterally and the needle is passed through the displaced skin and subcutaneous tissue into the muscle. The plunger of the syringe is withdrawn to ensure that the needle is not in a vein and the dose injected. On withdrawal of the needle, the displaced skin and subcutaneous tissue are released and return to their normal position, thus sealing the needle track and preventing any backflow of iron along the track.

Iron-dextran may also be given intravenously, either in one dose as a total dose infusion, or in several smaller doses spaced over a period of time. In either case, it is advocated that a small initial test dose of about 0.25 ml be given slowly over a period of a few minutes to test for the presence of sensitivity to the drug before larger amounts are administered. Since allergic reactions may be delayed, it is recommended that a period of at least 3 hours elapse between administering the test dose and any subsequent dose.

Dosage

One gram of hemoglobin contains 3.4 mg of iron. Therefore to increase the circulating hemoglobin concentration by 1 g per 100 milliliters (10 g per liter) the amount of iron required is given by the formula:

$$\frac{3.4 \times V \times W}{100}$$

where W is body weight in kilograms and V is blood volume per kilogram body weight (in adult males this is approximately 75 ml and in adult females about 66 ml). Very approximately, the number of milligrams of iron required to raise the hemoglobin 1 g per 100 milliliters is equal to 2.5 times the body weight in kilograms. In addition to the iron required to raise the hemoglobin concentration to normal, extra iron, say 5 mg per kilogram of body weight, should be given to replenish body stores. The total amount is best given by repeated intramuscular injections of 2 ml (100 mg of iron) over a period of days or weeks. Intravenously, following a successful test dose, iron-dextran can be given either by repeated injections of 100 mg over a period of time, or alternatively, the whole amount can be added to a liter of 5 percent dextrose and given by slow intravenous drip over a period of several hours (so-called total dose infusion).

Side Effects

Intramuscular iron may produce staining of the skin at the site of injection, but this can be minimized by using the Z technique referred to above. There may be pain at the site of injection and sometimes pain and swelling in the regional lymph nodes, but these are usually transient and relatively minor. Occasionally, there may be signs of a systemic reaction, such as fever, chills, arthralgia, urticaria, and vomiting, and in rare cases fatal anaphylaxis may occur. The intravenous administration of iron dextran appears to carry a greater risk of anaphylactic reaction than does administration by the intramuscular route. The former should, therefore, be used only when intramuscular injection is not possible. Because of the risk of allergic reaction, parenteral iron should be administered only in situations where resuscitation equipment is available.

With some parenteral iron preparations, a proportion of the dose may be excreted in the urine, making it appear dark. Despite this discoloration there is no detrimental effect on the kidneys.

In animals, sarcomas have been produced by the administration of subcutaneous or intramuscular iron-dextran. However, in spite of an occasional anecdotal report, there is no evidence that this is so in humans.

COMPLICATIONS

Although not strictly a complication of therapy, mention must be made of the possibility of accidental poisoning of infants and young children who ingest large amounts or iron pills. Often the pills are brightly colored and children are attracted to them and eat them in the misapprehension that they are sweets. Patients should always be warned to keep tablets well out of the reach of children.

Theoretically, long-term iron supplementation, or the excessive administration of intravenous iron, may lead to iron overload. This is particularly likely if the initial diagnosis of iron deficiency has been in error as may occur, for instance, in subjects with thalassemia who already have excessive body iron and who are misdiagnosed as suffering from iron deficiency anemia.

There is some evidence that parenteral iron therapy in infants and young children may predispose them to develop infections. However, since there is seldom, if ever, any justification for employing parenteral iron therapy in this age group, this is not a question of practical concern. There is also some suggestion that treating iron-deficient adults with oral iron may reactivate latent infections, but the evidence in support of this concept is not good. In any case, iron deficiency, when present, should be treated, and if infections are present or develop they also should be treated.

OTHER MEASURES

In addition to giving the patient iron supplements, it is essential to determine the cause of the iron deficiency and to treat it appropriately. At times the cause may be obvious, but at other times an extensive search must be made to determine the presence and cause of occult hemorrhage or to rule out conditions such as gluten-induced enteropathy that may present with iron deficiency as the sole clinical manifestation.

In patients with very severe iron-deficiency anemia, where there is an immediate need to raise the hemoglobin concentration (e.g., when a woman is about to deliver or when life-saving surgery is needed), blood transfusion may be necessary. In such circumstances great care must be taken not to overload the circulation. Intravenous furosemide should be given before starting the transfusion, and packed red cells rather than whole blood should be used, and the transfusion given slowly. If cardiac failure is present or develops, an exchange transfusion should be performed to prevent further increase in the circulating blood volume.

On occasion, when iron requirements are known to be high relative to the amounts that can be absorbed from the diet, prophylactic iron therapy is indicated to prevent the development of iron deficiency, particularly in infants and pregnant women. The best strategy for infants is to give them iron-fortified formulas and weaning foods. In pregnant women a strong case can be made for the routine administration of iron supplements in the form of one tablet of ferrous sulfate (300 mg, containing 60 mg of elemental iron) a day throughout the last two trimesters of pregnancy.

ASSESSMENT OF THERAPEUTIC RESPONSE

If a person is anemic, the simplest way of following the response to iron therapy is by serial hematologic measurements. The earliest sign of response is a rise in the reticulocyte count, which with optimal therapy, reaches a peak on the fifth to eighth day. This is followed by a progressive increase in hemoglobin concentration. The initial rate of rise in hemoglobin concentration is greater in more anemic subjects, and as the anemia improves the rate of increase decreases. Serial measurements of other parameters of iron nutrition may also be used to monitor the progress of therapy, but these are usually unnecessary unless there is doubt about the diagnosis. Once normal hemoglobin concentration has been achieved progress in repletion of iron stores can best be monitored by serial measurements of serum ferritin (providing there is no chronic disease present that can cause an elevation of serum ferritin even in the presence of depleted iron stores). An individual with iron deficiency anemia who is treated with oral iron is likely to need 4 to 6 months of therapy to ensure that iron stores are repleted.

SUGGESTED READING

Baker SJ, DeMaeyer EM. Nutritional anemia: its understanding and control with special reference to the work of the World Health Organization. Am J Clin Nutr 1979; 32:368–417.

Bothwell TH, Charlton RW, Cook JD, et al. Iron metabolism in man. Oxford: Blackwell, 1979.

International Anemia Consultative Group. Guidelines for the eradication of iron deficiency anemia. Washington, DC: The Nutrition Foundation, 1979.

MEGALOBLASTIC ANEMIA

ELIZABETH JACOB, M.B., B.S.(Madras), F.R.C.Path., F.R.C.P.C.
SELWYN J. BAKER, M.B., B.S., M.D.(Melb), F.R.A.C.P., F.R.C.P.C.

Megaloblastic anemia is a morphologically distinct type of anemia that results from a biochemical defect in DNA synthesis. From a practical point of view, the two common causes of megaloblastic anemia are folate and vitamin B_{12} deficiency. Folate coenzymes are essential in the synthesis of purine and pyrimidine nucleotides. With folate deficiency, nucleotide synthesis is impaired and this in turn leads to deranged DNA synthesis. A vitamin B_{12} coenzyme is an essential component of the folate cycle, and in vitamin B_{12} deficiency there is an accumulation of $N5$-methyltetrahydrofolate and a consequent deficiency of tetrahydrofolate. Thus, both folate and vitamin B_{12} deficiency have closely similar effects on the hematopoietic system, resulting in megaloblastic anemia. However, vitamin B_{12} also has other biochemical roles that are not related to folate metabolism. These include its action as methylmalonyl-CoA-mutase in the conversion of methylmalonyl-CoA to succinyl-CoA, and its action in maintenance of the integrity of myelin.

Folate is present in many foods, but particularly in green leafy vegetables, yeast, fruits, grains, and some animal products, especially liver. It is, however, fairly heat labile, and prolonged cooking may result in considerable loss of folate content. The folate in food is largely in the form of polyglutamates, which are broken down to monoglutamates during digestion and absorption. Absorption of folate normally occurs mainly in the duodenum and upper jejunum but can also occur in the more distal areas of the small intestine if for any reason absorption does not occur proximally. Entry of folate into the enterocyte appears to be mediated by a specific carrier. A normal adult requires about 500 μg of food folate a day to maintain health. In pregnancy, infections, and periods or rapid cell regeneration or growth, requirements are increased. When daily requirements exceed the amount absorbed, folate deficiency will supervene. However, a well-nourished adult has sufficient body stores to prevent the occurrence of anemia for up to 3 months if oral intake is nil.

All vitamin B_{12} in nature is derived from bacterial synthesis. For man, the chief sources are meat, fish, milk, and other animal products.

Vegetables, cereals, and fruit contain no vitamin B_{12} unless they are contaminated with soil or other sources of bacteria. The absorption of vitamin B_{12} is complicated and involves (1) the liberation of the vitamin from its binding to foods; (2) its combination with intrinsic factor (IF) secreted by the gastric parietal cells; (3) the combination of the IF-B_{12} complex with a specific carrier that is present only in the brush border of the cells in the terminal 100 cm or so of the ileum; (4) the passage of vitamin B_{12} through the enterocyte; and (5) its transport from the enterocyte to all cells of the body via the transport protein transcobalamin II. A normal adult requires about 0.2 μg per day to maintain health. An adult who eats meat, fish, and animal products has sufficient body stores to meet requirements for a number of years even after all absorption of the vitamin ceases.

PATHOGENESIS

As with any nutrient, deficiency of folate and vitamin B_{12} may be brought about by inadequate dietary intake, defective absorption, defective utilization, increased metabolic requirements, or increased losses from the body. Determining the cause of the deficiency may be crucial in deciding what type of therapy to employ.

DIAGNOSIS

The diagnosis of megaloblastic anemia can usually be suspected from a peripheral blood examination. Often the first indication will be an elevation of the erythrocyte mean corpuscular volume, which is reflected by the presence of macrocytic blood cells in the peripheral smear. An even earlier indication is the presence of an increased number of hypersegmented polymorphs in the peripheral blood. There may also be leukopenia and thrombocytopenia. Final confirmation is best made by a bone marrow examination demonstrating the presence of megaloblastic changes in the developing red cells.

Once megaloblastic anemia has been diagnosed, a decision must be made as to whether it is likely due to folate or vitamin B_{12} deficiency or even a combination of both. In some situations such as pregnancy, alcoholism, hemolytic anemia complicated by megaloblastic anemia, acute infections, and infants fed on goat's milk (which is low in folate), the megaloblastosis is almost certainly due to folate deficiency; in other situations, such as after gastric or ileal resection, it is almost certainly due to vitamin B_{12} deficiency. If the situation is not urgent, it is advisable to determine serum and red cell folate and serum vitamin B_{12} concentrations before starting therapy. A low serum vitamin B_{12} concentration with normal or high serum and red cell folates is indicative of vitamin B_{12} deficiency. Likewise, a normal serum vitamin B_{12} concentration with low serum and red cell folate is diagnostic of folate deficiency. However, when both serum vitamin B_{12} concentration and serum and red cell folate concentrations are low, the interpretation is more difficult, since in some cases of vitamin B_{12} deficiency folates may be low, and in some cases of folate deficiency serum vitamin B_{12} may be low. Other tests, such as urinary methylmalonic acid excretion and vitamin B_{12} and folic acid absorption, may help to clarify the issue. Further, a therapeutic trial with physiologic doses of either nutrient can usually decide the matter, but such trials are tedious and time consuming, and the practical approach in such cases is to treat with both agents.

FOLIC ACID

Dietary Management

Although seldom used in practice, it is theoretically possible to treat folate deficiency megaloblastic anemia that is not due to folate malabsorption by increasing the consumption of folate-rich foods. The most important indication for this type of therapy is in infants fed on goat's milk, which is deficient in folate. Here, the substitution of formulae fortified with folate will correct the deficiency.

Oral Therapy

Most patients with folate deficiency megaloblastic anemia will respond to small oral doses (e.g., 500 μg per day) of pteroylmonoglutamic acid (PGA). Possible exceptions are patients with severe malabsorption and those with markedly increased demands for folate. However, since the usual commercially available tablets contain 5 mg of PGA, excessive doses are not toxic, and the chief cost for the tablets is in the manufacturing rather than in the raw materials, almost all cases of folate deficiency megaloblastic anemia can be treated with the administration of a single tablet of folic acid once a day. Since in physiologic terms, this provides a relatively enormous dose, it is also adequate for those people with defective absorption or increased demands. In children who can swallow tablets, the dose can be the same. In infants, liquid preparations are easier to administer and a dose of 0.5 to 1.0 mg is more than adequate.

Parenteral Therapy

PGA is also available for parenteral administration. Indications are very few, and include total parenteral nutrition, severe generalized malabsorption, and isolated selective folate malabsorption, a very rare condition. Unless there is reason to suspect that demands are increased, the parenteral administration of 0.5 mg of PGA per day will provide adequate amounts of folate.

Side Effects

Folate has virtually no side effects, regardless of route of administration. There are a few anecdotal case reports that suggest an allergic response to PGA, but these are so rare that the risk is negligible.

Complications

Folic acid (PGA), given in the above therapeutic doses, will produce a hematologic response even in patients who have primary vitamin B_{12} deficiency megaloblastic anemia. The probable explanation is that the relatively large amount of folate overcomes the block in the conversion of $N5$-methyltetrahydrofolate to tetrahydrofolate caused by the deficiency of vitamin B_{12}. However, folate cannot substitute for the other functions of vitamin B_{12}, particularly those associated with maintaining the integrity of the nervous system. There is, therefore, a risk, albeit slight, of precipitating neural damage by mistakenly treating vitamin B_{12} deficiency megaloblastic anemia with folic acid. In order to prevent this, whenever there is a possibility of vitamin B_{12} deficiency coexisting with folate deficiency, it is wise to give vitamin B_{12} together with the folate until such time as vitamin B_{12} deficiency can be excluded.

On rare occasions, folate deficient patients with epilepsy may develop seizures when treated with PGA. Such patients should be carefully observed when initiating PGA therapy, and if necessary, the dose of anticonvulsant should be adjusted.

VITAMIN B$_{12}$

Dietary Management

When megaloblastic anemia is due to defective dietary intake of vitamin B$_{12}$, the addition of foods rich in the vitamin can bring about a cure. The outstanding example of this is the breast-fed child of a vitamin B$_{12}$-deficient mother who develops megaloblastic anemia, hyperpigmentation, and neurologic involvement. Such a child can be completely cured by increasing the vitamin B$_{12}$ content of the breast milk by treating the mother with the vitamin. In a similar way, strict vegetarians who develop vitamin B$_{12}$ deficiency can be cured if they are prepared to alter their diet to include adequate amounts of foods rich in vitamin B$_{12}$, such as dairy products and eggs.

Oral Therapy

As with dietary manipulation, oral therapy is usually considered appropriate only when the deficiency is caused by inadequate dietary intake of the vitamin. In such instances an oral daily supplement of 1 to 2 μg is sufficient. However, in North America such small doses are not readily obtainable except as a component of multivitamin preparations, which are unnecessarily expensive.

It is not well recognized that when large amounts of the vitamin (say 1,000 μg) are given by mouth, absorption occurs by diffusion in the duodenum and upper jejunum, quite independently of the intrinsic factor mechanism. High-dose daily oral vitamin B$_{12}$ therapy is, therefore, an acceptable way of treating patients with pernicious anemia or vitamin B$_{12}$ deficiency anemia due to other malabsorptive states such as ileal resection. However, if neurologic damage is present it is preferable to be certain that adequate amounts of the vitamin are available for the nervous system by giving it parenterally.

In the past, oral therapy with a combination of vitamin B$_{12}$ and intrinsic factor was employed for the treatment of pernicious anemia. Such preparations are expensive and may lead to the formation of circulating intrinsic factor antibodies. There is no place for such preparations in present day therapy.

Parenteral Therapy

Since the majority of patients with vitamin B$_{12}$ deficiency megaloblastic anemia have developed the deficiency because of a defect in the absorptive process, parenteral administration of the vitamin is usually appropriate. A wide variety of dosage schedules are recommended by different workers. In uncomplicated vitamin B_{12} deficiency, an injection of 1 μg a day is adequate to produce an optimal response. But since such small amounts of the vitamin are not readily available for injection, initial intramuscular injections of 25 to 100 μg of vitamin B_{12} per day may be given for the first week to build up body stores, followed by a monthly injection of 100 μg as maintenance therapy. Many advocate maintenance injections of 1,000 μg a month, but such large doses are wasteful and usually provide no advantage. When such large amounts of the vitamin are injected, all circulating vitamin B_{12} binding proteins become saturated and the free vitamin B_{12} then readily passes through the glomerular membrane and is excreted in the urine. In the presence of neurologic disease, many advocate larger doses but there is little evidence of increased benefit.

The most widely used form of the vitamin is cyanocobalamin, and this is advantageous because of its increased stability. Hydroxocobalamin is somewhat better retained in the body than cyanocobalamin but is less stable and more expensive. However, if for any reason it is difficult for a patient to have monthly injections or if costs are a significant factor, it may be preferable to give injections of 500 to 1,000 μg of hydroxocobalamin every 3 months for maintenance therapy.

In some countries, depot preparations of vitamin B_{12} are available. Unfortunately, these are more expensive and have been associated with allergic reactions. They have little to recommend them.

Side Effects

Some of the depot preparations of vitamin B_{12} have produced allergic reactions, but for all practical purposes other preparations of cyanocobalamin and hydroxocobalamin produce no side effects.

ASSESSMENT OF THERAPEUTIC RESPONSE

With optimal treatment of megaloblastic anemia the bone marrow reverts from a megaloblastic to a normoblastic pattern of erythropoiesis within 48 hours; the reticulocyte count increases, reaching a peak on the fifth or sixth day after initiation of therapy (the lower the pretreatment hemoglobin concentration the greater the reticulocyte response), and this is followed by a sustained rise in hemoglobin concentration. If there was initial leukopenia and thrombocytopenia the white count and platelet count are normalized.

Successful treatment of vitamin B_{12} or folate deficiency may at times "unmask" previously inapparent iron deficiency. In the presence of megaloblastic anemia the serum iron concentration may be high, but with treatment this falls, and as new red cells are made there is an increased demand for iron for new hemoglobin formation. If iron stores are inadequate, overt iron deficiency may supervene. This is often first suspected when hemoglobin concentration fails to return to normal levels. In such cases, concomittant iron administration will also be necessary to ensure that the patient achieves a normal hemoglobin concentration.

Therapy can also be assessed by measuring serum and red cell folate and/or serum vitamin B_{12} concentrations. However, in routine practice it is not necessary to repeat these measurements after the initial diagnosis has been made, unless there is an inadequate hemoglobin response.

Once normal hemoglobin concentration has been achieved it is desirable to continue therapy to build up body stores. Folate stores are reflected by the concentration of folate in red cells. Vitamin B_{12} stores are not so readily estimated, but the serum B_{12} concentration can be measured and should be kept in the normal range (above 150 pmol per liter).

The duration of therapy will depend on the cause of the deficiency. In some cases it will need to be lifelong, as in patients with permanent absorptive defects or chronic hemolytic anemias. In other cases it may only need to be continued for as long as there are excessive demands for the nutrient. In pregnancy there is an increased demand for folate, and except for those in Burma, Thailand, and other areas where dietary folate content is high, all pregnant women should take supplemental folate throughout pregnancy.

OTHER MEASURES

Rarely, patients may present with severe megaloblastic anemia in situations where it is imperative to obtain a response as quickly as possible; for example, in pregnant women at term or in patients with associated congestive cardiac failure. In such situations it may be necessary to resort to blood transfusion. This, however, carries considerable danger of precipitating or exacerbating congestive cardiac failure. Transfusion should only be done using packed red cells given after the patient has been treated with intravenous furosemide (40 to 80 mg), or alternatively, an exchange transfusion should be performed with an equal or slightly greater volume of the patient's blood being withdrawn by venesection to prevent circulatory overload.

In each case, the cause of the deficiency must be established and other measures employed as necessary to remedy the situation; for example, in patients with celiac disease who present with folate deficiency, treatment with a gluten-free diet will restore folate absorption to normal and prevent recurrence of the deficiency.

SUGGESTED READING

Baker SJ, DeMaeyer EM. Nutritional anemia: its understanding and control with special reference to the work of the World Health Organization. Am J Clin Nutr 1979; 32:368–417.

Herbert V. Biology of disease: megaloblastic anemias. Lab Invest 1985; 52:3–19.

Herbert V, Colman N, Jacob E. Nutritional anemias overview; megaloblastic anemias. In: Gordon AS, Silber R, LoBue J, eds. The year in hematology—1977. New York: Plenum Press, 1977; 549.

NUTRITION AND METABOLIC DISORDERS

DIABETES

ANNE B. KENSHOLE, M.B., B.S., F.R.C.P.(C), F.A.C.P.

Diabetes mellitus is a group of conditions characterized by relative or absolute lack of insulin, which results in wide-spread disturbances of carbohydrate, lipid, and protein metabolism. It may also cause structural and functional alterations in many systems and is characterized by damage to small and large blood vessels. It is a major cause of disability and premature death. In North America, diabetic retinopathy is the commonest cause of blindness in adult life and one-third of those who require dialysis or renal transplantation have diabetes. Accelerated aggressive atherosclerosis is a hallmark of the diabetic state, so that the prevalence of coronary artery disease is increased thirteenfold, peripheral vascular disease fivefold, and cerebral vascular disease threefold. Living with diabetes is difficult; not only does the diabetic have to manage the disease on a day to day basis, he may experience employment discrimination and social stigmatization, and there is always the specter of long-term disability or premature death.

Several different types of diabetes exist but this article will focus on the two commonest types found in North America: type 1, or insulin-dependent diabetes mellitus (IDDM), and type 2, non–insulin-dependent diabetes mellitus (NIDDM).

INSULIN-DEPENDENT DIABETES MELLITUS

Insulin-dependent diabetes most commonly presents in adolescence but can occur at any age. It is characterized by destruction of the beta cells, resulting in total loss of insulin secretion. The cause is not yet fully understood, but it is believed to be an autoimmune process perhaps triggered by a viral infection in an individual with a genetic predisposition. When more than 90 percent of the beta cells have been destroyed, a characteristic syndrome of excess urination and increased thirst due to the diuretic effect of sustained hyperglycemia occurs, followed by weight loss and, if total insulin lack occurs, the development of ketonuria. The diagnosis is confirmed by the finding of glycosuria with or without ketonuria and an unequivocal elevation of blood glucose. Hospitalization is usually required for initiation of insulin treatment and the correction of dehydration. Goals of therapy in IDDM include freedom from repeated episodes of hypoglycemia, avoidance of glycemia-related infections (e.g., bacterial skin infections and fungal infections of the mucous membranes) and the maintenance of the optimum level of glycemic control that is individually attainable, taking into account the age of the individual, the duration of the diabetes, and the presence of other health problems. In that the type 1 diabetic is especially at risk for the development of microvascular complications, which are commonly found 10 years or so after diagnosis and with an increasing prevalence thereafter, and as there appears to be a correlation between the level of glycemic control achieved and the risk of such microvascular complications developing, optimal management stresses striving for the best glycemic control realistically possible in each individual's case. This will vary from time to time in the same individual and from person to person depending on whether or not some residual insulin secretion is retained and the time and effort put in by the individual in balancing insulin availability against the impact of carbohydrate ingestion and exercise on glycemic flux.

The mainstay of management in type 1 diabetes is diet. Although the ideal diabetic diet remains to be determined, current practice endorsed by the American, Canadian, and British Diabetes Associations advocates the provision of 50 percent of total calories in the form of carbohydrates, chiefly complex carbohydrates with a high fiber content, with a restriction of calories derived from fat to 30 to 35 percent and protein representing 20 to 25 percent of calorie intake. Simple sugar should be restricted because of the rapid rise in plasma glucose that will result, which cannot readily be counteracted by insulin derived from subcutaneous injection. The current move toward a higher proportion of calories derived from complex carbohydrates and a reduction in calories from fat is prompted by the recognition that the blood glucose level in most diabetics is not increased with this change and a reduction in fat, especially saturated fat, may help to reduce the risk of atherosclerosis. The total calories required are established for each individual taking into account their sex, height, weight, age, and level of physical activity. It is important that enough calories are provided to allow for normal growth and development during childhood and adolescence and during pregnancy and lactation, but it is equally important that an overly generous calorie allocation, contributing to obesity, be avoided; thus repeated reassessment is needed during growth spurts in childhood and as physical activity declines with increasing age. The availability of a dietician able to translate energy requirements into a meal plan, understandable by and satisfactory to the individual with diabetes is invaluable. Individual likes and dislikes can and should be incorporated into an individual diet plan wherever possible. Lists of ethnic foods and cookbooks listing the caloric content of dishes together with the carbohydrate, fat, and protein proportions are widely available.

The role of dietary fiber has sparked considerable interest. It has been shown that doubling the traditional daily intake of 15 g can mute the glycemic excursion that occurs after carbohydrate ingestion and may actually result in a slight reduction in blood glucose and triglyceride levels. However, it is frequently difficult to incorporate the rather large quantities of fiber that are suggested into a meal plan that is both acceptable and practical.

It is now clear that varying postprandial increases in plasma glucose can follow ingestion of meals containing standard amounts of fat, carbohydrates, and protein. The "glycemic index" measures the mean plasma glucose over a 2- to 3-hour period after ingestion of a test food and compares this response with a reference standard of defined composition such as bread. Though of theoretical interest, the practical application of these findings in the management of diabetes remains to be determined.

The substitution of polyunsaturated fat for saturated fat is recommended not only for those diabetics who have a documented elevation of plasma cholesterol but also as part of the "prudent" diet that is widely recommended as offering some protection against atherosclerosis. This is not difficult to incorporate into the traditional diabetic way of eating.

In insulin-requiring diabetics the distribution of calories throughout the day is important in reducing the risk of hypoglycemia. A typical pattern includes 20 percent of total calories at breakfast, 25 percent at lunch,

30 percent at dinner and the remainder divided between one, two, or three midmorning, midafternoon and prebed snacks, depending on the number of insulin injections used, timing of physical activity, and intervals between main meals.

Insulin

By definition insulin is required daily and forever by the type 1, insulin-dependent diabetic. Insulin has traditionally been derived from the pancreas of pigs and cows, but human insulin is now manufactured, either by recombinant DNA technology or by the chemical conversion of the pork to the human insulin molecule. Insulin has to be given by subcutaneous injection, and a variety of preparations are available that differ in their peak and duration of action as well as immunogenicity. Many different patterns of insulin use have been devised, and each individual with diabetes may require several different patterns throughout his life as the specific level of desirable and achievable control and individual response to an injection of insulin change with time. The simplest regimen consists of one injection of intermediate-acting insulin each morning before breakfast. While this will prevent sustained hyperglycemia and may therefore be suitable for the small number of individuals in whom such a loose goal is acceptable, it will not produce adequate glycemic control for the majority of patients. The addition of a short-acting insulin such as crystalline or Regular with an intermediate-acting insulin such as Lente or NPH will improve glycemic control between breakfast and lunch. The use of a second injection containing a mixture of short- and intermediate-acting insulin before dinner will improve glycemic control afterwards and through the night; this "split mixed dose" is now a standard insulin regimen for the majority of type 1 diabetics of any age. Multiple injections using regular insulin before each meal with the addition of a small dose of a long-acting insulin such as Ultralente or Protamine Zinc, will further enhance glycemic control in some individuals though at the expense of considerable disruption in their day-to-day life. Continuous subcutaneous insulin infusion (CSII), using an insulin pump individually programmed to provide a basal infusion of insulin throughout the 24-hour period with premeal boluses of insulin being delivered by activation of the pump, will usually result in enhanced glycemic control, albeit at considerable expense. Unfortunately the cost of intensification of treatment rises proportionately with the degree, and as most or all of the costs of diabetes management is currently borne by the individual patient this remains a limiting factor in glycemic optimalization.

Monitoring

Though the diabetic state is associated with disturbances in many aspects of metabolism, monitoring of the blood sugar is an important and relatively easy parameter to follow. Traditionally diabetic control has been monitored by the presence or absence of glycosuria, but this is at best only an approximation of actual blood sugar levels and is often frankly misleading. Over the past decade, the practice of home blood glucose monitoring has become widely accepted. It is invasive, requiring a finger stick to obtain a drop of blood, and relatively expensive, but when properly performed it is an invaluable tool for the insulin-dependent diabetic who can, with its use attain a freedom of lifestyle with enhanced control never before attainable. Once they are accustomed to it, the majority of type 1 diabetics would not choose to monitor their diabetes in any other way. It can be used to test the blood sugar at different times throughout the day and, in need, during the night, for a better match of insulin dose to insulin need. The effect of exercise can be observed with this method. Though physical activity traditionally results in a fall in blood glucose, a paradoxical rise may occur on occasion as the result of the ratio of insulin to other hormones at that time. Home blood glucose monitoring can also be used for "problem solving," for example to discriminate between actual and pseudohypoglycemia, that is symptoms thought to be due to hypoglycemia but actually due to anxiety. In that some type 1 diabetics can experience asymptomatic nocturnal hypoglycemia, which is then followed by hyperglycemia due to the protective stimulation of the counter-regulatory hormones (the Somogyi effect), checking the blood sugar on occasion at 3 AM can result in the detection of this important phenomenon and its avoidance by appropriate adjustment of diet and insulin. Conversely, the dawn phenomenon may be documented. In this situation plasma glucose rises from the early morning hours onwards, again due to the anti-insulin effect of the counter-regulatory hormones. In this situation too, the prebreakfast blood sugar is elevated but the 3 AM blood sugar is not low.

The glycosylated hemoglobin ($HgbA_{1C}$) offers an integrated measurement of blood sugar levels over the preceding 2 months. The test is sensitive and inexpensive and can be obtained at any time of the day.

It provides patient and physician with an objective assessment of metabolic control.

The last decade has seen striking and important changes in the philosophy of diabetes management with the appropriately educated patient taking the major share of responsibility for self care, including using techniques and making decisions formerly the prerogative of the health professional. This approach can result not only in improved metabolic control but also in the diabetic feeling in control of his condition rather than being controlled by it.

NON-INSULIN-DEPENDENT DIABETES MELLITUS

By midlife 2 percent, and by age 70 close to 10 percent, of the population will have developed diabetes, usually of the non–insulin-dependent type. As longevity increases so does the prevalence of this type of diabetes. A family history of diabetes is frequently present and there is a strong association with obesity. There is considerable heterogeneity in phenotype and genotype with evidence of a primary abnormality in insulin secretion in some individuals and reduced insulin effect on target tissues in others. Impaired receptor function and postreceptor dysfunction are common and hyperinsulinemia is often present.

The clinical presentation tends to be subtle and the diagnosis is often suggested only by the finding of glycosuria or an elevated blood sugar on routine testing. The demonstration of a sustained elevation of the fasting blood sugar greater than 7.8 mmol per liter confirms the diagnosis; thus a glucose tolerance test is rarely necessary to establish the diagnosis.

The prognosis for the type 2 diabetic depends on the arterial system, as accelerated atherosclerosis commonly occurs. Management is therefore directed toward controlling those factors known to contribute to atherosclerosis, including detecting and maintaining good control of hypertension, avoidance of cigarettes and excessive alcohol, control of hyperlipidemia, weight reduction when indicated, and maintenance of reasonable glycemic control. This frequently involves a rather radical change in lifestyle that is particularly difficult to achieve in a middle aged or older individual, and this underlines the need for setting rational and realistic goals for each individual patient.

Wherever possible, the type 2 diabetic should be managed by diet alone with the addition of oral hypoglycemic agents or insulin only after diet therapy alone has clearly failed. Even a few pounds of weight loss in the obese hyperinsulinemic diabetic may result in significant improvement of glycemic control, as receptor function improves. Conversely, the lean type 2 diabetic with impaired insulin secretion frequently requires the addition of small doses of insulin to supplement declining endogenous production, and weight maintenance or increase rather than weight loss is desirable in this subgroup. To be successful, any diet prescription has to be tailored to the individual patient, taking into account age, activity, need to gain, maintain, or lose weight, personal likes and dislikes, and overall state of health. Even when all these factors are taken into careful consideration it is nevertheless recognized that dietary compliance is generally poor.

THE AGES AND STAGES OF DIABETES

Childhood

Diabetes in childhood is a rare condition affecting 12 per 100,000 under the age of 10. The expertise of a health care team experienced in dealing with the physical and emotional problems inevitably experienced by the family as well as the child is invaluable in managing this difficult condition. Parent groups offer support and practical tips for day-to-day management.

Children are naturally erratic in their activity and appetite so that it is frequently impossible to get a good match between insulin availability and glycemic flux. It is important that realistic expectations for metabolic control are accepted. Children are particularly prone to develop infections, which may rapidly and dangerously precipitate ketoacidosis.

Ketoacidosis should be avoided whenever possible, or at the very least, it should be detected rapidly and appropriate intervention implemented without delay. Conversely, nocturnal hypoglycemia, which may go undetected or be suggested by enuresis or nightmares, is undesirable but home blood glucose monitoring has helped considerably in its identification. As with any chronic illness, it is important that children with diabetes be allowed to develop normally, socially as well as physically.

The child usually knows instinctively how many calories he requires for normal growth. Flexibility is a must and battles between parents and child over finishing the last crumb on the plate should be avoided. Provision of snacks between meals will help to avoid hypoglycemic episodes and reduce "cheating." During intercurrent infection, dehydration can be prevented and energy supplied by the liberal use of regular (not diet) carbonated beverages, juices, and milk. Vitamin supplements are not generally required.

Adolescence

The peak age at which type 1 diabetes develops is around puberty and by age 20, 1 in 3,000 has diabetes. Adolescence is normally a period of turmoil, and it is not made any easier by the development of a chronic illness. Fear of future complications is not a good motivator, and in general an adolescent's main concern is to not appear "different" from his peer group. Growth spurts and the changing hormonal milieu make for metabolic instability, and ketoacidosis all too readily occurs. Repeated episodes, however, almost always result from failure to take insulin, though this is usually denied. The gradual taking over of responsibility for self management at a rate appropriate to the individual's developing maturity should be the goal, requiring a nice balance between authoritarianism and "looking the other way" on the part of the parents.

Management should emphasize "can" rather than "cannot." Participation in sports and social activities should be encouraged. Growth and development should be monitored and enough calories provided at each stage; however, when linear growth has ceased, an appropriate reduction in calories should be recommended. Though a diet made up exclusively of "fast foods" is undesirable, with appropriate education it is possible and practical to include typical teenage food choices in the diabetic diet. As it is likely that many teenagers will drink alcohol, they should be taught how to build this into their diabetic regimen while avoiding the hypoglycemia that can result. An erratic lifestyle is a hallmark of adolescence and the introduction of a split mixed insulin regimen, if not utilized before, will allow much needed flexibility; for example, with its use there will be less disruption of metabolic control when the teenager sleeps in later some mornings than others. There is a natural tendency to experiment at this time, and home blood glucose monitoring, though often sporadically performed, will allow the individual to discover his own glycemic response to "forbiddden foods." Fear of reaction during or as the result of physical activity can be diminished by appropriate size, type, and timing of carbohydrate snacks.

Young Adulthood

Although new-onset type 1 diabetes is not uncommon in the third and fourth decades, the majority of individuals will have type 1 diabetes of several years duration. Early microvascular complications are not uncommon in this age group, with attendant concern and frequently self-recrimination. The turmoil of adolescence has ceased and individuals are beginning to plan for the rest of their life.

It is at this age that a more intensified regimen with resulting improvement in glycemic control can often be achieved as a more regular lifestyle is established. Ketoacidosis is uncommon, but frequent hypoglycemia is more commonly seen as the individual strives to improve control. Repeated episodes of major hypoglycemia requiring external intervention are to be avoided.

Educating the spouse, especially if he or she is responsible for marketing and cooking, is important, and as many meals are likely to be eaten out of the home the appropriate choice of restaurant foods should be taught. Adjustment for shift work and travelling through time zones may be required.

Pregnancy

The outlook for a successful pregnancy in the diabetic woman has never been better, but as the outcome is greatly influenced by the level of diabetic control from conception until delivery, pregnancy management should start prior to conception with the goal of achieving a normal or near normal glycosylated hemoglobin at the time of conception. Fortunately the level of motivation in these patients is usually very high and excellent control can be achieved, albeit with the use of multiple injections or an insulin pump.

The addition of 100 calories per day in early pregnancy and 300 calories per day in late pregnancy is adequate, with an expected total weight gain of 10½ to 12½ kilograms. No attempt should be made to achieve weight reduction in pregnancy, though a smaller weight gain may be satisfactory in the obese woman. The diet should be adjusted to provide adequate calcium, iron, and folic acid and enough carbohydrates in the evening to avoid starvation ketonuria overnight. Home blood glucose monitoring is mandatory, aiming for fasting plasma glucose in the 3 to 5 mmol range and postprandial levels no higher than 6 mmol. Postpartum breast feeding is encouraged and drinking 1 liter of milk per day will supply the extra calories, protein, and carbohydrate required for lactation.

Middle Age

This group comprises two subgroups: the majority of patients, who are non–insulin-dependent, and a significant minority with type 1 disease, often of many years duration. Each group requires different management goals and strategies. Small and large vessel complications have by now become commonplace among the type 1 diabetics (though 25 percent appear genetically protected against such complications) and management has to be modified for control of hypertension, progressive renal insufficiency, or physical limitations imposed by claudication or ischemic heart disease. Visual impairment may limit self-care, including the ability to inject insulin or care for the feet. The majority, type 2 diabetics, are faced with having to adjust their long accustomed lifestyle and with no immediately perceptible benefit as they are frequently asymptomatic at diagnosis. Realistic if necessarily limited goals such as weight loss or increased physical activity are preferable to unrealistic goals that are doomed to failure. Education concentrating on the specific goals of management for the type 2 diabetic whether they are treated with diet alone or with oral agents or insulin is fundamental for effective self-care, while avoiding "information overload."

Old Age

In this age group, diabetes is frequently only one of several physical, emotional, social, and economic problems that the individual has to deal with, and its significance should be kept in proper perspective. The primary aim should be symptom control rather than tight metabolic control, the maintenance of a well-balanced nutritional intake rather than specific dietary restrictions, a minimum of blood and urine testing consistent with symptom-free control, and provision of appropriate services such as regular podiatric care when self-care is limited. It is especially important that those responsible for the care of the institutionalized elderly diabetic be acquainted with the specific goals of management for elderly diabetics, thus avoiding unnecessary lifestyle restrictions. Hypoglycemia induced by either insulin or oral agents should be avoided as it often presents atypically in the aged and may have a devastating consequence for the neurologic and cardiac systems. If a diabetic has reached the age of 80, he must be doing something right, and nonintervention is frequently preferable to the implementation of a formal diabetes regimen.

SUGGESTED READING

Guidelines for the nutritional management of diabetes mellitus. Toronto: The Canadian Diabetes Association, 1980.

Nuttall F. Diet and the diabetic patient. Diabetes Care 1983; 6:197–207.

OBESITY

THEODORE B. VAN ITALLIE, M.D.

It is generally agreed that most patients with moderate or severe obesity are best treated by dietary restriction of energy intake. However, some of the more drastic methods by which this goal is accomplished (e.g., starvation, very-low-calorie diets) are controversial and potentially hazardous. There is also wide consensus that the induction of substantial weight loss is pointless unless the patient is willing to make a commitment to long-term weight maintenance. Thus, the fact that an individual is obese does not automatically make him a suitable candidate for treatment.

The physician must use his clinical judgment to determine whether any given obese patient has both the motivation and the capacity to succeed in a weight control program. The basic motivation to undergo treatment must originate within the patient. If the impetus to seek help arises primarily from a referring physician, an employer, or a member of the patient's family, the outlook is not very favorable. Capacity to succeed is best demonstrated by deeds rather than words. Thus, if a patient will regularly and punctually attend treatment sessions, conscientiously keep food intake records, and cooperate in carrying out assignments given by the therapist, a successful outcome is much more likely. Patients who are excessively preoccupied with personal problems of various kinds (e.g., marital, drugs, alcohol, financial) probably should defer treatment until the problem in question is under better control.

ATTITUDE OF THE PHYSICIAN

Toward the Problem of Obesity

All physicians are therapy-minded but too few are prevention-minded. The fact that obesity is associated with a substantially increased risk of developing a variety of illnesses, including diabetes, hypertension, stroke, premature coronary heart disease, gallbladder disease, and certain forms of cancer is not yet taken seriously enough by many physicians. Simply

314

advising the patient to lose weight is rarely effective. If any success is to be achieved, the patient must be highly motivated to lose weight. The physician is strategically placed to reinforce and sustain a patient's determination to adhere to a weight control program. If the physician is unable to provide the kind of multidisciplinary treatment generally required by severely overweight patients, he should help the patient enroll in a weight control program that provides sophisticated nutritional and exercise counseling, behavior therapy, and psychologic support. The physician can contribute materially to the success of the undertaking by following his patient's progress and reinforcing his efforts to lose excess fat and thereafter remain at his reduced weight.

Toward the Obese Patient

Most obese patients are extremely sensitive about their overweight condition even though they may exhibit a facade of joviality or candor about the problem. Indeed, it should be kept in mind that many obese persons have been the victims of social and economic discrimination because of their physical appearance. The physician should be alert to such sensitivity and should go out of his way to treat the obese patient with respect, courtesy, and kindness. A lack of respect and regard for the patient is hard to conceal and is quickly noticed by obese patients who are acutely sensitive to slights.

As physicians learn more about obesity and its causes, and as they come to know obese patients better, any residual prejudice against obese individuals is likely to be dispelled and replaced by the understanding and warmth that are indispensable to the maintenance of a good doctor-patient relationship.

Since obese patients are not likely to remain under the care of a physician who appears to be insensitive or unsympathetic, the effect of giving such an impression is usually to drive the patient away and thereby frustrate the entire therapeutic process.

THERAPEUTIC OPTIONS

The nature of the treatment that should be offered to the obese patient is in large part determined by the severity of his obesity. Weight status is most easily evaluated by the use of the body mass index (BMI), which is calculated by dividing body weight (in kg) by the square of the height (in meters). This index normalizes for stature, thereby obviating the need for height-weight tables. Severity of overweight can be roughly categorized according to BMI, as shown in Table 1.

Morbidity and mortality ratios increase in accelerating fashion with increasing overweight; however, these risks appear to be exacerbated in individuals with upper body segment or abdominal (android) obesity and mitigated in individuals with lower body segment or femoral-gluteal (gynoid) obesity. The waist to hip ratio (WHR) is a useful index of type of obesity; thus, a WHR of 1.0 or greater in men (.80 or greater in women) is associated with an enhanced risk of certain obesity-related illnesses, including stroke, premature coronary heart disease, hypertension, and diabetes. Waist circumference should be measured at the natural waist or, if there is no natural waist, at the level of the umbilicus. Hip circumference is taken to be the largest circumference of the lower trunk between waist and thighs.

Age also modifies the adverse effects of obesity on health. If adults become overweight prior to middle age their relative risk of developing hypertension, diabetes, and hypercholesterolemia is quite high (Table 2). During middle age and subsequently, the health risks of being overweight are increasingly diluted by other health problems associated with aging.

Accordingly, obesity-related health hazards increase as overweight increases and are in many instances exacerbated in men and women with the android type of obesity, as indicated by a high WHR. Overweight in the young adult (aged 20 to 44 years) is of particular concern because it greatly enhances risk of developing diabetes and cardiovascular diseases. Knowledge of the determinants of risk can be used by the physician to estimate the urgency and importance of achieving weight control in a given patient.

In caring for their obese patients, physicians will have to rely

TABLE 1 Categories of Severity of Overweight

	Body Mass Index (kg/m²)
Acceptable range	20–24.9
Mild overweight	25–27.9
Moderate overweight	28–31.9
Severe overweight	32–41.9
Morbid obesity	42–

TABLE 2 Relative Risk Ratios* for Overweight American Adults

	Age ranges in years		
	20–74	*20–44*	*45–74*
Hypertension	2.9	5.6	1.9
Diabetes mellitus	2.9	3.8	2.1
Hypercholesterolemia	1.5	2.1	1.1

* Prevalence of health problem (%) among overweight persons divided by prevalence of the same problem among nonoverweight persons within the same age range. From Van Hallie TB. Health implications of overweight and obesity in the United States. Ann Int Med 1985; 103(6 pt 2):938–988.

increasingly upon the therapeutic assistance of various organized programs that are specifically concerned with treatment of obesity. Some programs may be directed and staffed by health-care professionals, including physicians; others may be operated by self-help groups or commercial organizations. The physician must know enough about the treatment of obesity to be able to determine which of these programs is most suitable for a given patient. Although individuals who are mildly overweight may be helped by attending certain nonprofessional programs, programs staffed by accredited health-care professionals are preferable for treatment of the more severe forms of obesity.

Dietary Treatment

Energy Content and Composition of the Low-Calorie Diet. With the exception of calorie content, diets used to induce weight loss should provide all of the essential nutrients in the amounts recommended by the Food and Nutrition Board's Committee on Recommended Dietary Allowances (RDA). An exception to this principle must be made for the protein content of the diet. The RDA for protein is based on the assumptions that the protein is of good quality and that the concurrent energy intake is adequate to meet daily energy needs. When energy intake falls well below maintenance requirements, an amount of dietary protein sufficient to meet RDA standards no longer may be able to sustain nitrogen equilibrium. Unfortunately, systematic studies have not been done to show what level of protein intake is optimal for any given percent energy deficit. Thus, most workers in the field have preferred to err on the side of caution and have used low-calorie diets that provide 75 g per day or more of a high-quality protein. Although this level of protein appears to be prudent, such diets also should contain sufficient carbohydrate (at least 50 g) to minimize or prevent ketosis.

Weight reduction diets should be tailored to the individual needs of the patient; it makes no sense to offer the same diet to all overweight patients. Several principles have to be kept in mind when a calorie-reduced regimen is prescribed. First, the ability of an overweight individual to tolerate calorie restriction (that is, to conserve body protein during weight loss) depends in considerable part on the degree of severity of his obesity. Thus, morbidly obese individuals generally can tolerate very-low-calorie diets (providing 300 to 500 kcal per day) far better than moderately obese persons can. As individuals lose more and more fat during treatment, their ability to conserve protein during caloric restriction is increasingly compromised. Thus, during therapeutic weight loss, the percent energy deficit that is prescribed should be periodically adjusted to percent body fat or some index of fatness such as BMI.

Percent energy deficit is the percent reduction from maintenance energy intake represented by a prescribed low-calorie diet. Thus, if the daily energy intake needed to maintain the weight of an obese patient is 2,400 kcal, a 600 kcal weight-reduction diet would create a 75 percent energy deficit. In most clinical settings, the energy intake required to maintain weight (in effect, the daily energy expenditure) must be determined from the estimated resting energy expenditure and the estimated level of physical activity.

The rationale for prescribing a "percent calorie deficit" rather than some arbitrary calorie intake arises from the simple fact that people often differ widely in their daily energy requirements for weight maintenance (ERWM). Thus, an 800 kcal diet will produce a far greater nutritional stress in a large, physically active man whose daily requirement for weight maintenance (ERWM) is 3,200 kcal than it will in a small physically inactive women whose ERWM is 1,800 kcal. In addition, the ERWM progressively decreases as more and more weight is lost.

Because the severity of a calorically restricted diet is best expressed in terms of percent energy deficit, it seems reasonable to characterize weight reduction diets in this fashion. Thus, as shown in Table 3, the most severely obese patients are permitted the most drastic caloric restriction.

As obesity becomes less severe, the percent energy deficit permitted is correspondingly smaller. It seems prudent to set a limit below which energy intake cannot be further reduced. The treatment method described herein sets that limit at 600 kcal per day. In this regard, the patient needs to understand (at least roughly) the physiologic rationale for controlling

TABLE 3 Example of How Calorie Prescription (Percent Energy Deficit) Might Be Geared to Body Mass Index

Body Mass Index	Calorie Prescription* (as % energy deficit)
25–27.9	50
28–31.9	60
32–35.9	70
36–39.9	75
40–43.9	80
44–	85

* In this model, an energy intake lower than 600 kcal per day is not recommended.

rate of weight loss; in effect, the difference between "quality" of loss and mere quantity.

It is important to emphasize that the system for prescribing calorie reduction shown in Table 3 is only a guide (not a guarantee) to help the patient lose weight of acceptable quality; namely, a weight loss that, on the average, is at least 75 percent and no more than 25 percent lean body mass (LBM). Whether this goal is actually achieved in any given case can only be ascertained if the body composition of the obese patient is monitored during weight loss. Thus, if the proportion of weight lost as LBM is persistently too high, an upward adjustment of the energy content of the diet is called for. Recently, two convenient methods for estimating lean body mass have become available—total body electrical conductivity (TOBEC) and bioelectrical impedance analysis.

Dietary Format. Low-calorie diets can take a variety of forms, as shown in Table 4. When calorie restriction is severe (ca. 60 to 80 percent deficit), either a liquid formula or a diet consisting of lean meat and fish supplemented with essential vitamins and minerals (in the amounts recommended by the Committee on RDA can be utilized. Both of these formats appear to favor improved adherence to the prescribed level of energy intake; however, the liquid formula is easier to prepare, is portable, and is more readily controlled as regards precise energy and nutrient content.

A wider range of formats is available when calorie restriction is mild to moderate (ca. 20 to 60 percent deficit). In this case, use of regular foods is generally to be preferred since the patient must ultimately learn to maintain his reduced weight on a diet consisting of everyday foods.

TABLE 4   Formats of Calorically Restricted Diets

Mild to Moderate Caloric Restriction		Severe Caloric Restriction	
Regular Foods	Formula	Regular Foods	Formula
Normal distribution of macro-nutrients	Normal distribution of macronutrients	High protein, low fat, low carbohydrate (diet limited to lean meat, fish and noncaloric drinks supplemented with vitamins and minerals)	High protein, low-to-moderate carbohydrate, low fat (usually supplemented with potassium and, if necessary, trace elements and other macrominerals)
Low in fat	Low in fat		
Low in carbo-hydrate	Intermittent meal replacement by formula		

Patients who are unable to adhere to a calorically restricted diet long enough to lose an appreciable amount of weight tend to become discouraged and drop out at an early stage of treatment. Such individuals may do better with a formula diet; however, eventually they must learn to deal with regular foods. Nevertheless, the reinforcement they obtain from successfully losing weight on a formula diet should help to keep them in a weight-control program long enough to permit the development of new habits of eating and exercise.

A formula diet should never be permitted to become the keystone of a weight control program. However, it can be an effective tool in helping severely obese individuals achieve a substantial loss of excess fat. A critical time for the formerly obese patient comes when he must undergo the transition from an exclusively liquid diet to a diet of normal foods.

Safety Considerations.   Ventricular arrhythmias and sudden death, although rare, can occur in obese dieters who undergo rapid, massive weight loss. Rapid weight loss (0.5 to 1.0 lb per day), if sustained for many weeks, is associated with an excessive loss of lean body mass and protein depletion of the heart. Such malnutrition of the heart may result in QTc interval prolongation, which renders the individual susceptible to the onset of a sudden ventricular tachydysrrhythmia. Ability to conserve body protein in the face of drastic caloric restriction varies directly with degree of fatness; thus, mildly and moderately overweight individuals are at high risk of becoming protein depleted during rapid weight loss. Morbidly obese persons are better able to tolerate prolonged, drastic caloric restriction.

Less severe side effects of drastic caloric restriction are listed in Table 5. Many of these untoward effects can be obviated or mitigated by individualizing caloric prescription, as shown in Table 3, and by taking measures to avoid inducing dehydration and ketosis.

All patients enrolled in a program designed to induce prudently rapid weight loss for a prolonged period should be carefully monitored by a knowledgeable physician on a weekly basis. The physician should ensure that the patient is adhering faithfully to the prescribed diet, including supplements such as potassium. After the first 2 weeks of caloric restriction, when the patient is more likely to be in water equilibrium, rate of weight loss should not appreciably exceed 138 g or 0.3 lb per 1,000 kcal deficit. This rate is consistent with a loss composed of approximately 75 percent fat and 25 percent lean body mass.

Electrocardiograms, with special attention to the QTc interval, should be taken every 2 to 4 weeks, depending on the clinical circumstances.

TABLE 5 Common Side Effects of Drastic Calorie Restriction*

Gastrointestinal disturbances: nausea, vomiting, diarrhea, constipation

Fatigue

Orthostatic dizziness—occasional syncope

Cold intolerance

Dry skin

Brittle nails

Hair loss

Muscle cramps

Amenorrhea

Decreased libido

Euphoria

Insomnia

Anxiety, irritability, depression

* Less commonly reported side effects include occult arrhythmias, cholecystitis and/or pancreatitis early in refeeding, and disorientation with regard to self-identity and body image.)

Blood chemistries must be obtained periodically (particularly for potassium, uric acid, blood glucose, and serum lipids). If possible, body composition should be measured every 4 to 6 weeks.

Changing Lifestyle

Roughly speaking, the fat content of the body is the consequence of an equilibrium achieved between the individual and his environment. In this equilibrium, genetic factors that influence maintenance energy requirements and the efficiency of energy storage interact with environmental factors that affect energy intake and expenditure (including physical activity level). The result is a degree of fatness that can be changed only by voluntarily altering lifestyle (dietary intake and/or physical activity) or by an alteration in the physiology of the body (illness, medication).

The usual therapeutic goal in weight loss and subsequent weight maintenance is to change lifestyle permanently. Since the environment cannot readily be altered, the focus of treatment is to help the patient create a microhabitat for himself that favors weight reduction. Thus, the patient must learn how to make appropriate food selections (nutritional counseling), how to implement them (behavior modification), and how to incorporate an increased level of physical activity into everyday life (exercise instruction). It is also important that he understand the metabolic and behavioral principles that underlie the treatment he is receiving. Comprehension of these principles will promote adherence to the treatment program and, at a later time, may help the patient to avoid falling prey to charlatanistic weight loss methods. As many support systems as possible (i.e., involving the spouse, close friends, and other family members) must be enlisted to reinforce and sustain the patient's determination to remain in a weight control program and to achieve the lifestyle changes necessary for permanent weight maintenance. As patients lose weight, new interpersonal problems may occur, arising from a favorable change in physical appearance.

Medication

The role of appetite suppressing drugs in the treatment of obesity remains controversial. When such a drug is used as part of a comprehensive treatment program, adherence to the prescribed diet may improve. However, the concurrent use of the drug may actually interfere with the ability of a course of behavior therapy to induce lasting effects on lifestyle.

There is growing interest in the possibility that certain antiobesity medications (for example, dexfenfluramine or fluoxetine) might be used for very long periods of time to promote weight maintenance. However, use of centrally acting drugs for this purpose at the present time would be premature.

To summarize this discussion, the following dicta are suggested to guide the physician in the treatment of the obese patient:

- Treat the obese patient with respect, kindness, and patience, but also with firmness.
- Take the problem of obesity and its associated health risks very seriously.
- Become educated about obesity as a health problem and as a therapeutic challenge.
- Before advising treatment, assess carefully the motivation and capacity of the patient to adhere to a demanding weight loss and maintenance program.
- Adapt treatment to the patient's particular needs and problems.
- Be pragmatic and flexible in treatment and be willing to call on experts from other disciplines (nutrition, clinical psychology, exercise physiology) to provide help.
- Be greatly concerned about the safety of the weight-loss regimen offered the patient and monitor his progress regularly and thoroughly.
- Focus on the problem of weight maintenance after weight loss and make sure the patient understands at the outset that, while losing weight is a tactical victory, the strategic problem is to maintain the reduced weight indefinitely.

SUGGESTED READING

Bjorntorp P. Regional patterns of fat distribution. Ann Int Med 1985; 103(6 pt 2):994-995.

Lukaski HC, Johnson PE, Bolonchuk WW, Lykken GI. Assessment of fat-free mass using bioelectrical impedance measurements of the human body. Am J Clin Nutr 1985; 41:810-817.

National Research Council Food and Nutrition Board. Recommended dietary allowances. 9th ed. Washington DC: National Academy of Sciences, 1980.

Van Itallie TB, Yang M-U. Cardiac dysfunction in obese dieters: a potentially lethal complication of rapid, massive weight loss. Am J Clin Nutr 1984; 39:695-702.

Van Loan M, Mayclin P. A new TOBEC instrument and procedure for the assessment of body composition: use of Fourier coefficients to predict lean body mass and total body water. Am J Clin Nutr 1987; 45:131-137.

Webster JD, Hesp R, Garrow JS. Composition of excess weight in obese women estimated by body density, total body water, and total body potassium. Hum Nutr: Clin Nutr 1984; 38C:299-306.

COMMON HYPERLIPOPROTEINEMIAS

GEORGE STEINER, B.A., M.D., F.R.C.P.(C)
KATHRYN M. CAMELON, B.A.Sc., R.P.Dt.

AIMS OF THERAPY

This chapter will focus on the common and clinically important forms of hyperlipoproteinemia. The importance of these hyperlipoproteinemias arises from their association with accelerated arteriosclerotic disease. The major aim of treatment is not merely to correct a plasma lipid abnormality, but more importantly, to prevent or slow the development of atherosclerosis. In this context, the chapter will not discuss rarer forms of hyperlipidemia such as hyperchylomicronemia, in which the major reason for treatment is to prevent attacks of abdominal pain. Because the ultimate aim of treatment is to prevent atherosclerosis, it must be recognized that one cannot treat hyperlipidemia in isolation from other atherogenic factors. Thus, an overall approach to the prevention of atherosclerosis must include assessment for and treatment of other atherogenic factors, such as smoking, hypertension, obesity, and diabetes. Hyperlipidemia may, on occasion, be secondary to an underlying disorder such as hypothyroidism, nephrotic syndrome, or diabetes. In any such situation, the treatment must be directed at the underlying disorder. More commonly, hyperlipidemia is not associated with such underlying disorders and may arise from a monogenic or polygenic background. Clearly, these are life-long abnormalities, and therefore treatment should be started at the earliest possible time and continued throughout the individual's life.

HYPERLIPOPROTEINEMIAS

The group of disorders known as hyperlipoproteinemias comprises many different disorders, each characterized by an abnormal accumulation of a different lipoprotein. Because of the differences in the compositions of the different lipoproteins, these disorders are manifested as elevations of plasma cholesterol or plasma triglyceride or both. The following are the circulating lipoproteins and their essential functions:

1. *Chylomicron*. These are very large, extremely low density, triglyceride-rich lipoproteins that transport fat absorbed from the intestine.
2. *Very Low-Density Lipoprotein (VLDL)*. These are large, very low-density, triglyceride-rich lipoproteins that transport triglyceride made in the liver from nondietary precursors.
3. *Intermediate-Density Lipoprotein (IDL)*. These are slightly more dense lipoproteins than the very low-density lipoproteins. They are derived from the very low-density lipoprotein and are somewhat poorer in triglyceride and richer in cholesterol than their precursor, the very low-density lipoprotein. They lie intermediate in the pathway of conversion of very low-density lipoprotein to low-density lipoprotein.
4. *Low-Density Lipoprotein (LDL)*. These lipoproteins have a low density but are heavier than any of the preceding ones. Their major lipid is cholesterol. Low-density lipoprotein is the catabolic product of intermediate-density lipoprotein, which in turn is the product of very low-density lipoprotein catabolism.
5. *High-Density Lipoprotein (HDL)*. These lipoproteins constitute a metabolically distinct family that are the highest in density and poorest in lipid. Much of their lipid is phospholipid; a great deal of the remainder is cholesterol.

Elevations of low-density lipoprotein are manifested primarily as hypercholesterolemia and are associated with an accelerated risk of coronary arteriosclerosis. Occasionally, hypercholesterolemia may also result from an elevation of high-density lipoprotein. Because high-density lipoproteins appear to confer protection from coronary artery disease, clearly this less frequent form of hypercholesterolemia is indicative of benefit rather than risk. Hence, it is important to consider the lipoprotein that has accumulated and not just the lipid (triglyceride or cholesterol) that is elevated. An increase in very low-density lipoprotein is manifested primarily as hypertriglyceridemia. An association between this and coronary artery disease has been suggested but has not been clearly demonstrated. An elevation of intermediate-density lipoprotein is frequently accompanied by both hypercholesterolemia and hypertriglyceridemia. This reflects the nature of the particle, which although poorer in triglyceride than very low-density lipoprotein still contains moderate amounts of triglyceride and cholesterol. There is increasing evidence to implicate elevated concentrations of intermediate-density lipoprotein in early arteriosclerotic disease. The reader is referred to standard textbooks of endocrinology and metabolism for more details about the clinical and metabolic abnormalities associated with hyperlipoproteinemias.

EVIDENCE RELATING LIPID-LOWERING TO THE REDUCTION OF CORONARY RISK

A number of studies have demonstrated an increased incidence of coronary arteriosclerosis, in association with hypercholesterolemia. Furthermore, experimental induction of hypercholesterolemia in animals has produced arterial lesions resembling human atherosclerosis. Although these studies clearly suggested a role for hypercholesterolemia in atherogenesis, they did not provide any information with respect to the effectiveness of cholesterol reduction on the prevention of atherosclerosis.

The recent completion of the Lipid Research Clinic-Coronary Primary Prevention Trial has provided evidence that the reduction of plasma (low-density lipoprotein) cholesterol will reduce the risk of coronary artery disease. There has been some debate about the ability to extrapolate from the specific study population examined in the Coronary Primary Prevention Trial to the general population. However, both on the basis of that study's data and the data from other pathophysiologic and epidemiologic studies, it is reasonable to conclude that the benefits of cholesterol reduction will be seen in the general population.

There is more controversy with respect to HDL and the triglyceride-rich lipoproteins (VLDL and IDL). As noted above, increased levels of HDL appear to be associated with protection from arteriosclerosis. It is possible that the relationship between LDL and HDL is even more important than the absolute level of either one. In spite of this, to date no evidence has been produced to indicate that increasing the level of HDL in an individual who has previously had a low level of HDL will reduce the risk of coronary artery disease. With respect to hypertriglyceridemia, there is also general agreement that it is associated with early atherosclerosis. However, there is debate as to whether this effect is independent of alterations in other plasma lipoproteins. To date, no studies have definitively demonstrated that reducing elevated plasma triglycerides will reduce the risk of coronary artery disease. Despite this, in the case of either reduced HDL or elevated triglyceride-rich lipoprotein levels, such evidence as exists does make it reasonable to give advice aimed at normalizing them as long as the treatment method does not bear an inordinate risk.

AIMS IN LIPID REDUCTION

In deciding on the aims in reducing plasma lipids, one should differentiate between the general population and the high-risk population. It should be recognized that the risk of atherosclerosis increases as the concentration of cholesterol increases, and that there is no threshold level for this association. Hence, it is reasonable to advise the general population that its risk of atherosclerosis would be decreased by reduction of cholesterol regardless of the level from which the cholesterol is reduced. Obviously, such advice cannot be given in a physician's office but must be effected through public health measures. In the physician's office, the treatment of hyperlipidemia is more appropriately restricted to those who are at highest risk. For practical purposes, this means that one should aim to treat the top 5 percent of the population by intensive physician/dietitian intervention. In the next 20 percent (i.e., those between the 75th and 95th percentile), one should aim to institute such general public health measures as would reduce the cholesterol levels.

The reader may notice that this chapter refers to the percentile of the population into which an individual falls. This is because there is no distinct separation between normal and abnormal for the plasma lipids as there would be for a patient with a genetic disorder such as phenylketonuria. Hence, in considering plasma lipid levels, one must have a knowledge of the lipid concentrations in the general population. These differ according to age and sex and each individual must be considered in relation to those of the same sex and age. Tables giving such population values may be found in the Lipid Research Clinics Population Studies Data Book and as a resumé in a special report of the American Heart Association. In general, it is reasonable to suggest that individuals who have an LDL cholesterol exceeding 200 mg per deciliter or those who have an LDL cholesterol lower than this but have an LDL cholesterol/HDL cholesterol ratio exceeding 5 should be treated with the aim of reducing the LDL cholesterol to below 150 mg per deciliter and reducing the LDL cholesterol/HDL cholesterol ratio to a value less than 3. With respect to plasma triglyceride, the aims of therapy are less clearly defined. There is general agreement that those with a plasma triglyceride over 10 g per liter have an increased likelihood of developing acute attacks of abdominal pain and should be treated in order to avoid them. There is also general agreement that those who have plasma triglycerides exceeding 500 mg per deciliter might benefit from triglyceride reduction, at least by dietary means, in an attempt to reduce coronary disease risk. There is less agreement about the necessity for treatment in individuals whose triglyceride concentrations lie between 250 and 500 mg per deciliter. It is not within the scope of this chapter to discuss the various arguments relating to the treatment of plasma triglyceride concentrations within this range.

TREATMENT STRATEGIES

As noted above, there are two approaches to the treatment of hyperlipidemia. One is the reduction of plasma lipids in the general population and the other is the reduction of plasma lipids in specific high-risk individuals. As far as the general population is concerned, as noted earlier, the approach advocated here is the use of public health measures to alter the behavior and diet patterns of the population. The high-risk population requires more specific physician/dietitian intervention. Such high-risk individuals are those who have markedly elevated plasma lipoproteins, who have family histories of early heart disease, who have had premature vascular disease themselves, or who have other risk factors, such as diabetes hypertension, obesity, or smoking.

A general and common strategy may be applied to any patient with hyperlipidemia. The first step is to determine whether the hyperlipidemia is secondary to another disorder such as obesity, diabetes, or hypothyroidism. If it is, then the initial treatment should be directed at this underlying disorder. If this does not correct the problem or if the hyperlipidemia is not attributable to an underlying disorder, then it should be treated by appropriate dietary alterations. If diet alone is not sufficient to normalize the hyperlipoproteinemia, then an ancillary drug may be used. It must be recognized that drug treatment is an addition to, rather than a substitution for, dietary treatment programs.

GENERAL THERAPEUTIC APPROACHES

In approaching the dietary treatment of hyperlipidemia, the first step is to restrict the energy content of the diet to that which will return an individual to his ideal body weight and maintain that weight. In addition, the dietary content of fat and cholesterol should be controlled. Fat intake can be controlled with respect to quantity and the proportion of polyunsaturated to saturated fats. In addition, certain individuals with hypertriglyceridemia may need to regulate the type of carbohydrates and the amount of alcohol they consume. The basic procedure involved in managing a patient by dietary methods is to start him on a given diet after at least two baseline plasma lipoprotein evaluations. After a period of 2 to 3 months, the effectiveness of the particular diet is assessed both clinically and by laboratory tests. Should the desired result not have been attained, the individual is then placed on the next stage of dietary treatment and once again reevaluated in 2 to 3 months.

Drug treatment should be reserved for those individuals who have had full dietary treatment and have not yet reached the target lipoprotein value. Drugs that are particularly useful in reducing cholesterol include the bile acid binding resins (cholestyramine, or colestipol) and/or nicotinic acid. A new class of drugs that inhibits hydroxymethylglutaryl coenzyme A reductase, the rate-limiting enzyme of cholesterol synthesis, are currently undergoing clinical trial and have the potential for being extremely useful agents. The most useful drugs in reducing plasma triglyceride are derivatives of fibric acid; the two currently available in Canada are gemfibrozil and clofibrate.

SPECIFIC DIETARY APPROACHES

Dietary recommendations for the general population are directed toward an overall reduction in plasma lipid levels. Energy consumption to attain and maintain ideal body weight throughout the adult years is a primary dietary goal. This can be achieved by the individual's commitment to weight control facilitated by a knowledge of food composition, food preparation, and meal and snack planning techniques. A reduction in average fat and cholesterol intake is desirable and compatible with weight control for most North Americans. Health education in schools and community information programs should provide, guidance about the macronutrients in foods, the constituents of a balanced diet, and how such a diet can be obtained from the local food supply. Dietary changes generally required are an increase in consumption of fruit, vegetables, grain, and cereal products and a decrease in consumption of alcohol, animal protein, high-fat dairy foods and baked goods, and concentrated sweets. Food manufacturers and the food service industry are encouraged to provide appealing low-fat, nutrient-dense, low-energy foods that consumers can find and identify in all eating situations. As there is a steadily increasing proportion of meals and snacks eaten away from home, and as more fully prepared foods are being purchased by consumers, the food industry can have a major impact on public health by consistently providing nutritious low-fat food choices.

Persons who are identified as being at high risk (i.e., have markedly elevated plasma lipids) require a sequential program of management aimed at normalizing plasma lipids. There are four steps to any such approach. The first step is an evaluation of the patient's usual diet and eating habits. The patient should be encouraged to maintain his typical and favored meals and snacks during the assessment period. Recent changes in food consumption or body weight should be noted. Some methods of assessment are self-completed food records, food frequency and habit questionnaires, and the diet history. Any method of assessment needs to allow the patient to discuss with the dietitian his feelings and concerns about changing the food eaten, family influences, and personal dietary goals. This provides information from which an individualized dietary prescription can be designed by the dietitian.

The second step is planning the dietary recommendations for each patient. The dietitian aims to produce a change in the patient's consumption of those foods and nutrients that alter plasma lipids, while keeping the overall diet balanced. First, energy intake is adjusted to achieve ideal body weight. Since many North Americans are overweight and even a small reduction (2 to 5 kg) in body weight will contribute to a decrease in plasma lipids, lowering energy intake is usual. Secondly, and in support of weight loss, the total fat content of the diet is reduced from the usual 35 to 40 percent of total energy to 20 to 30 percent. Meanwhile, the proportion of energy from carbohydrate increases by 5 to 10 percent and the protein contribution remains constant at about 15 percent.

Most of the reduction in dietary fat is in the form of saturated fat. Some of the saturated fat is replaced by polyunsaturated fat to achieve a polyunsaturated/saturated (P/S) ratio of 1/1. Dietary cholesterol is restricted to an average of 100 to 300 mg per day. These dietary alterations are described in the American Heart Association's three phase diet scheme, summarized in the table below:

TABLE 1   Composition of the American Heart Association Phase Diet for the Treatment of Hyperlipidemia

| | *Percent of Energy From* | | | | *Cholesterol (mg/day)* |
	Fat	*Carbohydrate*	*Protein*	*P/S*	
Phase I	30	55	15	1/1	<300
Phase II	25	60	15	1/1	200–250
Phase III	20	65	15	1/1	100–150

Adapted from the American Heart Association. Counseling the patient with hyperlipidemia, 1984. With permission.

This diet is a model for the progressive decrease in the amounts of total fat, saturated fat and cholesterol and is an extension of the advice to the general public. The exact characteristics of each individual's diet are determined by the nature and severity of the lipid disorder, composition of the baseline diet, and willingness to make changes in food habits.

Persons with hypercholesterolemia most often are advised to eat a diet modeled after the Phase II criteria. This generally represents sufficient change from the baseline meal pattern to produce a decrease in plasma cholesterol, yet it is reasonable for a patient to follow. While some people initially prefer a moderate diet (Phase I) that is then made more restrictive if necessary, we have been more successful in advising a stricter diet (Phase II) at the beginning of the treatment period when patient motivation to change eating habits is highest. Later, diet control can easily be "loosened" if warranted. A Phase III diet is instituted when the plasma cholesterol response on a less strict diet is less than desired *and* the patient is willing to consider further altering his diet to this semivegetarian regimen. As the diet becomes increasingly restrictive, greater care in planning and food preparation is required to ensure that the dietary goals are met. The availability of time for these activities may be a limiting factor in dietary compliance.

Persons with hypertriglyceridemia are treated with a diet having a slightly different orientation. If the patient is overweight, reduction to ideal body weight is imperative and often sufficient to normalize triglycerides. A weight reducing diet, particularly restricted in simple sugars and alcohol and designed after the Phase I model for fat alterations, is recommended. If the patient's body weight is appropriate for height, the sugar and alcohol restrictions assume greater importance. The extent of alcohol and sugar restrictions depends on the severity of the hypertriglyceridemia and the amount in the patient's typical diet. Advice about the amount of alcohol permitted often requires negotiation with the patient to establish a practical, yet significant, reduction in consumption.

After the dietitian has designed the diet, taking into account the baseline lipid and food pattern information, the third step is to instruct the patient and the household members involved with food handling in the principles of the diet. Since most people think of a diet in terms of specific foods rather than generalized dietary goals, adequate time must be allotted for a thorough discussion of all food products and preparation techniques. Follow-up counseling to the initial diet teaching is necessary to make required adjustments in the original diet prescription, to answer patient enquiries about new foods and eating situations encountered, and to assess and encourage dietary adherence. Learning to control weight and to eat a diet different from their customary one is a skill that patients acquire through practice, feedback from the dietitian and physician is needed to achieve best results. Two to three sessions to follow up initial teaching are usually sufficient to establish a person comfortably on a new diet. Where weight reduction is involved, regular contact is recommended until the weight goal is achieved.

Step four in the dietary approach to lipid reduction is an assessment of the effectiveness of the dietary treatment as indicated by the degree of plasma lipid change, and a decision by the physician about whether additional treatment is necessary. Because the management of hyperlipidemia is a lifelong challenge, and diet is always part of, if not the primary, treatment strategy, reviews of the patient's eating habits are warranted every 2 to 3 years in order to optimize dietary control.

There will always be a small number of patients who refuse to follow any special diet. For such persons a discussion of their self-imposed limitations on the number of treatment strategies is justified before moving on to drug therapy. These people may benefit from general population shifts in eating habits over a long period and dietary changes should always be open to them as an option.

SUGGESTED READING

American Heart Association Special Report. Recommendations for treatment of hyperlipidemia in adults. Circulation 1984; 69:1067A–1090A.

The Lipid Research Clinics Population Studies Data Book, Vol. 1. The prevalence study, lipid metabolism branch, division of heart and vascular diseases. National Heart, Lung and Blood Institute. National Institutes of Health. NIH Publication No. 80–1527. U.S. Government Printing Office, 1980.

Stanbury JB, Wyngaarden JB, Fredrickson DS. The metabolic basis of inherited disorders. New York: McGraw-Hill, 1978.

METABOLIC BONE DISEASE

JOAN E. HARRISON, M.D., F.R.C.P.(C)

Proper nutrition is essential for the growth and preservation of the skeleton, as for all other body tissues. This chapter examines the nutrients required for optimum bone health and under the special circumstances of bone disease.

THE STRUCTURE AND FUNCTION OF BONE

Bone is a living organ consisting of cells, organic matrix, and calcium phosphate deposited as apatite crystals. The organic matrix consists largely of collagen fibers that govern the shape of the bone. Apatite crystals provide rigidity. There are three types of cells concerned with (1) synthesis of new bone, (2) resorption of bone, and (3) the supply of nutrients to mature bone tissue. Throughout childhood, bone undergoes extensive modeling and remodeling as the skeleton increases in size. Throughout adult life, bone remodeling continues at a slower rate. This adult remodeling process maintains healthy bone by replacing old bone with new bone, and in addition, alters the mass and shape of bone in response to body requirements.

The skeleton has two quite different functions: to provide support for the body and to provide a reservoir for the storage of bone minerals. Bone mass and strength are controlled by the forces applied to bone through physical activity, increasing with strenuous physical activity and decreasing with relative inactivity. The bone minerals, calcium and phosphate, not only provide skeletal rigidity for support functions but also are essential for many vital body functions. In order to preserve these functions, bone will be resorbed, as required, to maintain normal soft tissue levels of calcium, at the expense of the support functions of bone. Bone mineral also can provide buffering for body fluids against excess acidity. The removal of bone mineral is always associated with resorption of total bone tissue (mineral and matrix).

METABOLIC BONE DISEASE

There are four basic types of metabolic bone disease. Listed in order of prevalence: (1) osteoporosis is defined as low bone mass with remaining bone of normal composition, (2) osteomalacia (or rickets in children), as defective bone mineralization, (3) osteitis fibrosa, as excessive bone remodeling associated with abnormally high levels of parathyroid hormone, and (4) osteosclerosis, as extensive bone overgrowth. Each of these types of bone disease has different causes and correspondingly, different therapeutic considerations. In individuals, multiple factors may contribute to the bone disease and in some situations, a mixed type of bone pathology may occur. In these complex situations, optimal nutritional and other therapeutic measures are difficult to establish.

THE IMPORTANCE OF NUTRITION

Malnutrition may cause or contribute to bone disease. With its satisfactory treatment, as with other underlying causes, the bone heals and no further dietary measures may be required. In general, nutritional therapy is directed toward preserving optimal bone health with modifications as required in various disease situations.

OSTEOPOROSIS

Osteoporosis is a problem of low bone mass and bone strength so that fractures occur with little or no abnormal force. The upper back hump, due to spinal fractures, and the geriatric hip fracture often seen in elderly women are typical of this disease.

Primary Osteoporosis

There are many known causes of osteoporosis, but, for most patients, no underlying cause can be identified. This primary osteoporosis can occur in men and women of all ages, including children, but is most common in older women. One in three women over 65 have vertebral fractures, and extreme old age (over 85 years), one in three will have hip fractures.

This primary osteoporosis may well be multifactorial. Risk factors include loss of estrogen at menopause, reduced physical activity with aging, and possibly, genetic or racial factors. Osteoporosis is more common in whites than in blacks or orientals and is particularly prevalent in short, thin, fair women. Suboptimal nutrition is an additional risk factor. Conventional treatment for primary osteoporosis is supplemental calcium (1 g per day). In post menopausal women, estrogen may be prescribed. Appropriate exercise programs and attention to diet are of additional benefit.

Secondary Osteoporosis

This type of osteoporosis is associated with dietary deficiencies or malabsorption of essential nutrients. Some hormonal abnormalities, including over activity of the thyroid or adrenal glands and loss of sex hormones (hypogonadism) are known causes of osteoporosis. With inactivity, due to paralysis or to prolonged immobilization, profound bone loss occurs. Renal disease, some cancers (e.g., multiple myeloma), and prolonged medication with steroids or anticonvulsant drugs may cause osteoporosis. The coexistence of the various risk factors for primary osteoporosis will further contribute to bone loss in secondary osteoporosis.

Medical treatment for secondary osteoporosis is directed to correction of the underlying disease or to any additional risk factors. In most cases, however, the underlying disease cannot be treated successfully and treatment for primary osteoporosis is prescribed.

Nutritional Factors

General Considerations. To establish an optimal diet for bone growth, consideration must be given to the optimal dietary levels of the bone minerals, bone mineral vitamins, total calories, protein, drug foods (caffeine, nicotine, and alcohol), and some trace elements. The requirements for these nutrients may vary, depending on other components of the diet, on other risk factors for primary or secondary osteoporosis, and on other underlying disease.

For prevention of osteoporosis, these nutritional considerations are most important for those at risk of osteoporosis, i.e., white women, particularly small, thin, fair subjects or women with a strong family history of osteoporosis. For males and for women of nonwhite racial groups, nutrition appears to be less important. It should be stressed that, for subjects at risk, attention to nutrition should be a life-long commitment.

Although osteoporotic fractures occur in the elderly, the bone disease may be a problem of childhood or young adult life. Suboptimal bone mass at maturity or accelerated bone loss in premenopausal years will increase the risk of fractures after menopause, when further bone loss is known to occur.

In addition to those most at risk for primary osteoporosis, subjects with risk factors for secondary osteoporosis will require special nutritional considerations.

Calcium. In adults, the recommended level of dietary calcium is 700 mg per day. The recommended levels are increased to 1,000 mg per day with the increased demands of childhood growth, pregnancy, and lactation. Normal intestinal calcium absorption is incomplete. Fractional calcium absorption varies from 10 to 70 percent or above depending on intake and body requirements. Without the greater mineral requirements associated with pregnancy and lactation and with normal bowel function, calcium intake of 700 mg per day should be sufficient to offset normal daily losses in urine and bowel secretions of some 300 mg per day. The average North American diet in adults, however, does not provide this level of calcium, with amounts decreasing from 600 to 500 mg per day between young adulthood and old age. Every effort should be made to increase use of dairy products so that at least the recommended calcium levels are met.

Recently, arguments have been made for increasing dietary calcium to 1,000 mg per day and to 1,500 mg per day in pre- and postmenopausal women, respectively, but the value of these higher levels remains controversial. Nevertheless, they may well be helpful, at least for some individuals, and are not likely to be harmful. Additional dietary calcium would be helpful for patients with some inhibition of calcium absorption, associated, for example, with bowel disease or with such medications as antacids, steroids, and some antibiotics. Furthermore, the optimal level of dietary calcium may depend on other constituents of the diet. High levels of dietary fiber and phosphate inhibit calcium absorption, while protein excess appears to increase renal calcium losses. Additional calcium may be beneficial to offset the deleterious effects of these other nutrients. In some cases, however, high calcium intake can be harmful. With abnormally high urine calcium excretion (hypercalciuria) additional calcium intake would be contraindicated.

All sources of readily absorbed calcium, * given in equal amounts,

---

* Calcium in some vegetables may not be absorbed.

are considered of equal value, but intuitively, calcium-containing foods would seem preferable to pharmaceutical preparations. Of interest, calcium ingested in milk has been shown to cause less suppression of bone remodeling than the various calcium tablet preparations, but the significance of this finding is unclear. Use of calcium tablets may be more attractive than use of dairy foods but easy access to these non-prescription products may lead the nutritional enthusiasts to ingest such extraordinarily high levels of calcium that the deleterious effects of calcium overdoses (primarily soft tissue calcification) occur. Limitation of calcium intake to food products is unlikely to cause such calcium abuse. Nevertheless, with intolerance to dairy products (e.g., intestinal allergy, cultural practice, or taste preferences) calcium tablets should be considered.

Phosphate. Phosphate levels in North American diets are more than adequate for body requirements. Even with intestinal malabsorption, phosphate deficiency is rare. In the past, excess dietary phosphate was considered deleterious to bone health due to inhibition of calcium absorption and stimulation of secondary hyperparathyroidism. Animal data have supported this theoretic consideration but it has not been confirmed in clinical studies. At the present time, phosphate is considered more than adequate for body requirements and excessive intake is not considered deleterious.

Protein. Adequate dietary protein is essential for bone health. In the average North American diet protein is more than sufficient for body requirements, but such protein excess may be deleterious to bone. High protein intake appears to increase renal calcium absorption, and net losses of bone mineral have been observed. Sufficient calcium intake should offset the increased calcium losses associated with excessive protein intake, but some moderation in protein intake may be desirable, particularly for high-risk patients.

Total Calories. Osteoporosis is more common in underweight than in overweight individuals. Many factors may contribute to the development of osteoporosis in the underweight individual, including some nutrient deficiencies, loss of sex hormone activity (amenorrhea), and lack of energy and associated inactivity. Conversely, obesity appears to be protective, possibly due to additional stress put on the skeleton. Despite the common desire of young women for extreme thinness, made popular by the fashion and entertainment industries, adequate calories appear to be essential for bone health.

Vitamins. Vitamins A and C are essential for bone synthesis. Vitamin D deficiency causes osteomalacia, but suboptimal vitamin D may contribute to osteoporosis by inhibiting intestinal calcium absorption without the defective bone mineralization of complete deficiency. Adequate intake of these vitamins is essential, but there is no known additional benefit to excessive intake, and megadoses of vitamin D are deleterious to bone. Vitamin D requirements are discussed further in the section on osteomalacia.

Magnesium, Fluoride, and Essential Trace Elements. Adequate levels of magnesium, copper, manganese, zinc, and silicon are essential for normal bone metabolism. In the absence of fad diets or intestinal malabsorption such deficiencies do not occur and additional supplementation of these elements has no known value.

Fluoride is not considered an essential element, but, in trace amounts, may be beneficial for the preservation of bone mass. The incidence of osteoporosis has been reported to be higher in populations using water supplies with low fluoride content (less than 0.1 ppm) compared to populations using water with high fluoride levels (greater than 4.0 ppm). Furthermore, research treatment of osteoporotic patients with considerably higher fluoride levels (greater than 20 mg per day) has caused substantial increases in bone mass and appears to reduce the incidence of fractures. With the addition of fluoride to water supplies, at 1 ppm, the incidence of dental caries has been greatly reduced, but reductions in the incidence of osteoporosis have not been observed. Possibly, the low level of fluoride supplementation (1 ppm) is insufficient for any beneficial effects, but the follow-up period since fluoride supplementation may be insufficient to demonstrate beneficial effects. The possibility remains, however, that life-long intake of fluoride may well prove to have a protective effect against osteoporosis in later life.

Drug Foods. The popular drugs caffeine, nicotine, and alcohol have all been associated with osteoporosis. It is possible that use of these drugs may not be a cause or contributing factor in the development of osteoporosis but may instead reflect some other risk factor associated with drug use (e.g., a sedentary lifestyle or suboptimal intake of other nutrients). Nevertheless, moderation in the use of these drug foods is recommended.

Acidity. Bone may be resorbed to provide additional buffering against increased acidity in body fluids. Thus, excessive use of acidic foods may be undesirable.

Nutritional Considerations for Secondary Osteoporosis. Malnutrition will cause osteoporosis. In this situation, treatment is directed toward restoration of specific nutrient deficiencies, which may include calorie and protein starvation and deficiencies of calcium, vitamins, and the essential trace elements. These deficiencies occur with starvation, with intestinal malabsorption, and with some fad diets, particularly those designed for rapid weight reduction. The osteoporosis should heal with correction of the malnutrition unless other risk factors persist. With alcoholic liver disease, for example, osteoporosis may occur as a result of inadequate nutrition or malabsorption associated with the liver disease, but even with adequate nutrient intake, continued alcohol use, progressive liver disease, and relative inactivity may preclude satisfactory bone healing.

Hypercalcemia and hypercalciuria occur with rapid osteoporotic bone loss. This abnormal calcium metabolism is associated with disuse osteoporosis, particularly in the initial months following paralysis. It also occurs with osteoporosis related to cancer. In these situations, dietary calcium should be reduced (not increased) in order to minimize risk of urinary stone formation and soft tissue calcification.

OSTEOMALACIA AND RICKETS

Deficient Vitamin D Activity

Deficiency of vitamin D is known to cause osteomalacia, or rickets in children, and normally can be prevented or cured by proper diet. Vitamin D is synthesized in the skin by the action of sunlight, but in cases where sunlight exposure is inadequate (e.g., during the winter of the far northern and far southern parts of the world), dietary vitamin D must be provided to compensate for the deficiency.

Because the need for vitamin D is well established, it is perhaps surprising that vitamin D–deficient bone disease still occurs. In North America osteomalacia and rickets are largely prevented by the addition of vitamin D_2 to dairy products and margarine. The recommended daily intake for children is 10 μg per day. This level is also recommended for adults with additional bone mineral requirements (e.g., pregnancy and lactation). Throughout most of adult life, when the bone mass maintains a near steady state, it is believed that lower levels of vitamin D are sufficient, but vitamin D–deficient osteomalacia continues to occur in the adult population. Institutionalized subjects are particularly at risk since sunlight exposure is minimal and these elderly subjects or chronic invalids tend to avoid vitamin D–fortified foods. Similarly, the cultural patterns of some ethnic groups limit both skin and dietary sources of vitamin D. Patients with intestinal malabsorption of fats and fat-soluble vitamins, due to bowel or liver disease, are also at risk.

Osteomalacia and rickets can occur, in spite of normal body stores of vitamin D, as a result of abnormal vitamin D metabolism. Vitamin D at the physiologic level is not biologically active but undergoes metabolism to produce the active substance 1,25-dihydroxy vitamin D. A hereditary form of abnormal vitamin D metabolism (hereditary vitamin D–dependent rickets) can be satisfactorily cured by administration of the active form of vitamin D or with massive doses of vitamin D. (The pharmacologic doses are greater than 1,000 μg per day.) Abnormal vitamin D metabolism also occurs with prolonged use of anticonvulsant drugs but, in these cases, only modest increases in vitamin D are required.

Osteomalacia Unrelated to Deficient Vitamin D Activity

Vitamin D refractory rickets (or familial hypophosphatemia) is a hereditary disorder causing severe bone abnormalities associated with low blood levels of phosphate. The pathogenesis of this disorder is not understood. Treatment with phosphate supplements (4 g per day) together with small doses of the active form of vitamin D is of some benefit but does not cure the bone disease.

Osteomalacia also occurs with fluoride toxicity (or fluorosis) and with cadmium toxicity. The osteomalacia will heal when exposure to these toxins is eliminated. Curiously, mega doses of vitamin D will cause osteomalacia, together with abnormally high blood levels of calcium and phosphate and soft tissue deposits of calcium phosphate. Vitamine D toxicity usually occurs as a complication of medical treatment for diseases requiring pharmacologic doses of vitamin D, but it also can occur with use of mega doses of vitamin D as part of fad diets.

OSTEITIS FIBROSA

The rapid bone remodeling of osteitis fibrosa is caused by excessive parathyroid hormone activity (hyperparathyroidism).

Primary Hyperparathyroidism

This disease is caused by a tumor of the parathyroid gland and heals readily following surgical removal. Calcium supplements are commonly prescribed post-operatively in order to prevent or minimize a fall in blood calcium levels and to facilitate bone healing. In some post-operative cases a serious fall in blood calcium occurs, necessitating treatment with pharmacologic doses of vitamin D or, now more often, with the active vitamin D metabolite ($1,25(OH)_2D$). This hypocalcemia is usually transient (a few weeks) and is caused by a delay in hormone secretion from the remaining parathyroid tissue.

Secondary Hyperparathyroidism

Parathyroid activity will increase in response to any situation in which calcium intake is insufficient to meet body requirements. For example, with insufficient dietary calcium combined with the increased requirements of pregnancy and lactation, parathyroid activity will increase to preserve normal soft tissue levels of calcium by bone mineral resorption. In most cases, such secondary hyperparathyroidism can be corrected by additional calcium intake, by use of either dairy products or calcium tablets. The importance of dietary calcium was discussed further in the previous section.

OSTEOSCLEROSIS

Osteopetrosis is a genetic defect of osteosclerosis, due to defective bone resorption. There is no satisfactory medical or nutritional treatment.

Other osteosclerotic conditions are associated with such osteomalacic conditions as familial hypophosphatemic rickets, fluorosis, and vitamin D toxicity. Treatment for these conditions was discussed in the section on osteomalacia.

MIXED BONE PATHOLOGY

Renal Osteodystrophy

Osteosclerosis, osteomalacia, and also osteitis fibrosa may occur in varying degrees with this bone disease of end-stage renal failure. Renal osteodystrophy has a multifactorial etiology. Loss of renal function causes phosphate retention and secondary hyperparathyroidism. In addition, the synthesis of the active form of vitamin D may be defective. Excessive retention of aluminum and fluoride may cause further complications.

Treatment for these various problems is not entirely satisfactory. Protein and phosphate restriction and calcium supplementation are commonly prescribed. Administration of vitamin D (or the active metabolite) may be beneficial. The antacid aluminum hydroxide is widely used to further inhibit phosphate absorption but may result in aluminum toxicity. Fluoride-free water is used for dialysis, but the dietary intake of fluoride in drinking water and in some foods (e.g., tea) may cause extensive fluoride retention and fluorosis.

Total Parenteral Nutrition

Osteomalacia has been observed with prolonged total parenteral nutrition and has been attributed either to aluminum toxicity or to hypersensitivity to physiologic levels of vitamin D. Aluminum contamination occurs with use of casein hydrolysates and can be eliminated by use of synthetic amino acids as the only source of protein. Reduction in vitamin D intake and prevention of aluminum toxicity will cure the osteomalacia, but osteoporotic fractures continue to be a significant problem. The cause of this osteopenia remains obscure.

In conclusion, when possible, treatment of metabolic bone disease is directed to elimination of the underlying cause or causes of the disease. In some cases malnutrition is the primary cause and appropriate correction of nutrient deficiencies will cure the bone disease.

In situations where the cause of the bone disease is unknown or treatment for known etiology is unsatisfactory, optimal nutrition is desirable.Nutritional considerations for optimal bone health will vary, depending on the cause or contributing factors of the disease. In general, attention should be given to (1) sufficient dietary calcium to meet or exceed Canadian guidelines (although excess calcium intake can be deleterious), (2) sufficient calories to maintain or exceed ideal body weight, (3) moderation in protein intake, and (4) adequate intake of other minerals and vitamins. The usually high levels of dietary phosphate are not considered deleterious. There is no known advantage to excessive intake of magnesium, trace elements, or essential vitamins, and mega doses of vitamin D are deleterious to bone health. In specific disease situations, modification of these general recommendations is required.

Nutrition undoubtedly plays an important role in the prevention and treatment of bone disease, but our knowledge in this area is far from satisfactory. Extensive research is required to establish, definitively, the optimal levels of various nutrients in relation to interacting effects of other dietary components, of underlying diseases, and of medications. With further understanding, current guidelines will likely be revised.

SUGGESTED READING

Frame B, Potts JT, eds. Clinical disorders of bone and mineral metabolism. Excerpta Medica, International Congress Series 617, 1983.

Harrison JE, McNeill KG. The skeletal system. In: Kinney KN, Jeejeebhoy GL, Owen QE, eds. Nutrition and metabolism in patient care. Philadelphia: WB Saunders, in press.

Heaney RP, Gallagher JC, Johnston CC, et al. Calcium nutrition and bone health in the elderly. Am J Clin Nutr 1982; 36:986–1013.

Nordin BEC, ed. Metabolic bone and stone disease. New York: Churchill Livingstone, 1984.

Parfitt AM. Dietary risk factors for age-related bone loss and fractures. Lancet 1983; 36:1181–1185.

NUTRITION AND CANCER

HEAD AND NECK CANCER

ABBY S. BLOCH, M.S., R.D.
MOSHE SHIKE, M.D.

Nutritional therapy is an important component in the management of patients with head and neck cancer. As in other types of cancer, malnutrition can contribute significantly to morbidity and mortality in these patients. Major nutritional problems may arise from a variety of causes including (1) diminished nutrient intake because of the effects of the tumor and its therapy on the ability to eat and swallow, (2) metabolic derangements associated with cancer, and (3) preexisting nutritional status.

The normal process of swallowing is a complex mechanism requiring a well-coordinated chain of events involving oral, pharyngeal, laryngeal, and esophageal function. Thus, cancer of the head and neck and its therapy can diminish nutrient intake for a number of reasons, including (1) obstructive and structural changes secondary to tumor or surgery, (2) disturbances in motility and sphincteric function, (3) loss of motor and sensory function, (4) persistent ulceration and fistula formation, (5) fear of aspiration, and (6) anorexia. In spite of recent advances in the rehabilitation of the swallowing process in patients with head and neck cancer, dysphagia is still common and active nutritional support is necessary.

It is now suggested that cancer-induced metabolic aberrations may contribute significantly to cancer cachexia. Such aberrations, observed in patients with a variety of tumors, include increased energy expenditure, accelerated protein turnover, and a high rate of gluconeogenesis. It has not been determined whether such metabolic abnormalities play an important role in patients with head and neck cancer and whether they contribute to malnutrition. A large proportion of patients with head and neck cancer have a long-standing history of excessive alcohol intake and heavy smoking, and thus are predisposed to the nutritional deficiencies of alcoholism.

The patient with head and neck cancer is at high risk for malnutrition and its consequences. The appropriate approach to prevention and treatment of malnutrition in these patients initially requires a thorough evaluation of the nutritional status, the causes of malnutrition, the potential for rehabilitation, and the anticipated length of disability. In addition, a general medical evaluation is necessary, particularly in relation to problems that may directly affect nutritional therapy, such as diabetes and the status of the gastrointestinal tract and renal and liver function.

MODALITIES OF NUTRITIONAL SUPPORT

Among the methods that can be utilized for nutritional therapy in patients with head and neck cancer are dietary therapy and manipulations, gastroenteral feeding through a variety of feeding tubes (nasopharyngeal, nasogastric, endoscopic gastrostomy, surgical gastrostomy), and parenteral nutrition. In most patients the gastrointestinal tract functions normally and therefore should be utilized. Only in rare cases is parenteral nutrition required, usually when a concomitant illness precludes utilization of the gastrointestinal tract for feeding.

In choosing the appropriate modality of nutritional support, an evaluation has to be made of the patient's ability to chew and swallow and to consume a normal diet, soft textured foods, or only liquids.

In patients with tumors and surgical procedures that do not grossly affect the upper alimentary passages, liquid diets can be used. Thus, following thyroidectomy, lip excision, removal of small lesions in the oral cavity (palate, gum, tongue), excision of the palate with insertion of an obturator, parotidectomy, tracheostomy, mandibular surgery, and radical neck dissection, patients can be given a liquid diet. Within days or weeks these patients are usually able to ingest a regular meal and do not require further nutritional therapy.

Patients with head and neck cancer who undergo surgery or radiation may experience insufficient salivation and thus have difficulty in swallowing. By selecting soft, moist foods, adding gravies and sauces, or preparing foods in liquids, patients can overcome the dryness during eating. Using liquids in conjunction with the solids also aids in chewing and swallowing. Foods with high water content such as gelatin, mousses, soft cooked eggs, and soups ease the problem considerably. Rinsing the mouth frequently or using artificial saliva can also alleviate the problem to some degree.

A group of patients requiring specific dietary manipulations are those who have dysphagia for liquids. For these patients, textured soft foods, purees, and thick liquids such as nectar, custards, thickened soups, thinned yogurt, and ice cream should be used. Such patients can usually control a large bolus more easily than small pieces of food, which become lost in the mouth. Foods that form a bolus in the mouth, such as moist meatloaf with gravy, or foods that do not break apart such as macaroni and cheese, are more easily handled. Some foods like cottage cheese and dry hamburger break up into small pieces and are very difficult for the patient with dysphagia to chew and swallow. The small pieces of food may stick in the throat or collect in the cheeks, causing coughing and aspiration. In extreme cases of liquid dysphagia, the patient can consume sufficient food but may require gastric or enteral administration of fluids.

In patients with excessive mucus formation or drooling, foods that tend to increase salivation should be restricted. Such foods include milk products, chocolates, citrus juices, and sweets.

If the patient is able to meet nutritional requirements with these therapeutic diets and can maintain normal nutritional status, no other intervention is required. When the patient is unable to meet nutritional needs, more aggressive nutritional support measures have to be instituted.

For patients whose diets progress from clear liquids to pureed or soft foods, reassessment of nutritional status must be ongoing to assure appropriateness of the current dietary regimen. If at any time the patient is unable to consume adequate amounts of food and begins to lose weight, dietary management must be altered.

For those patients who on initial assessment are determined to be at risk for malnutrition due to an inability to chew or swallow adequately, enteral feeding should be implemented as soon as possible to prevent deterioration of the patient's nutritional status. This is especially true when further therapy (surgery, radiotherapy, or chemotherapy) is contemplated. It is desirable that the patient be in the best possible nutritional condition to withstand these procedures.

Short-term or temporary enteral feeding may be used by patients who are extremely anorectic, are experiencing severe pain, or have limited ability to consume foods by mouth due to the effects of the disease. Enteral feeding in the immediate postoperative period is required in patients who undergo supraglottic partial laryngectomy, pharyngectomy, extensive excision of the floor of the mouth, radical tonsillectomy, extensive glossectomy, mandibular or maxillary resection, gum excision, palatectomy, extensive cheek reconstruction, or mandibulotomy.

For short-term tube feeding, a nasopharyngeal or nasogastric tube can be utilized. In patients with anomalies of the throat and neck, difficulty may arise in passing a small diameter, soft silastic or polyurethane tube even with an introducer or stylet. For these patients, a tube made of firmer material such as rubber (Rob Nel tube) may be more successful although not as well tolerated or as comfortable as the smaller diameter tubes made of softer materials.

When no gastric or intestinal disorders exist, bolus or gravity feeding of the nutrient formula through the feeding tube is well tolerated. In such cases, 300 to 400 cc of the feeding formula can be given over 15 to 20 minutes. More rapid administration of the formula should be avoided since it may result in a sensation of fullness, abdominal discomfort, vomiting, or aspiration. For patients who do not tolerate rapid feeding, a simple enteral feeding pump providing controlled, constant infusion at a tolerable rate can be helpful.

As the patient regains the ability to eat and swallow and tolerates oral intake, tube feeding can be discontinued gradually. The clinician and the dietitian should ensure that the patient is capable of taking sufficient nutrients orally before discontinuing enteral support completely. This can be done by calorie count or diet history.

After a partial or supraglottic laryngectomy, patients may be able to swallow solids but experience difficulty in swallowing liquids. The management of their problems has been discussed earlier. After partial glossectomy, patients have difficulty in passing food to the back of the throat. Special utensils such as long-handled spoons can aid in placing the food far enough back in the mouth to allow uninterrupted swallowing. After total glossectomy, a patient may tolerate liquids and thin pureed foods. A large syringe may be helpful for these patients, and special equipment is available to aid the transport of food to the back of the mouth and throat area.

Long-term or permanent tube feeding may be required in patients with glossectomy, mandibulectomy, severe mucositis from ongoing radiation therapy, and recurrent aspiration secondary to tumor or surgery.

In these patients, nutrient solutions can be administered through nasopharyngeal or nasogastric tubes or through gastrostomies placed surgically or endoscopically. Percutaneous endoscopic gastrostomy and jejunostomy facilitate enteral feeding. A feeding gastrostomy with a tube up to 18 F can be placed endoscopically in a procedure requiring only a local anesthetic and mild sedation. Such a procedure can be performed in an outpatient setting or during a day admission with minimal complications. In our experience with the first 100 endoscopically placed gastrostomies in cancer patients, the complication rate was 15 percent and all were minor. This approach is preferable to a surgically placed gastrostomy, which has a higher morbidity and cost. Because the endoscopically placed gastrostomy is better tolerated and more effective than the nasogastric or nasopharyngeal tube, it is currently the method of choice when long-term or permanent enteral feeding is required.

The method of feeding must be based on the patient's clinical condition. If the patient can tolerate bolus feedings of 300 to 400 cc, this method is preferable to a continuous drip, which is time consuming. In the hospital, the best time for enteral feeding is during the day and evening when supervision by the nursing staff is maximal. If the patient is to be fed enterally at home, night-time feeding is sometimes more convenient since it allows freedom during the day. If night-time feeding is used, an enteral feeding pump that controls the infusion is desirable.

The enteral feeding formula can be prepared at home by blenderizing regular food or a nutritionally complete ready-made commercial formula can be used. In the absence of gastric, intestinal, or pancreatic problems, polymeric nutrient solutions can be employed. In these solutions, the macronutrients are in the form of whole proteins, polysaccharides, and triglycerides, and their use requires that digestive and absorptive mechanisms be intact. They are generally iso-osmolar with reference to plasma and therefore are well tolerated. In the presence of pancreatic insufficiency or partial intestinal resection, consideration can be given to the use of monomeric enteral feeding solutions in which the protein is partially or completely predigested, the carbohydrates are in the form of monosaccharides, and the amount of fat is minimal. These solutions tend to be hyperosmolar compared with plasma.

Blenderized natural foods offer the benefit of complete nutrition providing both the known and the as yet unidentified nutrients in food. Foods also offer natural bulk and residue to stimulate gastrointestinal motility and bowel function. Since milk is usually added to the natural food formulas, lactose intolerance must be excluded before recommending them. The home-prepared formula may be adjusted to reduce or omit milk or lactose and to substitute other ingredients to provide the necessary calcium intake. Lactose-free formulas are available commercially. The diet must be balanced and complete if a blenderized home-prepared formula is used.

Currently there are over 75 commercial products for enteral feeding. With their varying nutrient sources and composition, they offer the clinician a wide choice so that the formula can be specifically chosen to fit the patient's clinical and metabolic needs. Tables comparing the products and their nutrient contents have been published and they can aid the clinician in choosing an appropriate product.

PARENTERAL NUTRITION

In most patients with head and neck cancer the gastrointestinal tract is intact and can be utilized for feeding. Such patients rarely require parenteral nutrition. When a concomitant intestinal problem precludes oral or enteral feeding, parenteral nutrition can be utilized. In such cases, parenteral feeding can be given with the usual care and precautions that have been published. There have been numerous reports regarding the utilization of parenteral nutrition in head and neck cancer patients without severe gastrointestinal problems. However, it must be emphasized that because of the higher cost and the potential for complications with parenteral nutrition, preference should always be given to enteral feeding. Even in the patient with cancer of the head and neck who is malnourished and who is facing radical surgery, a feeding tube can usually be passed so that enteral feeding can be given preoperatively.

SUGGESTED READING

Aguiler NV, Olson ML, Shedd DP. Rehabilitation of deglutition problems in patient with head and neck cancer. Am J Surg 1979; 138:501–507.

Bloch AS, Shils ME. In: Shils ME, Young V, eds. Modern nutrition in health and disease. 7th ed. Philadelphia: Lea & Febiger, 1988:Tables A40–A42.

Brennan MF. Total parenteral nutrition in the cancer patient. N Engl J Med 1982; 305:375–382.

DeWys WD, Begg C, Lavin PT, et al. Prognostic effect of weight loss prior to chemotherapy in cancer patients. Am J Med 1980; 69:491–497.

Schroy P, Ritchie M, Shike M. Home enteral nutrition via endoscopically placed percutaneous gastrostomies. Am Soc Clin Oncology Proceedings 1987:263.

METASTATIC CANCER

ANN T. FOLTZ, R.N., D.N.S.
DANIEL W. NIXON, M.D.

Many nutritional problems can accompany metastatic cancer and its treatment. Common patient complaints that can affect food intake include anorexia, hypogeusia, dysgeusia, nausea with or without vomiting, fatigue, mucositis, constipation, abdominal discomfort, and pain. Each problem area will be discussed in conjuction with approaches that are clinically effective.

ANOREXIA

Loss of appetite is a major concern among cancer patients and their families. The etiologies of cancer-related anorexia include the cancer itself, cancer treatment, and the accompanying emotional upset. The origin of anorexia should be sought on a patient-by-patient basis, since intervention depends upon the source of the problem.

Anorexia associated with metastatic disease is poorly understood; cancer-secreted products, such as cachexin and tumor metabolites, and metabolic derangements have been identified as precursors. Unfortunately, the only intervention for cancer-induced anorexia is effective cancer treatment. Indeed, patients will often note improved appetite even before objective response to therapy is achieved. For the majority of patients with advanced disease, however, this magnitude of response is not possible. For these patients, aggressive nutritional counseling can often increase oral intake to caloric levels 1.7 times the amount of needed calories estimated by the Harris-Benedict equation. Successful counseling requires the cooperation of both the patient and at least one care provider in the home. Even when effective, however, the dietary improvements have not been associated with improvement of survival or response to treatment. Moreover, studies have suggested that undernourished tumor-bearing animals live longer than well-nourished animals. Thus, the role of nutritional repletion in the cancer patient with advanced disease remains uncertain. Our preferred treatment of patients with anorexia due

351

to disease progression is to (1) reduce the emphasis placed on dietary intake by the family and (2) offer relatively easy methods to increase intake (e.g., provide a variety of commercial supplements, have snacks easily available to patient, etc). With selected patients, a small amount of sherry or alcohol-containing vitamin preparation (Gevrabon, Lederle) before meals may improve appetite and intake. Very often, deemphasizing the importance of eating in relation to improving longevity reduces stress on both patient and family, and this may, in itself, be accompanied by improved intake.

Aggressive nutritional counseling can be effective in management of anorexia associated with cancer treatment. Such counseling should take into account patterns of anorexia, as well as preferred foods and dietary habits. Increasing intake at breakfast, for example, can take advantage of the common phenomenon of better morning appetite, while adding a high-calorie snack at bedtime may reduce metabolic costs and improve weight gain. Investigation of such treatment-related problems as lactose intolerance can also be carried out during counseling session. Appropriate use of commercial supplements can be instituted. Effective nutritional counseling requires not only a nutritionist who is knowledgeable about cancer but also a commitment from both the patient and a family member. The patient and family must be willing to keep dietary records, so that calorie counts and nutritional adequacy can be monitored.

The psychological impact of cancer and its treatment may also affect nutritional status. Depression and anxiety have been shown to both decrease and increase dietary intake. Assisting patients to find counseling, either individual or group, may improve the patient's coping skills and reduce the effect of disease on eating habits. Short-term use of psychotropic drugs, in conjunction with counseling, may also be helpful.

HYPOGEUSIA AND DYSGEUSIA

Loss of taste and taste perversion can accompany both advanced disease and cancer treatment. Decreased salt and bitter perception have been reported in some studies, and patients so affected may be able to increase intake by using additional salt, soy sauce, and other seasonings. Increasing salt intake may not be advisable in patients with edema or ascites, however. Some taste perversion is associated with decreased zinc levels; zinc supplementation may reverse the taste anomaly. Such supplementation should be monitored carefully. In addition, all medicines being taken by patients complaining of taste alteration should be reviewed. Some patients put themselves on high doses of vitamins and minerals, which can produce taste alterations.

NAUSEA AND VOMITING

Nausea and vomiting are among the most common side effects of cancer chemotherapy. There are actually little data to indicate that nausea and vomiting interfere with nutrition for the majority of patients, but the potential for dehydration, electrolyte imbalance, and undernutrition does exist and must be evaluated in patients receiving chemotherapy. Prevention is the best treatment. Unfortunately, the mechanisms of nausea stimulation and blockade are not well understood, making it difficult to develop effective antiemetic regimens. We ordinarily provide prophylactic antiemetic medication prior to all chemotherapy administration and suggest that patients continue to take medication around the clock for 24 to 48 hours after administration, depending on the emetic potential of the chemotherapeutic agent(s) involved. We currently premedicate with metoclopromide, 10 to 20 mg by mouth and dexamethasone, 10 mg intravenously, for most drug combinations given on an outpatient basis. Phenothiazines are added as needed. For patients with only mild nausea, we have used concentrated carbohydrate solution (Coke syrup; Emetrol, Rorer) for nausea control. In outpatients with severe nausea and vomiting, chlorpromazine suppositories can be helpful. Antiemetic regimens for inpatients are usually more aggressive and may include combinations of intravenous glucocorticoids, lorazepam, diphenhydramine, and high-dose metoclopromide given prior to chemotherapy administration and at set intervals afterward. There have been a few studies that employed nonpharmacologic treatment, such as self-hypnosis, music, and guided imagery, with antiemetic drugs. These interventions may improve antiemetic control in a subset of patients.

Patients receiving abdominal or cranial irradiation may also have nausea and/or vomiting. These symptoms are usually managed by the radiotherapist, using techniques similar to those employed to minimize chemotherapy-induced nausea and vomiting: premedication and combination drug therapy. Nausea associated with radiation-induced cerebral edema is very effectively controlled with dexamethasone, given around the clock.

Another source of nausea and vomiting in patients with advanced cancer is metastasis of disease to the colon or liver. If the nausea and vomiting is caused by intestinal obstruction, we usually consider conservative therapy first. Intestinal decompression with a short nasogastric tube or longer Miller-Abbott or Cantor tube may be sufficient for relief. A decompression colostomy or similar bypass procedure may be required when conservative measures fail. Once the initial episode of obstruction resolves, the patient can then slowly progress from chemically defined diets to low residue as tolerated. The patient may eventually be placed on a high-residue diet if colon activity is sufficiently restored. If an obstruction occurs that is not amenable to either conservative or surgical means, a decision concerning the degree of aggressiveness of treatment must be made by the patient and family, with assistance from the physician. We have, on rare occasions, supplied peripheral parenteral nutrition for patients at home. The more usual procedure is to supply dextrose and water or saline at varying rates. We tend to give solutions at low rates, especially to patients with ascites, edema, heart disease, or lung involvement. Patients may be managed at home if sufficient resources are available.

Liver metastasis may produce feelings of queasiness or nausea in some patients. Relief from this distress is difficult to achieve, but concentrated carbohydrates or low-dose dexamethasone may relieve distress in some patients.

FATIGUE

Fatigue is a common complaint with nutritional implications; it can interfere with the patient's ability to buy, prepare, and even ingest food. Fatigue associated with hypoxia related to pleural effusion, loss of lung volume, lymphangiatic spread, or obstructive changes may improve with bronchodilator therapy or oxygen administration. Fatigue resulting from anemia may be reversed by transfusion. However, we rarely transfuse if the hematocrit is 25 percent or above. In many cases, fatigue may not be reversible. Fatigue is especially problematic for persons living alone or with another disabled person. There are often resources that can be mobilized, including relatives, friends, church groups, hospice workers, and community services (Meals-on-Wheels). This area can be explored by social workers through hospitals and local governmental agencies. In addition, identifying energy-saving methods of self-care and instructing patients on balancing periods of rest and activity may be helpful.

MUCOSITIS

Mucositis can occur in patients with advanced cancer as a result of chemotherapy and can be severe. In addition, candidiasis and herpetic infection can follow antibiotic administration. Preventive care, including instructions on oral care and dietary intake of yogurt and buttermilk, can be helpful. Once superinfection has developed, nystatin and acyclovir can be prescribed. Anesthetic mouthwashes may be required in patients with severe ulcerations. One common and effective mouthrinse is the combination of equal parts antacid, viscous xylocaine, and liquid diphenhydramine hydrochloride. Occasionally, oral mucositis is accompanied by irritation of other portions of the gastrointestinal tract. Management is the same, although additional treatment of symptoms such as diarrhea may be needed. There are many antidiarrheal agents available, including diphenoxylate hydrochloride, loperamide hydrochloride, and tincture of opium.

CONSTIPATION

Although constipation is a common problem among patients with advanced cancer, it usually does not interfere with nutrition. However, nutritional intervention can be helpful. There are a number of newer products on the market that provide added fiber; regular use of these dietary aids and increased intake of juices, raw fruit, and vegetables improve bowel function and reduce reliance on laxatives.

ABDOMINAL DISCOMFORT

Abdominal discomfort ranges from severe pain to feelings of fullness among patients with advanced cancer, especially in the presence of hepatomegaly or ascites. Severe pain following intake is often the result of reflux and can be managed with antacids. A product with simethecone is preferable, since gas pain is another common problem. Feelings of fullness can be reduced in some measure by taking several small meals, separating the intake of solid and liquid foods, and remaining sitting or in a semi-Fowler's position after eating. For some patients, using metoclopromide to improve gastrointestinal motility may be beneficial. For patients with abdominal cramping, a combination of phenobarbital, hyoscyamine, atropine, and scopolamine (Donnatal) may be more effective.

PAIN

Both pain and pain medicine can interfere with the perception of hunger. Treatment of pain in advanced cancer requires the same evaluation as treatment of pain in any patient. Acute onset of pain can accompany pathologic fractures, thrombophlebitis, and other conditions that are amenable to curative or palliative treatment that may provide complete pain relief. Chronic pain related to the presence of disease demands creative use of all disciplines. A consult with a pain clinic may provide interventions that have little effect on the patient's appetite. Such interventions include nerve blocks, cordotomy, and transcutaneous nerve stimulation. Psychological interventions such as self-hypnosis, distraction, music, and guided imagery can be useful. When nonpharmacologic treatment is not successful, drugs can be added to combat chronic cancer pain. For mild pain, aspirin, acetaminophen, and nonsteroidal anti-inflammatory products can be effective. As pain increases, codeine and oxycodone may be added to aspirin and acetaminophen products. The new, sustained action narcotics may be very helpful for patients with severe pain and have the benefit of providing 8 to 12 hours of relief without interim medication administration. Combinations of narcotics and psychotropic drugs can be helpful in improving rest and pain control. Combination therapy can also be effective with particular sources of pain, such as the addition of diuretics with lymphedema and antibiotics with infected malignant ulcerations. Patients are instructed to take pain medication on a regular, rather than on an "as needed" basis. Patients are also told to take all narcotic medication with food to reduce the incidence of nausea. In cases of intractable pain, intravenous analgesia can be arranged on both an inpatient and an outpatient setting. Nutritional intake is usually no longer a major concern by the time intravenous pain medication is needed.

Pain may also result from cancer treatment. Discomfort following thoracotomy, mastectomy, axillary node dissection, and radical neck dissection are common. Nonpharmacologic treatments, particularly gentle exercise, massage, and heat application can be helpful in combination with aspirin or nonsteroidal anti-inflammatory agents. Radiation-associated tenesmus and other radiation-linked side effects can also occur and respond well to short-term steroids. Pain associated with radiation-induced fibrotic changes is less amenable to steroid treatment and may require neurologic intervention and/or pharmacologic management.

SUGGESTED READING

DeWys W. Abnormalities of taste as a remote effect of a neoplasm. Ann NY Acad Sci 1974; 230:427–434.

Nixon D, Daly J, Jeejeebhoy K, et al. Augmented or standard nutritional intervention in advanced colorectal and nonsmall cell lung carcinoma. Proc AACR 1984; 25:172.

Theologides A. Cancer cachexia. Cancer 1979; 43:2004–2012

OTHER CONSIDERATIONS

NUTRITION IN PREGNANCY

NICHOLAS A. LEYLAND, B.A.Sc., M.D.
JERRY SHIME, B.A., M.D., F.R.C.S.(C)

During pregnancy, certain nutritional demands are created by the growing conceptus and altered maternal physiology. In this chapter, we will provide an approach to dietary assessment and counseling in pregnancy designed to optimize maternal nutrient intake and assist in the achievement of a favorable perinatal outcome. Fortunately, the receptiveness of the gravid woman on behalf of her fetus often facilitates the necessary dietary adjustments. Nevertheless, certain groups will be identified who, by virtue of medical conditions, socioreligious factors or personal habits must be considered nutritionally at risk.

NUTRITIONAL ASSESSMENT

Nutritional assessment and counseling commence with the first prenatal office visit. In addition to a general prenatal assessment, we obtain a dietary history. The basis for enquiry is Canada's Food Guide (Table 1). Consumption of the appropriate numbers of servings from each of the four major food groups can be established, or alternatively, areas of inadequate intake can be identified. In general, these center on neglect of one or more of the food groups, commonly milk or milk products. More complicated problems may require consultation with a dietitian who can provide a detailed nutritional assessment and recommend the appropriate dietary modifications.

TABLE 1 Food Guide for Pregnancy*

Milk and milk products:
  Calcium, protein, riboflavin, vitamin A, vitamin D
  Choose 3–4 servings
  Some examples of a serving:
  250 ml (1 cup) skim, 2% whole, reconstituted dry or evaporated milk,
    buttermilk
  175 ml (3/4 cup) yogurt
  45 g (1 1/2 oz) cheddar or process cheese

Meat, fish, poultry and alternates:
  Protein, iron, B vitamins
  Choose 2 servings
  Some examples of a serving:
    60–90 g (203 oz) cooked poultry, fish, liver, or lean meat
    60 ml (4 tbsp) peanut butter
    250 ml (1 cup) cooked dried peas, dried beans, or lentils
    125 ml (1/2 cup) nuts or seeds
    60 g (2 oz) cheddar cheese
    2 eggs

Fruits and vegetables:
  Vitamin A, vitamin C, folic acid, fiber
  Choose 4–5 servings
  Include at least two vegetables. Try a variety of cooked or raw fruits and vegetables
    or their juices. Include yellow, green, or green leafy vegetables.
  Some examples of a serving:
  125 ml (1/2 cup) vegetables or fruits
  125 ml (1/2 cup) juice, fresh/canned/frozen
  1 medium potato, carrot, tomato, peach, apple, orange, or banana

Breads and cereals:
  Carbohydrate, iron, B vitamins, fiber
  Choose 3–5 servings
  Whole grains are best
  Some examples of a serving:
    1 slice whole grain or enriched bread
    125 ml (1/2 cup) cooked or
    175 ml (3/4 cup), ready-to-eat whole grain or enriched cereal
    125–175 ml (1/2–3/4 cup) cooked converted or brown rice, whole grain
      or enriched macaroni or spaghetti
    1 roll or muffin

---

* Adapted from ''Canada's Food Guide,'' Health and Welfare Canada, 1983 with permission of the
Minister of Supply and Services Canada.

TABLE 2   Foods Rich in Iron, Calcium, and Folic Acid*

Good sources of iron:

Liver, any kind
Red meat—beef, pork, lamb, veal
Dried beans, peas, lentils—pork and beans, split pea soup, chili con carne
Whole grain or enriched breads and cereals—all kinds
Dried fruits—apricots, dates, raisins, peaches, prunes, and prune juice
Dark green vegetables—spinach, Brussels sprouts, broccoli, peas
Other good sources of iron—clams, sardines, seeds (pumpkin, squash, sesame,
    sunflower), nuts (almonds, cashews)

Good sources of calcium:

Milk, any kind
Yogurt
Cheese
Cottage cheese
Ice cream
Milk pudding
Canned salmon (with bones)
Sardines
Soybean curd (tofu)
Dark green leafy vegetables
Cream soup made with milk

Good sources of folic acid:

Liver or kidney
Spinach
Broccoli, asparagus
Brussels sprouts, beets
Beans, peas, squash
Turnips, corn
Avocados
Cantaloupes, bananas
Oranges or orange juice
Grapefruit or grapefruit juice
Dried beans (cooked)
Nuts (almonds, cashews, peanuts, walnuts)

* Health and Welfare Canada, 1983.

TABLE 3 Recommended Daily Nutrient Intake for the Reproductive Years and Pregnancy

Age	19–24 Years	25–49 Years	Pregnancy
Energy (kcal)*	2,100	1,900	+300 (100 kcal/0.4 mJ 1st trimester)
(mJ)	8.8	8.0	+1.3
Protein (g)	43	44	+ 15 (1st trimester) + 20 (2nd trimester) + 25 (3rd trimester)
Thiamin (mg)	.8	.8	+.04 (1st trimester) +.12 (⅔ trimester)
Niacin (NE)†	15	14	+ 0
Riboflavin (mg)	1	1	+0.3
Vitamin B₆ (mg)	0.6	0.7	+.2 (1st trimester) +.3 (2nd trimester) +.4 (3rd trimester)
Folate (μg)‡	175	175	+295
Vitamin B₁₂ (μg)	2	2	+1.0
Vitamin C (mg)	45	45	+ 0 (1st trimester) + 20 (2/3 trimesters)
Vitamin A (RE)§	800	800	+100
Vitamin D (μg)#	2.5	2.5	+2.5
Calcium (mg)	700	700	+500
Iron (mg)**	14	14	+ 6

* Increased energy intake recommended during second and third trimesters. An increase of 100 kcal (0.4 mJ) per day is recommended during the first trimester.

† 1 NE (niacin equivalent) is equal to 1 mg of niacin or 60 mg of tryptophan.

‡ Recommendation given in terms of free folate.

§ 1 RE (retinol equivalent) corresponds to a biologic activity in humans equal to 1 mg retinol (3.33 IU) or 6 μg beta-carotene (10 IU).

\# One μg cholecalciferol is equivalent to 1 μg ergocalciferol (40 IU vitamin D activity). This intake should be increased to 5.0 μg daily during pregnancy and lactation.

** A recommended total intake of 20 mg daily during pregnancy and lactation assumes the presence of adequate stores of iron. If stores are suspected of being inadequate, additional iron as a supplement is recommended.

A well-balanced diet planned according to Canada's Food Guide provides the basis for the expectant mother's nutrient intake during pregnancy. At the first prenatal visit, we provide our patients with a copy of Canada's Food Guide. In addidition, we encourage the consumption of foods containing iron, calcium, and folic acid (Table 2), the nutrients most commonly found to be lacking in a pregnant woman's diet. The following information represents an overview of nutritional requirements during pregnancy. References to nutrient requirements in pregnancy are based on the Recommended Nutrient Intakes for Canadians, Health and Welfare Canada, 1983, (Table 3).

NUTRITIONAL REQUIREMENTS IN PREGNANCY

Weight Gain and Caloric Requirements

The average weight gain in pregnancy is 13 kg, with a range of 9 to 16 kg. The American College of Obstetricians and Gynecologists' Committee on Nutrition has recommended a gain of 10 to 12 kg during pregnancy as optimum. Gains of this order have been associated with the most favorable perinatal outcome in epidemiologic studies. For the individual patient, the pattern of weight gain may be more significant than the absolute increase in weight. Close monitoring of maternal weight at each office visit will ensure an acceptable pattern. In the first trimester, a gain of approximately 1 kg can be anticipated. For the second and third trimesters, a linear increase in weight of approximately 0.3 to 0.4 kg per week should be observed. Significant deviations from this pattern should alert the physician to initiate a more detailed assessment. For example, a weight gain of 1 kg or less each month has been defined as inadequate and may be evidence of poor maternal nutrition and/or poor fetal growth. Excessive weight gain can be an early indicator of pre-eclampsia and should alert the clinician to check for signs of abnormal fluid retention.

Caloric requirements of pregnancy are increased due to the physiologic demands of the developing fetus and placenta as well as changes in maternal tissue. Health and Welfare Canada (1983) has recommended an increase of 400 kJ (100 kcal) per day during the first trimester and 1,300 kJ (300 kcal) per day during the second and third trimesters over the nonpregnant state. Generally, this translates into a small increase in the amount of food consumed by the mother and may be provided by the addition of two servings of milk or a milk product from group one plus modest increases from the other food groups. It is likely that if the pregnant patient selects foods as recommended by Canada's Food Guide and eats according to her appetite her additional caloric needs will be satisfied.

Protein

The amount of protein required during the average gestation to meet the demands of the developing conceptus and the changes in maternal tissues has been established as an additional 15 to 25 g daily throughout pregnancy. The requirement for the first trimester is an additional 15 g per day, increasing to 20 g and 25 g per day for the second and third trimesters, respectively. In actuality, most North American diets provide the requisite protein for pregnancy, even during the nonpregnant state. Diets providing inadequate amounts of protein are unusual and, in general, are restricted to vegetarian patients (see below).

Minerals

Iron. Dietary iron deficiency and iron deficiency anemia are the most frequently encountered nutritional problems in pregnancy. It may be difficult to differentiate the physiologic dilutional anemia of pregnancy from true iron deficiency anemia. Pregnancy results in the expansion of plasma volume in excess of the increase in red cell mass. Hemoglobin levels invariably decrease, but this may not represent true anemia. The World Health Organization has set the lower limit of hemoglobin level in pregnancy as 110 g per liter, and it is estimated that 20 to 80 percent of females are anemic during pregnancy, depending on the population screened. The accurate diagnosis of iron deficiency anemia is best established by an abnormal serum ferritin, i.e., less than 9 mg per liter.

Approximately 500 mg of iron are needed for the increase in maternal red blood cell volume, and an additional 400 mg are required to meet the needs of fetal erythropoiesis. Therefore, nearly 1 g of elemental iron is required over the course of pregnancy to meet the needs of the developing maternal-fetal unit. During pregnancy, the recommended daily intake of iron is 20 mg of elemental iron, assuming the presence of adequate stores. Since many North American women have neither the stores nor an adequate dietary intake to meet this need, some authors recommend, daily supplementation of 30 to 60 mg of elemental iron for all gravid women. However, iron supplementation may be associated with considerable gastrointestinal upset and reduced bioavailability of other nutrients, in particular vitamins A and C. For this reason, our practice is to reserve iron supplementation for those patients with inadequate dietary intake, or those with a documented deficiency state.

Heme iron is readily absorbed from the gastrointestinal tract. Non-heme iron is derived from vegetable sources, and its absorption may be impaired by chelating agents such as tea, milk, phytates, and calcium salts, which tend to bind iron in the gut, reducing its bioavailability. Thus, pregnant women should be apprised of the best nutritional sources of heme iron, such as red meats and liver (see Table 2). Women unable to ingest sufficient dietary iron should have supplementation with 60 mg of elemental iron daily, provided by one 300 mg tablet of ferrous sulfate. This should be ingested 2 hours before meals or on an empty stomach to maximize absorption.

For women actually found to have iron deficiency anemia, we administer iron in therapeutic doses, that is ferrous sulfate, 300 mg two to three times daily. Those experiencing significant dyspepsia with this regimen can be advised to ingest the iron with meals, recognizing that absorption will be suboptimal.

Calcium. Over the course of pregnancy, a total of approximately 30 g (750 mmol) of calcium is required to meet the needs of the developing fetus and provide for maternal calcium homeostasis. The daily requirement of 1,200 mg can be provided by approximately 1 L of milk. In addition, this amount of fortified milk will provide appropriate amounts of vitamin D and high-quality protein. However, this volume of milk or milk itself may not be an acceptable food for some gravid patients, particularly those with lactase deficiency (common in individuals of Asian, African, and Middle Eastern descent). Women not taking milk for reasons of personal preference or because of lactose intolerance should be counseled regarding acceptable alternate food sources and/or supplementation with calcium and vitamin D (see Tables 1 and 2).

Vitamins

Table 3 shows the recommended daily nutrient intake for the reproductive years and the increase in requirements for pregnancy. Requirements for most, if not all, vitamins are increased during pregnancy to meet the demands of the growing conceptus as well as the changes in maternal tissues. In general, North American diets are sufficient to provide for these increased demands.

Folic acid requirements are increased during pregnancy in relation to the increased demands of erythropoiesis as well as to fetal and placental growth. Folic acid, along with vitamin B_{12} is required for DNA synthesis. Its dietary sources are ubiquitous and include meats, vegetables, and fruits. In spite of this, many pregnant women consume diets with inadequate amounts of this vitamin. In addition, the vitamin is heat labile and therefore is destroyed by prolonged cooking.

During pregnancy, the daily requirement for Folicin is 470 μg per day. The World Health Organization has recommended supplementation for all pregnant women with 500 μg per day. Many authors recommend prenatal supplementation with folic acid since toxicity is not a problem and deficiency may be associated with neural tube defects, abruptio placentae, spontaneous abortion, and fetal growth retardation.

Serum levels of all the water-soluble vitamins have been shown to decline during pregnancy, secondary to hemodilution from expansion of plasma volume. These declines should not be interpreted as deficiency states.

Requirements for fat-soluble vitamins are increased during pregnancy by up to 25 percent. These vitamins cross the placenta slowly and thus accumulate in the fetus at lower levels than maternal serum. Despite this, vitamin A in excessive amounts is suspected to be teratogenic, and therefore, supplementation should be avoided.

Prenatal Vitamin Supplementation. Vitamin and mineral deficiencies are uncommon in North American women. The role of supplementation during pregnancy is controversial, yet many physicians routinely recommend one of many prenatal vitamins available on the market. There is no evidence that a woman consuming a diet as outlined by Canada's Food Guide requires vitamin and mineral supplementation, with the possible exceptions of iron and folic acid. Generally speaking, the use of supplements may be justified for those patients whose compliance with nutritional advice is questionable or when available food choices are limited for whatever reason. Otherwise, a more appropriate approach would be to identify nutritional problems early in pregnancy to allow for proper counseling and supplementation with specific nutrients found to be deficient.

SPECIFIC NUTRITIONAL CONCERNS

Special consideration may be necessary for women identified as having particular medical or psychosocial problems that may preclude optimum nutritional status during pregnancy.

High-risk Pregnancy

The Society of Obstetricians and Gynecologists of Canada (SOGC) has developed a list of nutritional risk factors (Table 4) to enable the practitioner to identify patients who need nutritional counseling.

The Overweight Patient. The obese patient, defined as weighing in excess of 20 percent of the standard weight for height, requires special consideration. A weight gain of not less than 7 to 9 kg has been associated epidemiologically with the most favorable perinatal outcome for

TABLE 4 Nutritional Risk Groups in Pregnancy*

Adolescents

Patients with anemia before and/or during pregnancy (Hb less than 100 g/L)

Patients with abnormal prepregnant weight (excessive or low) and/or inappropriate weight gain during pregnancy

Patients following vegetarian diets that exclude milk and eggs, fad diets, reducing diets, and other diets liable to result in nutritional deficiencies

Patients with multifetal gestation

Patients suffering from a medical illness or condition that may compromise absorption, digestion, or utilization of food (e.g., diabetes, bowel or liver disease including bowel bypass, malabsorption syndromes) and those taking drugs interfering with absorption or liver function (e.g., diphenylhydantoin)

Cigarette smokers and/or those with significant intake of alcohol or nonprescription drugs

* Adapted from The Perinatal Medicine Committee of the S.O.G.C. The Society of Obstetricians & Gynaecologists of Canada Bulletin, 1984; 6(5).

these patients. Overzealous attempts to correct weight problems during pregnancy by caloric restriction may adversely affect fetal development. We recommend that no patient consume less than 1,600 kcal per day, and we encourage the consumption of foods of high nutrient content but moderate caloric density in order to support a normal pattern of weight gain of at least 9 kg. Conversely "empty-calorie" foods, such as sweets and alcohol should be avoided.

The Underweight Patient. Women commencing pregnancy underweight (defined as less than 95 percent of ideal body weight for height) are at increased risk of delivering small-for-gestational age infants. Optimal obstetric outcome can be anticipated if, in addition to the recommended pregnancy weight gain of 10 to 12 kg, the patient gains the amount necessary to achieve her ideal weight for height.

A more general approach for the underweight patient is to recommend a gain of 13 to 14 kg to ensure the best perinatal outcome. Consultation with a dietitian may be necessary to ensure adequate nutritional support for these patients.

The Adolescent Patient. Many teenage girls have poor nutritional habits with diets deficient in iron, calcium, and vitamins A and C. The average birthweight of infants born to adolescent patients is substantially lower than that of infants born to older mothers and perinatal mortality is greater.

With considerable societal and peer pressure to maintain fashionable slimness, the pregnant adolescent may persist in consuming too few calories. The best assurance of sufficient caloric intake is an acceptable pattern of weight gain. This goal may be accomplished by an aggressive team approach to prenatal nutritional counseling and emphasis on a healthy lifestyle for pregnancy and postnatal life.

Vegetarian Patients. Lacto-ovo vegetarians should be advised that with properly planned diets their pregnancy can have a successful outcome. Protein requirements can easily be met following Canada's Food Guide.

Strict vegetarians (vegans), who omit eggs and milk from their diet, will have difficulty consuming a sufficient volume of food to meet the additional caloric requirements of pregnancy. They are likely to have iron, calcium, and vitamin B_{12} deficiencies. Protein will be preferentially catabolized when a caloric deficit is maintained. Strict vegans need specific counseling on complementary proteins needed to supply adequate amounts of essential amino acids to the developing fetus (Table 5).

TABLE 5 Complementary Proteins in Vegetarian Diets*

Food Group	Complement	Limiting Amino Acids
Legumes	Seeds and Nuts Cereals and Grains Milk	Tryptophan Methionine
Seeds and Nuts	Legumes Milk	Isoleucine Lysine
Cereals and Grains	Legumes Milk Brewer's yeast	Isoleucine Lysine

* To ensure the consumption of all the essential amino acids complementary protein sources need to be ingested.
Modified after Lappé FM. Diet for a small planet. New York: Raines and Raines, 1977:100.

Since there are no plant sources of vitamin B_{12}, supplementation or vitamin B_{12}–fortified soybean milk must be used to avoid deficiency. Careful meal planning with the help of a dietitian and judicious use of supplements are necessary for those women who wish to follow strict vegetarian diets during pregnancy. Certain therapeutic nutrients, such as Ensure Plus, provide vitamins, minerals, calories and, most importantly, protein from a soybean isolate, which is acceptable by vegans.

Non-nutritional Foods

Research into the effects of ethanol on fetal development has yet to determine a safe level of alcohol intake during pregnancy. The fetal alcohol syndrome (FAS) has been clearly linked to heavy consumption of alcohol during pregnancy, but other adverse perinatal events have been associated with more modest ethanol use. Further, peak blood levels reached on single occasions may be as important as total consumption over an extended period of time. As of this writing, to our knowledge, there have been no reported incidences of FAS in mothers who consumed less than 40 g of absolute alcohol per week which is the equivalent of four drinks (one drink equals one glass of wine, one bottle of beer, or one ounce of spirits). At this juncture, we advocate the guidelines prepared by the Perinatal Medicine Committee of the SOGC (September 1984), which recommend that patients abstain from alcohol from the time of conception until after delivery and lactation. Patients who find this regimen unacceptable should at least be encouraged to limit consumption to less than four drinks per week.

Caffeine has not been associated with fetal defects. Moreover, this substance is consumed at least once during pregnancy by more than 90 percent of women. Notwithstanding, heavy caffeine usage frequently coexists with cigarette smoking and poor health habits in general and should alert the physician to focus special attention on nutritional and lifestyle counseling.

A well-balanced diet in accordance with Canada's Food Guide recommendations provides the basis for nutritional counseling in pregnancy. The consumption of a diet providing adequate milk and milk products and emphasizing whole grains, fruits and vegetables, and sufficient fiber should ensure that the increased nutrient requirements for pregnancy are met. The use of supplementation during pregnancy should be limited to those patients at risk of specific deficiencies or those with a documented deficiency state.

SUGGESTED READING

Health and Welfare Canada. National guidelines on nutrition in pregnancy. Ottawa, 1986. The Society of Obstetricians & Gynaecologists of Canada Bulletin, 1986; 8(5).

Perinatal Medicine Committee of the SOGC. The Society of Obstetricians & Gynaecologists of Canada Bulletin, 1984; 6(5).

ANOREXIA NERVOSA AND BULIMIA NERVOSA

DAVID S. GOLDBLOOM, M.D., F.R.C.P.(C)
PAUL E. GARFINKEL, M.D., F.R.C.P.(C)

Anorexia nervosa is characterized by self-imposed starvation due to relentless pursuit of thinness and fear of fatness; this leads to varying degrees of emaciation and significant medical and psychiatric complications. It occurs in a serious form in about 1 percent of Western adolescent and young adult women, with more mild variants found in approximately 5 percent of the female population. About 5 percent of reported cases occur among men. Its morbidity emanates from the starvation and the variety of means used to pursue and maintain thinness. It continues to carry a significant mortality of roughly 5 percent despite increased diagnostic awareness and improved treatment.

Bulimia nervosa exists as a symptom of a variety of medical disorders, as a subtype of anorexia nervosa, and as an autonomous syndrome—bulimia nervosa—in women at relatively normal weight. As a syndrome, it describes a pattern of binge eating involving ingestion of large quantities of food with a feeling of being out of control, which is associated with a desire to be thinner and depressive moods. This is often complicated and perpetuated by purging behavior, including self-induced vomiting and diuretic and laxative abuse. It occurs in 2 to 5 percent of adolescent and young adult women in a form associated with significant medical and psychiatric complications. As in the related disorder of anorexia nervosa, individuals with bulimia nervosa are preponderantly female. The last decade has witnessed a dramatic increase in the incidence of bulimia nervosa, more so than anorexia nervosa; doubtless, this reflects a confluence of factors from heightened diagnostic awareness to mounting sociocultural pressures leading to the almost universal tendency toward dieting among women. Current standard diagnostic criteria for anorexia nervosa and bulimia nervosa are presented in Table 1.

ETIOLOGY

The etiology of these disorders is unknown. Most clinicians and

TABLE 1 Diagnostic Criteria*

Anorexia nervosa:

Refusal to maintain body weight over a minimal normal weight for age and height, e.g., weight loss leading to maintenance of body weight 15% below expected; failure to make expected weight gain during period of growth, leading to body weight 15% below expected.

Intense fear of gaining weight or becoming fat, even though underweight.

Disturbance in the way in which one's body weight, size, or shape is experienced, e.g., the individual claims to "feel fat" even when emaciated, believes that one area of the body is "too fat" even when obviously underweight.

In females, absence of at least three consecutive menstrual cycles when otherwise expected to occur (primary or secondary amenorrhea). (A woman is considered to have amenorrhea if her periods occur only following hormone, e.g., estrogen, administration.)

Bulimia nervosa:

Recurrent episodes of binge-eating (rapid consumption of a large amount of food in a discrete period of time).

A feeling of lack of control over the eating behavior during the eating binges.

The person regularly engages in either self-induced vomiting, use of laxatives strict dieting or diuretics, fasting, or vigorous exercise in order to prevent weight gain.

A minimum average of two binge-eating episodes per week for at least 3 months.

Persistent overconcern with body shape and weight.

* From American Psychiatric Association. Diagnostic and statistical manual of mental disorders. 3rd ed, revised. Washington, DC: American Psychiatric Association 1987:63–64.

researchers embrace a multideterminant model that acknowledges risk factors at several levels. Culturally, prejudice against obesity is strong and exaltation of thinness is high. Conflict between pressures on women to perform and to be nurturing may highlight concerns about personal control that are manifested in weight regulation. A family history of depression, alcoholism, obesity, or anorexia nervosa may augment risk for development of an eating disorder. At an individual level, predisposing factors include a sense of personal helplessness, fear of losing control, self-esteem highly dependent on the opinions of others, and an all-or-nothing way of thinking. Triggering events include the onset of puberty, separations and losses, and dieting itself. A variety of circumstances may coalesce to provide the individual with a maladaptive sense of personal meaning through the pursuit of thinness and avoidance of weight gain. Physiologic factors may then intercede to perpetuate the disorder. Many of the signs and symptoms attributed to anorexia nervosa and bulimia nervosa reflect the pathology of starvation due to any cause.

DIAGNOSIS

In terms of treatment, the obvious initial step is accurate diagnosis. Because of secrecy and shame in the patient and lack of awareness of these disorders among physicians, diagnosis may be delayed until medical complications emerge; these are summarized in Table 2. Even within psychiatry, eating disorders must be distinguished from other illnesses (Table 3).

Treatment begins with the initial assessment, which includes a careful history of diet, weight, methods used to control weight, and any associated psychosocial stressors. An inquiry into attitudes regarding weight and shape, body image perceptions, typical behaviors such as compulsive exercising, preoccupation with food, and mood states regulated by food and weight may all contribute to a larger portrait of an eating-disordered patient. Medical investigations that should be used routinely to determine complications include determination of serum electrolytes and amylase levels, a complete blood count, and an electrocardiogram.

TREATMENT

Eating-disordered patients, particularly those with anorexia nervosa, often distrust physicians, whom they perceive as only wishing to control and refeed them. If this becomes the sole focus of treatment, then in a sense their perception is correct. The true goal is the relief of suffering, and this is reached in part through weight restoration but also through addressing other problems identified by the patient, such as food preoccupation, depression, or social isolation. Another potential roadblock to treatment is the feelings these patients produce in treating personnel. Eating disorders are usually chronic diseases under some degree of voluntary control; this may evoke both angry and puritanical responses in the physician. Treatment may then become punitive and confirm the patient's

TABLE 2 Complications of Anorexia Nervosa and Bulimia

Complication	Frequency	Cause	Treatment
Cardiovascular system:			
Bradycardia	Common	Starvation	Responds to weight restoration
Hypotension	Common	Starvation; fluid depletion	Responds to weight restoration
Arrhythmias	Infrequent	Usually provoked by exercise in starvation; may be due to hypokalemia	Responds to weight restoration or potassium supplements
Cardiomyopathy	Rare	Emetine toxicity from ipecac	Stop ipecac abuse
Central nervous system:			
Nonspecific EEG changes	Common	Starvation	Weight restoration
Reversible cortical atrophy	Uncommon	Starvation	Weight restoration
Renal/electrolytes:			
Hypokalemia	Common	Loss of potassium from multiple routes (vomiting, diarrhea, and diuretics), salt restriction, and water intoxication (to meet weight goals)	Prevent purging; may need a potassium supplement Well-balanced diet with appropriate amount of fluids
Increased BUN	Uncommon	Dehydration	Rehydration
Metabolic alkalosis	Common	Purging	Prevent purging
Edema:	Common	Not clearly understood	Elevate feet for 1 hour t.i.d., avoid salt; do not use diuretics
Gastrointestinal system:			
Parotitis	Common	Mechanical trauma; starvation	No specific treatment; stop binges and vomiting
Early satiety	Common	Delayed gastric emptying	Domperidone 20 mg t.i.d.
Gastric dilatation	Rare	Rapid refeeding	Avoid oral feeding; use IV feeding

TABLE 2 Complications of Anorexia Nervosa and Bulimia (Continued)

Complication	Frequency	Cause	Treatment
Constipation	Common	Starvation; reliance on laxatives	Use diet—emphasis on dietary bulk, fruits, vegetables and try to avoid laxatives
Dental caries	Common	Acidic nature of vomitus	Dental consultation
Hyperamylasemia	Common in bulimia nervosa	Unknown	Prevent purging
Gastric rupture	Rare	Binging	Surgery
Superior mesenteric artery syndrome	Rare	Weight loss	Weight restoration
Musculoskeletal system:			
Myopathy	Uncommon	Starvation; hypokalemia; emetine myotoxicity from ipecac	Weight restoration; stop ipecac abuse
Osteoporosis	Rare	Starvation	Weight restoration
Thyroid:			
Decreased serum T3 and increased reverse T3	Common	Starvation	Weight restoration
Persistent Amenorrhea	Infrequent	Low weight; emotional stress	Restore weight to 90% of average
Hematologic changes:			
Anemia	Infrequent	Bone marrow hypoplasia due to starvation	Weight restoration; may need iron
Thrombocytopenia	Rare	Starvation	Weight restoration
Hypercholesterolemia	Common	Unknown	Balanced diet
Hypercarotenemia	Infrequent	Ingestion of high carotene foods	Balanced diet

TABLE 3   Psychiatric Differential Diagnosis of
Anorexia Nervosa

Conversion Disorder
Depression
Schizophrenia
Anorectic drug abuse (e.g., amphetamines)

sense of control by the physician, such as in frequent tube feeding. In contrast, the wish on the part of the physician to be liked by these patients may lead to excessive tolerance of behaviors that perpetuate the eating disorder. This therapeutic tightrope requires a careful balancing of firmness, encouragement of normal eating and weight, discussion of attitudes toward weight and food, and tolerance of the frequent chronicity of these disorders.

When the patient remains involved with her family, a family assessment is appropriate. Diagnostically, it allows evaluation of how relationships and attitudes within the family may predispose to or perpetuate the illness. It offers an opportunity to reduce tensions, blame, and guilt for all involved and provide frequently needed education about eating disorders.

Educational input is extremely valuable in treatment and usually begins in the first encounter. Basic information about the epidemiology and contributing factors of eating disorders, as well as about the sequelae of starvation, helps patients to feel both more understood and less alone. For families who have usually exhausted their own resources in dealing with their affected member, it provides reassurance and information regarding a phenomenon that has overwhelmed them. A number of publications for patients and families are helpful in this education process.

Outpatient Management

All patients with eating disorders should have at least one psychiatric consultation by a physician knowledgable about anorexia nervosa and bulimia nervosa. However, continuing treatment can be carried out by a family physician, pediatrician, or internist, often in collaboration with a nutritionist.

For anorexic patients, a weight range must be set as a goal. This usually is about 90 percent of average for the person's age and height. A range of 3 to 5 pounds rather than a precise weight is selected both to recognize natural fluctuations in body weight and to counter the tendency of anorexics to become focused on precise numbers. Beyond the use of actuarial tables, however, it is important to know the patient's premorbid weight prior to onset of the anorexic episode and the weight at which secondary amenorrhea developed; these will provide guidance toward restoration of an appropriate weight for that individual.

For bulimic patients, the issue is not so much weight gain as regulation of eating patterns; this may lead more to a diminution of characteristic weight fluctuations than weight gain per se.

Patients must relinquish their subjugation to their body weight; this means throwing out the scales at home and being weighed weekly by the physician. At the same time, the physician must explain to the patient the importance of being at a higher body weight: to confront the phobia regarding body size, to relieve the symptoms of starvation, and ultimately to resume control in a disorder that has overtaken her.

Once a target weight range is agreed upon, the next step is the prescription of a regular eating plan. It is useful to have patients keep a daily diary of their eating in terms of content and associated thoughts, feelings and behaviors. While this may seem a facile technique, it often reveals the idiosyncratic rules, habits, and restrictions of the anorexic and the dietary chaos of the bulimic. Simple recommendations in terms of frequency, setting, and quantity of meals may allow the patient to gain weight gradually or regulate urges to binge.

For anorexic patients, an initial regimen of 1,800 calories per day is usually adequate to begin weight gain without causing gastric dilatation associated with intensive refeeding. This intake is usually increased by 200 to 300 calories per week toward a target of about 2,400 calories per day. A rate of weight gain of 0.5 to 1.0 kg per week is desirable; more rapid weight gain can be associated with medical complications including gastric dilatation, fluid overload, and edema as well as fear and distrust in a patient who remains at best ambivalent about weight gain. Given the propensity of these patients to think in catastrophic extremes, it is important to reassure them that while they have relinquished control of their weight to their physician, they will not be allowed to gain weight too rapidly.

For bulimic patients, there is often a history of significant daily dietary restriction between binge episodes. The prescription of three structured daily meals of adequate caloric value goes some way toward diminishing the chaos of their eating patterns and the intensity of their urges to binge. In addition, individualized recommendations of pleasurable alternatives to binging behaviors when the patient feels out of control may be helpful.

It is not practical to provide here details of psychotherapy that accompanies nutritional rehabilitation except to indicate that in our experience comprehensive treatment must include both psychological and caloric input. It must be remembered, however, that psychotherapy involves both learning and a trusting relationship and that cognitive processes needed for learning may be impaired in starvation. An important goal is learning to recognize feeling states, to trust oneself, and to untie one's sense of self-worth from the scales.

In terms of medications, the only recommended pharmacotherapy for the outpatient treatment of anorexia nervosa is food. Appetite stimulants such as cyproheptadine are not effective. Indeed, until the latter stages of the disorder, the patient is consumed with hunger she is trying to control. With regard to bulimia nervosa, there is increasing evidence for the efficacy of antidepressants for a subset of patients who fail to respond to more conservative approaches. A personal or family history of depression per se is not an indication, and the antibulimic effect of these drugs does not necessarily coincide with the antidepressant effect. The tricyclic antidepressant desipramine is an ideal choice because of its relatively low anticholinergic toxicity and established efficacy. Practical guidelines for its use are illustrated in Table 4. There is comparable efficacy literature on another group of antidepressants, the monoamine oxidase inhibitors. However, because of the dietary restrictions they require, they should be prescribed only by a physician well familiar with their use.

Abuse of medications in eating disorders emanates from both the patient's drive for thinness and the physician's misunderstanding of symptoms and complications. Table 5 indicates a number of drugs to be avoided by eating-disordered patients.

Inpatient Management

Increasingly, anorexia nervosa and bulimia nervosa are managed on an outpatient basis. Nevertheless, there remains a set of indications for hospitalization.

TABLE 4 Practical Guidelines for the Use of Desipramine in Bulimia Nervosa

Initial dose	50–75 mg PO q.h.s.
Dose increase	25–50 mg every 3–4 days as tolerated
Therapeutic dose	Up to 250 mg per day in outpatients
Maintenance dose	Same as therapeutic dose
Response lag	2–4 weeks after initiation of treatment
Response failure	Check plasma level for evidence of poor absorption or noncompliance Consider trial of MAO inhibitor Consider psychotherapy alternatives
Complications	Anticholinergic toxicity Overdose potential
Maintenance dose duration	4–6 months (as in depression)

1. Rapid weight loss of greater than 30 percent within a 6-month period.
2. Significant hypokalemia (less than 3.0 mmol per liter despite potassium supplementation).
3. Depressed mood with active suicidality.
4. Failure of outpatient management either to break a cycle of binge eating, purging, and restriction or to restore body weight adequately.

Inpatient treatment consists of a team approach, including physicians, nurses, occupational therapists, psychologists, and nutritionists. As in outpatient management, a target weight range is set for anorexic patients. Following a preadmission interview with the patient and other family members where appropriate, bedrest with supervised meals begins. During the first week of hospitalization, a detailed assessment of the patient's psychological and nutritional state is made so that a program can be tailored to her needs.

Bedrest tends to counter the patient's denial by emphasizing that she is ill; it restricts activities such as compulsive exercising that are used to perpetuate emaciation and serves as a starting point for a behavioral

TABLE 5 Drugs to Avoid in Eating Disorders

Insulin

Thyroxine

Diuretics

Laxatives

Appetite stimulants

Benzodiazepines
(in bulimia nervosa)

reward program to encourage weight gain. Close nursing monitoring both fosters a trusting relationship and limits the degree of behaviors such as concealing or vomiting food. Dietary education helps dispel myths and misconceptions about food en route to an appropriate diet. As with outpatients, an initial daily intake of 1,500 calories is commenced. Because inpatients are often more emaciated than outpatients, weight gain of 1 to 2 kg per week and a gradual increase in intake up to 3,500 calories per day are acceptable.

As weight gain progresses, the patient spends increasing time out of bed, engaged in a variety of activities from occupational therapy to group meetings. Construction of a highly detailed reward system is usually unnecessary and can often play into a patient's preoccupation with rules and minutiae.

It is, in our experience, the rare patient who requires either nasogastric feeding or total parenteral nutrition—less than 1 percent of anorexic inpatients. These techniques should be used only in life-threatening circumstances or when all other means have failed; while they restore weight, they do not represent the normalization of eating that a treatment program should encourage. In the initial phases of hospitalization, severe anticipatory anxiety may interfere with the patient's beginning to eat. When this does not respond to group and nursing support or relaxation techniques, the temporary use of lorazepam, a short-acting benzodiazepine, 0.5 to 1.0 mg an hour prior to meals, may be used. Because of serious reversible and permanent side effects, the use of antipsychotic medications is not advocated.

Patients are weighed three times weekly at a standard time (in the morning before breakfast and after voiding) and in standard clothing. We provide patients with information about their weight changes and encourage them to discuss their perceptions of and reactions to them.

Once the patient reaches her target weight range, a process that may take 6 to 8 weeks, hospitalization or a day-treatment program continues for about 2 weeks to ensure consolidation of the gains made and to allow resumption of autonomy by the patient. This means giving the patient more control over food choice, decreasing supervision, and allowing psychotherapy to focus more sharply on the psychological issues associated with the eating disorder.

For the bulimic inpatient, mere environmental constraints on binging and vomiting are insufficient therapeutically. Diminishing the urge to binge through regular meal patterns as opposed to characteristic prebinge restriction, introducing "forbidden" foods that are associated with binges, and working on other deficits in impulse control are also important. Care must be taken to prevent the simple conversion of a bulimic patient to a restricting one; this would reflect management purely at a target behavior level, ignoring the core pathology of fear of fatness that is common to both anorexia nervosa and bulimia nervosa.

Outpatient follow-up after discharge is strongly recommended for these patients. Some anorexic patients will be compliant with an inpatient program in order to be free of it, without relinquishing any of the perceptual and conceptual distortions that gave rise to the disorder. Bulimics may relapse without the structure of a hospital program. Further, a significant number of eating-disordered patients proceed to manifest other psychiatric disorders, chiefly depression and anxiety states.

Even today, mortality from anorexia nervosa remains at 5 percent; long-term studies of the outcome of bulimia nervosa have not been performed. Twenty-five percent of anorexics have a chronic form of the illness but two-thirds do well. Further research in the nutritional, psychological, and medical management of these patients will hopefully improve the outcome of these disorders.

SUGGESTED READING

Garfinkel PE, Garner DM. Anorexia nervosa: multidimensional perspective. New York: Brunner/Mazel, 1982.

Garfinkel PE, Garner DM, eds. The role of drug treatments for eating disorders. New York: Brunner/Mazel, 1987.

Garner DM, Garfinkel PE, eds. Handbook of psychotherapy for anorexia nervosa and bulimia. New York: Guilford Press, 1985.

DRUG-NUTRIENT INTERACTIONS AND DRUG-INDUCED NUTRIENT DEFICIENCIES

NORMAN STEINHART, B.Sc., M.D.

Interest in drug-nutrient interactions (DNI) and drug-induced nutrient deficiencies (DIND) is increasing. These iatrogenic problems are more common than previously estimated in our heavily medicated society; recent concerns about the safety and necessity of many medications are leading practitioners to examine more closely the relationship between drugs and nutrients. The issue of DNI has been given little or no attention in most medical schools and by pharmaceutical companies; however, the ever-increasing use of powerful, and sometimes toxic, drugs on a chronic basis and the uncontrolled use of nonprescription medications also raise the risk of developing such deficiencies. The factors that increase the difficulty of detecting DIND are listed in Table 1.

MECHANISMS OF DRUG-NUTRIENT INTERACTIONS

The classification of DNI by mechanism is useful, since it relates the pharmacologic activity of drugs to nutrient metabolism and can be used to remember common causes of DIND and predict drug effects on

TABLE 1 Factors Interfering with Diagnosis of Drug-Induced Nutrient Deficiencies

Multiple drug regimens

Lack of clinical suspicion and knowledge by practitioners

Lack of information concerning most drugs' effects on nutritional status

Interaction of disease, diet, and drugs in producing nutrient depletion

Variable nature of drug effects on nutriture in individuals due to differences in compliance, pharmacogenetics, drug metabolism in liver and kidney, initial nutrient status, etc.

nutrient status when reported information is lacking. Table 2 describes the types of DNI and the drugs and nutrients commonly involved in each type of interaction.

Any agent that disrupts one or more of the steps of nutrient intake, digestion, absorption, binding, activation, catabolism, or elimination has the potential for causing possible depletion. Malabsorption is a common and important DNI. Besides the agents listed here, any drug that causes prolonged diarrhea or is known to interfere with gastrointestinal function has the potential for causing nutrient malabsorption. When drugs such as sulfasalazine are being used to treat inflammatory bowel disease, the primary symptoms already involve the bowel, and knowledge of its specific effect on folate is essential. The use of nonprescription anorexiants, laxatives, and antacids may be concealed or underestimated in patients with eating disorders, obesity, or anxiety neuroses, making diagnosis of DNI very difficult. Any unexpected nutrient deficiency should raise suspicion of a DIND.

The other important mechanism of DNI involves antinutrients. These drugs structurally resemble nutrients and either compete directly for enzymes needed for active conversion of precursors, such as folate reductase and pyridoxal kinase, or are analogues that compete with the cofactor or combine and antagonize the active nutrient. Because these agents are so specific, they can cause significant deficiencies, especially in the presence of a marginal diet. Because the antagonism is competitive, increasing the nutrient intake can prevent the deficiency.

DRUG-INDUCED NUTRIENT DEFICIENCIES

Since DNI refers to a biochemical relationship and not a clinical event, it is important to remember that only those interactions that cause depletion or antagonism in excess of body stores or nutrient intake will produce a deficiency state. In addition, different levels of deficiency can occur from the same medication and dosage, ranging from subclinical to grossly abnormal, with very different clinical significance. The time frame and severity of deficiency develop very differently in certain individuals despite similar regimens. Thus, a concept of host susceptibility to DIND can be developed and various risk factors that often contribute to depletion are listed in Table 3.

TABLE 2 Mechanisms of Drug-Nutrient Interactions

Mechanism	Drug	Nutrients
Reduced intake	Anorexiants (obesity) Stimulants (children)	Protein, calories
Reduction of synthesis	Topical agents, PABA Oral antibiotics	Vitamin D Vitamin K
Malabsorption		
Intestinal hurry	Laxatives (phenol)	Vitamin D, Ca
Solubilization	Mineral oil	Carotene, Fat-soluble vitamins
Chelation	Tetracycline	Magnesium, cations
Insoluble precipitates	Antacids (AlOH, MgOH)	Phosphate
Lipase inactivation and mucosal damage	Neomycin	Fat, nitrogen, Ca, K, Fe, lactose, sucrose
Bile salt binding	Cholestyramine	Fat, vitamins A, K, D, B_{12}, Fe
Lowered ileal pH	KCl supplements	Vitamin B_{12}
Mucosal damage and enzyme damage	Colchicine	Fat, carotene, vitamins K and B_{12} and Na+ Lactose
Competitive inhibition of uptake	Oral hypoglycemics	Vitamin B_{12}
Block of mucosal uptake	p-Amino salicylate, sulphasalazine	Fat, folate, vitamin B_{12}, Folate
Elevated pH	NaHCO	Folate
Gastric acid secretion	H_2 receptor antagonists	Vitamin B_{12}
Unknown	Oral contraceptives	Folate
Displacement from binding site and increased excretion	INH	Vitamin B_6
	Glucocorticoids	Potassium (K+), Ca
	Borate	Vitamin B_2
	Penicillamine	Cu, Zn
	Antibiotics	Mg
	Oral contraceptives	Folate
Increased catabolism	Phenobarbitol	Vitamin D
	Glucocorticoids	Vitamin D
	Oral contraceptives*	Vitamin B_6
Antinutrients (see Table 4)		
Inhibition of activating enzyme (folate reductase)	Methotrexate	Folate
Increase of inactive form	Coumarin	Vitamin K
Complex with active form	Isoniazid	Vitamin B_6

* Suspected mechanism of action
Compiled in part from Roe D. Drug-induced nutritional deficiencies. 2nd ed. Westport, CT:AVI, 1985.

TABLE 3   Risk Factors for Drug-Induced Nutrient Deficiencies

Host Factors	Drug Factors
Increased nutrient needs:	Unknown nutrient effect
Pregnancy, lactation	Multiple drug regimen
Growth	Chronic usage
Catabolism, trauma	High dosage
Neoplasia	Significant DNI
Marginal diet	
Predisposing diseases:	
Chronic disease	
GI disease, especially malabsorption	
Malnutrition of disease	
Hepatic or renal disease	
Pharmacogenetics:	
Slow drug elimination	
Drug abuse:	
Alcohol	
Illicit (street) drugs	
Nonprescription drugs	

Adapted from Roe D, Campbell C, eds. Drugs and nutrients. New York: Marcel Dekker, 1984.

The first three host factors are all important in raising the risk of DIND. If any of these are combined with significant DNI such as malabsorption or antagonism, then clinical suspicion should arise and intensive monitoring of the patient is indicated.

There are three major models of development of depletion from a DNI: the sequential model, the continuous use model, and the interactive model. The sequential model supposes that one DIND predisposes for other deficiencies and/or increased toxicity. For example, hypomagnesemia initially caused by aminoglycoside nephrotoxicity may lead to hypocalcemic symptoms and further nephrotoxicity. As well, a subclinical DIND followed by or causing a change in disease status may result in a clinical DIND. Thus practitioners should monitor patients at regular intervals and be aware of changes in nutrient status due to sequential events. The continuous model suggests that nutrient depletion occurs slowly over time; this could occur when a patient starts with a marginal intake or increased needs. The interactive model recognizes that many host, dietary, and drug factors interact simultaneously to cause DIND. While all three methods of depletion occur, it is the interactive concept that resembles the clinical situation most closely.

CLINICAL ASPECTS

A solid knowledge of clinical nutrition is necessary to diagnose or prevent DIND. Nutritional assessment must be done with regard to the nutrients that are commonly affected, drug history, and physical symptoms commonly found with DNI. Many symptoms can be related to a single nutrient, such as vitamin B_6 deficiency, which can cause symptoms of pellagra through reduced niacin synthesis, neuropathy, and anemia. The most common DINDs involve vitamins, especially B_6, B_{12}, and folate, probably because of the specific antinutrients that antagonize these three vitamins (Table 4).

Multiple deficiencies can exist, and lack of one nutrient often exacerbates deficiencies of others; for example, vitamin B_6 deficiency increases that of vitamin B_3; vitamin B_2 depletion worsens a vitamin B_6 deficiency; and folate or vitamin B_{12} depletion decreases serum vitamin C levels.

History

A history of drug intake concurrent with or immediately preceding the diagnosis of nutrient deficiency must be obtained to consider an incident as a DIND. Any symptoms not explainable by either the disease itself or drug toxicity or hypersensitivity require assessment of nutritional status. This is especially true if multiple or chronic pharmacotherapy is being administered, or the patient is at high risk (Table 3). In addition, suspicion or diagnosis of a nutrient deficiency unusual in the clinical set-

TABLE 4   Vitamin Antagonists

Folate antinutrients:	Vitamin B_6 antinutrients:	Vitamin B_{12} antinutrients:
Methotrexate	INH	Nitrous oxide
Pyrimethamine	Hydrazine	
Triamterene	Cycloserine	
Trimethoprin	L-Dopa	**Vitamin K antinutrients:**
Sulfasalazine		Coumarin anticoagulants

ting (i.e., a vitamin B_1 deficiency without alcohol abuse) should lead to a review of drug intake.

Specific symptoms suggesting DIND include weight loss and/or growth retardation due to protein-calorie malnutrition, diarrhea or steatorrhea of malabsorption, and symptoms of vitamin B_6, B_{12}, D, or K, folate, potassium, or calcium deficiency.

A thorough drug history should be taken, of course, including nonprescription agents, especially laxatives, antacids, anorectic agents, and vitamin supplements. A proper dietary history is an important but overlooked aspect of most clinical histories. A single 24-hour recall is not representative of the usual diet; either three separate 24-hour recall histories or a food frequency recall is the minimum information needed to obtain reliable dietary data.

Physical Examination

Physical signs of deficiency of commonly depleted nutrients (vitamins B_6, B_{12}, D, or folate) should be sought. Signs of massive malabsorption, such as weight loss, muscle wasting, abdominal abnormalities, or bone tenderness, should be checked. Signs of dermatitis (vitamins B_3 and B_6), anemia (vitamins B_6 and B_{12}, folate, Fe), or neuropathy (vitamins B_6 and B_{12}) should be sought.

Laboratory Tests

Tests of malabsorption, specific nutrient status, and skeletal metabolism and density should be done routinely in high-risk situations or as indicated by other findings. These procedures may include fecal fat, carotene, breath H_2 (malabsorption); blood count and iron indices; Ca, Mg, P, protein albumin, RBC, serum folate, serum vitamin B_{12}, alkaline phosphatase, and prothrombin time; and skeletal bone density and radiographs.

PHARMACOLOGIC ASPECTS

There are a limited number of medications that commonly cause DIND, and any practitioner licensed to prescribe these drugs should be aware of these potential effects. Table 2 demonstrates the multiple effects of some agents. Practitioners should also be aware that the information on DNI and DIND is quite incomplete and that absence of reported deficiencies with a specific drug should not provide a false sense of security. The high-risk patient can present with rapid depletion from unexpected medications. The influx of new pharmacologic agents with unknown effects on nutrition provides further challenge to practitioners.

PREVENTION OF DRUG-INDUCED DEFICIENCIES

The integration of the information presented in this chapter on drug (Tables 2 and 4) and host factors (Table 3) of DNI, combined with a knowledge of pharmacology and clinical nutrition will allow practitioners to gain proficiency in this area of medicine. This information will help them to foresee or recognize most interactions in the early stage. The use of nutritional supplements during pharmacotherapy, as suggested in Table 5, will prevent many DINDs from occurring. Further research on and attention to this topic are needed to minimize the adverse effects of our pill-oriented society.

TABLE 5 Supplementation to Prevent Drug-Induced Deficiencies

Drug	Supplement—Daily Dose
Anticonvulsants	Vitamin D 400–800 IU Vitamin K 1–5 mg Folate 400–1,000 μg (< 2,000 μg)
Nonsteroidal anti-inflammatory agents	Folate 400–1,000 μg Ascorbic acid 50–100 mg
Cholesterol-lowering, bile-binding agents	Vitamin A 2,000–5,000 IU Vitamin D 200–800 IU Vitamin K 2–25 mg Folic acid 400–1,000 μg
Antituberculous agents	Vitamin B_6 26–50 mg Vitamin B_3 15–25 mg Vitamin D 400–800 IU
Hydralazine	Vitamin B_6 25–100 mg
Oral contraceptives	Vitamin B_6 1–5 mg Folate 400–1,000 μg
Neuroleptics (phenothiazines)	Vitamin B_2 2–5 mg

With permission from Roe D. Drug-induced nutritional deficiencies. Westport, CT:AVI, 1985.

SUGGESTED READING

Roe D. Drug-induced nutritional deficiencies. 2nd ed. Westport, CT:AVI, 1985.
Roe D, Campbell C, eds. Drugs and nutrients. New York: Marcel Dekker, 1984.
Winick M, ed. Nutrition and drugs. New York: John Wiley & Sons, 1983.

DIET THERAPY COMPLICATIONS

KHURSHEED N. JEEJEEBHOY, M.B., B.S., Ph.D., F.R.C.P.(C)

Nutrition is commonly considered to be such a beneficial aspect of living that it is difficult to conceive of it being the source of complications. However in excess, or in a distorted form, nutrition is capable of causing problems.

COMPLICATIONS OF AN ORAL DIET

Natural foods can cause complications because of excessive intake, dietary imbalances, and mechanical factors in patients with bowel disease.

Excessive Intake

Calories. Excessive caloric intake results in obesity with its complications. This subject is discussed in detail in the chapter on *Obesity.*

Protein. Excessive protein intake causes increased urea production. The need to excrete extra urea increases the oxygen demands of the kidney, which then becomes vulnerable to injury. This theory has been proposed to explain the development of renal impairment with age. In addition, high-protein diets are poorly tolerated by patients with hepatic encephalopathy and may precipitate coma in that circumstance.

Electrolytes. High sodium intake, common in the average North American diet, can precipitate hypertension in susceptible persons. The current fad for taking large amounts of calcium cannot be supported on any rational basis. High calcium intake has not been shown in controlled trials to prevent bone loss with aging. On the other hand, high calcium intake increases urine calcium and may predispose to the formation of renal calculi. Excessive calcium in the diet also increases gastric acid secretion and may exacerbate heartburn and ulcer dyspepsia.

Vitamins. Fat-soluble vitamins are all toxic in excessive quantities. An excessive intake of vitamin A can cause fatigue, insomnia, pains in bones and joints, and even pathologic fractures. Headaches and vertigo can occur. In children, periosteitis may be noted. Vitamin D in excess causes decalcification of bones and metastatic calcification of arteries, together with muscular hypotonia, polyuria, pruritus, and renal failure. Anorexia, nausea, and vomiting may occur. The popular practice of taking vitamins in large doses is to be deplored.

Trace Elements. In limited quantities these elements are beneficial, but in excess they can be poisonous. Weight for weight, selenium is more poisonous than arsenic. If taken in excess, the results are a garlic taste, anorexia, nausea, and vomiting with diarrhea. Hair may fall out and a skin rash appear. This element is at present being considered as an anticancer nutrient, and it is important not to take excessive amounts with the notion that if a little is good, then more is better.

Unbalanced Diets and Complications

Nutrients are interdependent for complete utilization. For example, carbohydrate oxidation requires thiamine, and incorporation of protein into lean tissue requires potassium, phosphorus, magnesium, and zinc. Thus it is necessary to eat a diet that is balanced in all respects, and it is therefore not surprising that diets composed exclusively of single entities can cause metabolic complications.

Peptic Ulcer Diet. In the past, diets composed exclusively of milk were prescribed to soothe peptic ulcers. Such diets caused vitamin deficiencies such as scurvy.

Protein Diets for Obesity. These diets have caused cardiac arrhythmias and arrest. These complications are believed to result in part from the hypokalemia that follows ingestion of an exclusively protein diet.

Vegetarian Low-Protein, High-Fiber Diets. Vegetarian diets can be balanced and provide excellent nutrition as long as attention is paid to the need for various nutrients. However such diets can also be quite unbalanced. The so-called "macrobiotic" diets, in which due attention is not given to first-class proteins, can cause severe protein deficiencies, especially in growing children. High fiber intake without other sources of calcium and trace elements can cause deficiencies of calcium, magnesium, and zinc. Often these diets are deficient in vitamin B_{12} and may result in pernicious anemia. Iron deficiency can also occur because iron in cereals is bound to phytates and not available, while the heme iron that is most easily absorbed is found in animal products.

Starvation and Binge Eating. The practice of starvation, if followed by a large meal, can cause pancreatitis.

Hypocaloric Feeding Followed by a High-Carbohydrate Diet. This practice is seen in obese individuals on chronic low-calorie diets interrupted by periods of "going off the diet" by "cheating" with high carbohydrate foods. This process is associated with sodium retention and the occurrence of so-called "refeeding edema." Here the intake of carbohydrate results in sodium retention and a rise in insulin. The patient complains of water retention and is treated with a diuretic, which in turn causes potassium loss and a feeling of fatigue. The end result is an obese individual complaining of bloating and chronic fatigue.

Mechanical Factors and Complications. Fiber in moderation is excellent for proper colonic function. However, in patients with strictures of the intestine, as in patients with Crohn's disease, the ingestion of long fibers can cause bolus obstruction, and a high-vegetable diet can cause pain and even clinical obstruction. The same problem can arise in patients with a small intestinal stoma—eating a lot of fiber can cause stomal obstruction. Therefore, use of fiber in such individuals must be carefully regulated or eliminated in some cases. When very low-fiber diets are given, there is danger of deficiency of the vitamins derived from green vegetables such as folate and vitamin C. These vitamins should be supplemented when such diets are prescribed.

COMPLICATIONS OF ENTERAL NUTRITION

Misplaced Tube. This problem can be avoided by taking an x-ray film prior to infusion in all cases. If the catheter is misplaced, serious problems can arise if nutrients are infused into a bronchus or the peritoneum. In the case of jejunostomy and gastrostomy tubes, it is necessary to check during the first week after insertion for displacement from bowel into the peritoneum.

Gastric Retention and Aspiration. This is avoided by nasoenteral, rather than nasogastric, feeding of critically sick patients. If gastric feeding is used, then the residual volume is checked. If above 150 ml, infusion is resumed at half the rate and the residue determined every 4 hours. Intravenous metaclopramide may help gastric motility and reduce the residue. To minimize aspiration, the patient can be nursed with his head raised to 30 degrees, reducing gastric residues.

Diarrhea and GI Discomfort. This is due to a number of factors which include:

1. Lack of sodium in the feeding—as has been discussed by Halperin and colleagues. Add sodium.
2. Flow into the intestine is uncontrolled—use a pump to regulate its flow.
3. Bacterial contamination—change bags and sets every 24 hours. Reduce hang times to 8 hours. Use aseptic preparation for feedings.
4. Infusing ice cold feeds—warm to room temperature before feeding.
5. Broad-spectrum antibiotic administration—review use of antibiotics; culture stools for *C. difficile* and test for its toxin.
6. Intercurrent GI problem—examine patient for GI disease.

Nausea, Vomiting, and Cramps.   The causes of these problems are the same as for diarrhea and gastric retention and need the same attention.

Electrolyte Disturbance.   The special problem is that of osmotic diarrhea causing hypernatremia, hyperchloremia, and dehydration. Infusion of free water intravenously controls the problem. However the cause is lack of nutrient absorption, which causes osmotic diarrhea. This should be evaluated and the rate of infusion adjusted. Also water requirements should be assessed and met.

Metabolic Complications.   These are the same as with parenteral nutrition.

COMPLICATIONS OF PARENTERAL NUTRITION

The complications of parenteral nutrition (PN) can be divided into three categories: technical, septic, and metabolic. Many published reports have documented these complications, the most frequent of which are catheter-related. The following discussion presents the complications related to catheter insertion, catheter-related sepsis, and late complications of indwelling catheters, before proceeding to metabolic ones. Despite this array of problems, it should be understood that with proper patient monitoring, good observation, and good aseptic technique, most are preventable. The following are most commonly seen.

Technical Complications

Complications of Catheter Insertion

Injury to the Lung and Pleura.   Pneumothorax is the most common complication of catheter insertion. On occasion, a tension pneumothorax can develop. Usually this will be diagnosed by the chest film taken following catheter insertion. If small and causing no clinical symptoms, no treatment is required. The size of the pneumothorax can be documented by daily roentgenograms. If it enlarges, needle aspiration or insertion of a thoracostomy tube is indicated. On the other hand, if a patient presents with dyspnea, chest pain, or cyanosis following catheter insertion, a major complication of the pleural space should be suspected. If warranted, a large-bore needle or a thoracostomy tube should be inserted to relieve a probable pneumothorax, tension pneumothorax, or hemothorax. If the catheter is in the correct position within the superior vena cava and if the pneumothorax is simply treated, catheter removal is unnecessary.

Injury to the Artery and Vein. Injury to the subclavian artery with resultant external bleeding can be treated by removing the needle and/or catheter and applying direct pressure. The radial and ulnar pulses on the injured side should be checked frequently. Laceration of a major vein should be controlled by direct pressure. If the tip of the catheter lacerates the vein and terminates in the pleural space, infusion of fluid quickly produces chest pain, dyspnea, and possible shock. A chest film and aspiration of the chest confirms this diagnosis. This complication can be avoided if only normal saline is infused until the position of the catheter is confirmed radiologically. Treatment should include immediate discontinuation of the infusion, catheter removal, and monitoring of the pleural space by a thoracostomy tube if necessary.

Injury to the Brachial Plexus. Nerve damage reflected by radial, ulnar, or median nerve signs can be treated simply by removing the catheter.

Injury to the Thoracic Duct. Injury to the thoracic duct from a left subclavian catheter is obvious when clear lymph drains from the insertion site. Treatment involves removal of the catheter. Chylothorax has been reported and should be treated by evacuation and aspiration of the pleural space until lymphatic drainage ceases.

Injury to the Mediastinum. Insertion of a temporary catheter may occasionally result in the production of a mediastinal hematoma. If large, this can cause compression of the superior vena cava. In this situation, emergency surgery is required to evacuate the hematoma and relieve the obstruction.

Embolus. Air embolism can occur at the time of catheter insertion when the syringe is removed prior to threading of the catheter. It can be avoided by having the patient perform a Valsalva maneuver during this step in the technique. Embolism of the catheter can occur if it has been inserted through a needle, when the catheter is pulled back and its position adjusted while the needle is still in the vein. The catheter is sheared off by the bevelled tip of the needle and lodges in a vein. The treatment of choice for a catheter embolus is transvenous removal with a guidewire snare technique performed under image intensification in the cardiac catheterization unit.

Malposition of the Catheter. The catheter must be positioned low down in the superior vena cava (SVC). On occasion during insertion, the catheter will enter the ipsilateral internal jugular vein or cross over to the contralateral innominate vein. In either location, infusion of hypertonic solutions can cause thrombophlebitis. If malposition occurs, it should be corrected by repositioning under fluoroscopic control. If this is not possible, the catheter should be removed and a new catheter inserted on the contralateral side.

Cardiac Complications. Cardiac arrhythmias may occur if the catheter is positioned within the right atrium or ventricle. This complication can be avoided by correct positioning of the catheter within the SVC.

Complications of Catheter Maintenance

Clotted Catheter. If the catheter becomes clotted, an attempt should be made to unplug it. A 1-ml syringe containing sterile normal saline is attached directly to the hub of the catheter and an attempt is made to loosen the clot by irrigation. If this fails, the clotted catheter should be unplugged by instilling urokinase, which will dissolve the fibrin in the catheter and make it patent once again. The technique consists of dissolving 5,000 Ploug units (7,500 IU) of urokinase in 3 ml of normal saline and injecting as much as will go into the catheter, up to a maximum of 2.5 ml. Then the catheter is capped for 3 hours and flushed with 10 ml saline containing 1,000 units of heparin.

Venous (and Catheter) Thrombosis. Thrombosis of the SVC and its main tributaries can occur following long-term PN. The usual cause is malposition of the catheter and resultant phlebothrombosis and thrombophlebitis. This complication usually requires removal of the catheter. Streptokinase or urokinase is used to induce clot lysis.

Thrombi can also occur at the tip of the catheter. Catheter thrombosis and sepsis are closely related complications of indwelling dimethicone catheters. Glynn and colleagues described a procedure by which thrombi can be dispersed with urokinase while the catheter remains in situ. Urokinase was successful in clearing the catheter in all 20 patients treated. The concomitant use of antibiotics cleared the sepsis. The procedure resulted in no detectable fibrinolysis or other systemic complication.

Air Embolism. This can occur as a late complication if the intravenous tubing inadvertently becomes detached from the catheter or if the catheter itself is unwittingly removed. The patient is usually found collapsed with the intravenous line detached from the catheter. The physician or nurse should immediately cover the catheter tip and place the patient in the Trendelenburg position with the right side up. It is imperative that the patient be placed in the left lateral decubitus position to prevent air obstruction of the pulmonary artery. If cardiac arrest has occurred and the patient does not respond quickly, aspiration of the air from the right ventricle is indicated.

Septic Complications

Catheter sepsis can be defined as an episode of clinical sepsis in a patient receiving short- or long-term intravenous alimentation that resolves following removal of the catheter. Confirmatory evidence includes a positive culture from either blood or removed catheter tips. The incidence of catheter sepsis varies from 2 to 7 percent, depending on the care given to the catheter. Sepsis is a serious complication of PN, and patients receiving this therapy are susceptible to infection for various reasons. If a fever develops during the administration of PN, a close examination for focal sources must be carried out. In particular, injection abscesses, phlebitis, chest infection, urinary tract infection, and abdominal sepsis should be considered. The fever may also be associated with allergic reactions to the nutrients, an infected central venous line, and contaminated fluid or tubing.

The most common organisms involved in catheter sepsis are *Staphylococcus epidermidis* and *S. aureus*. Less frequently cultured are coliform, enteric, and fungal organisms, particularly *Candida*. Factors that may contribute to catheter sepsis include poor technique in catheter insertion, lack of adherence to postinsertion protocol, duration of catheterization, and patient population. Certain patients are at greater risk for catheter sepsis than others; these include anergic patients, those receiving steroids, and those with acute pancreatitis or severe inflammatory bowel disease.

The most common portals of infection are those around the entrance site or the hub connection of the catheter. While possible, infection via the infusion set or fluids rarely occurs.

A low-grade fever in the absence of a discernible source should alert the physician to the possibility of catheter sepsis. A fever spike to 102 °F or above may also occur.

If catheter sepsis is suspected and other sources of fever are ruled out, PN should be discontinued and the infusate and tubing sent for culture. Maintenance intravenous fluids should be substituted. Peripheral blood cultures and retrograde cultures through the catheter are obtained. The exit site of the catheter is swabbed and cultured. Routine cultures of urine, sputum, mouth, and drainage sites are also obtained. If the blood cultures are positive or if the fever continues, the temporary subclavian catheter should be removed and reinserted after subsidence of the fever for 48 hours. If the blood cultures are negative and the temperature returns to normal, Toronto General Hospital policy has been to resume PN through the same line after 48 hours. Sepsis related to a permanent silicone rubber line has been successfully treated without removal of the catheter in 66 percent of cases. In this situation, urokinase is used as described above for clotted catheters, and antibiotics given daily for 4 weeks. If the sepsis is not controlled or fever returns, the catheter must be removed.

Even after removal, in certain circumstances fever and positive blood cultures will persist. In this situation, antibiotics are used. The catheter should not be reinserted until at least 48 hours after the temperature has returned to normal. Patients with established and persistent fungemia should be treated appropriately with intravenous amphotericin B over a 4- to 6-week period depending on the total dose given.

Metabolic Complications

Hyperglycemia. This occurs when the rate of infusion exceeds the rate at which the body can metabolize glucose. It may be caused by infusing the amino acid–dextrose mixture too rapidly or by metabolic factors. The ability to utilize glucose may be decreased by trauma and sepsis. It should be noted that the sudden appearance of hyperglycemia in a patient who was previously euglycemic usually heralds infection. This ability may also be compromised by the following conditions: diabetes, pancreatitis, liver disease, some antibiotics (cephalosporins), and steroids.

The first sign of hyperglycemia is usually glucosuria (2+ or more by Clinitest). If this is allowed to continue and is not treated, it will lead to the development of osmotic diuresis, followed by hyperosmolar nonketotic acidosis and possibly coma. The patient should be watched carefully for glucose intolerance and if glucosuria, dry skin, oliguria, confusion, or lethargy are noted, the nurse should be instructed to call the physician. If hyperglycemia persists due to continuing glucose intolerance, the blood glucose levels should be measured regularly and exogenous insulin may be infused or the flow rate decreased.

When insulin is needed, it is more economically given by a constant infusion for several reasons. If the patient is acutely sick and has low blood pressure or poor peripheral circulation, then intravenous infusion (in contrast to subcutaneous administration) is the only way to ensure that injected insulin is available to the body. The intravenous route allows careful control of blood sugar in the unstable patient. Finally, the requirements for insulin with a constant infusion are low compared with the amounts required using intermittent dosage.

Hypoglycemia. This is less common but may occur if hypertonic glucose infusions flowing at a rapid rate are abruptly terminated or decreased. Mechanical causes, such as clogged filters, kinked tubing, or piggybacking of additional medications can lead to this phenomenon. Symptoms include weakness, trembling, diaphoresis, headache, chills, rapid pulse, and decreased consciousness.

Ensuring a constant flow of hypertonic glucose infusions prevents hypoglycemia. If the volume infused falls behind schedule, do not increase the rate to "catch up." The rate should be recalculated in order to infuse at a uniform rate the prescribed amount of solution over the remainder of the 24 hours, provided this rate does not exceed the original drip rate by more than 10 percent.

Electrolyte Imbalances. The most common imbalances involve potassium, phosphorus, and magnesium. During active protein synthesis and anabolism, the level of these ions in the plasma may fall. Careful monitoring of laboratory values and attention to the general condition of the patient (i.e., urine output, heart rate, etc.) will help to detect deficiencies and excesses. These should be corrected immediately, usually through a change in the PN prescription. Severe hypokalemia should be treated by discontinuing PN and giving boluses of potassium.

Trace Element Deficiencies. Trace element deficiencies can be avoided by daily supplementation with these elements. Zinc deficiency causes a rash and loss of hair and of taste. Copper deficiency causes anemia and leukopenia. Chromium deficiency causes persistent hyperglycemia, and selenium deficiency causes muscle pain.

Vitamin Deficiencies. Vitamins should be added to the PN solution daily, since most vitamin stores are depleted in malnourished patients. The input of fat-soluble vitamins should be carefully controlled; excessive intake of vitamins A and D can cause toxic effects, especially hypercalcemia.

Hyperlipoproteinemia. An elevation of blood lipids may occur as a result of overproduction of lipids from endogenous sources, overinfusion of exogenous lipids, or reduced utilization, singly or in combination. The overproduction of lipids causing hyperlipidemia may result from infusing carbohydrates in excess of needs. Correspondingly, excessively high infusion rates of lipid emulsions may also cause hyperlipidemia, despite the 500 IU of heparin added to 500 ml of lipid emulsion (in order to activate lipoprotein lipase). Under these circumstances, reducing total caloric intake, both the carbohydrate and lipid moieties, can restore blood lipid levels to normal. Even with an appropriate caloric intake however, a deficiency of lipoprotein lipase, as with the syndrome of Type I hyperlipoproteinemia, may impair lipid clearance. This may also occur with severe protein deficiency and diabetes.

Hypercholesterolemia. Hypercholesterolemia may be seen when lipid emulsions are infused at high rates, i.e., in excess of 2 g per kilogram per day. The elevation returns to normal within a few days of discontinuing the infusion.

Abnormalities of Liver Function. The most common abnormality of liver function is a slight rise in the alkaline phosphatase level, which returns to normal and has no clinical significance. Fatty liver is also a common problem due to the infusion of carbohydrate in excess of caloric needs, and/or to a deficiency of essential fatty acids. Clinically the patient presents with a large tender liver and an elevation of serum glutamic-oxaloacetic transaminase (SGOT).

The other hepatic clinical syndrome seen with PN is cholestatic jaundice with elevated serum bilirubin and alkaline phosphatase. This syndrome occurs commonly in children and bears a relation to the duration of PN. Interestingly, it is seldom seen in home PN patients despite the fact that they have been receiving PN for years. Hence, the condition does not result simply from prolonged PN, but is probably due to a combination of prolonged PN and acute illness. One such factor may be sepsis, since jaundice is most often seen clinically in adults who become septic or those with foci of infection.

Pancreatitis. When pancreatitis is seen in association with PN it may be due either to hypercalcemia or to hyperlipidemia. In practice, we have identified the former as being the main cause of pancreatitis.

Essential Fatty Acid Deficiency (EFAD). EFAD is manifested as dry, scaly skin and hair loss. This can be prevented or corrected by administration of a fat emulsion intravenously. When lipid is used as a source of calories this deficiency is never seen.

SUGGESTED READING

Brenner BM, Meyer TW, Hostetter TH. Dietary protein intake and the progressive nature of kidney disease: the role of hemodynamically mediated glomerular injury in the pathogenesis of progressive glomerular sclerosis in aging, renal ablation, and intrinsic renal disease. N Engl J Med 1982; 307:652–659.

Halperin ML, Wolman SL, Greenberg GR. Paracellular recirculation of sodium is essential to support nutrient absorption in the gastrointestinal tract: an hypothesis. Clin Invest Med 1986; 9:209–211.

Nilas L, Christiansen C, Rodboro P. Calcium supplementation and post-menopausal bone loss. Br Med J 1984; 289:1103–1106.

NUTRITION AND PEDIATRICS

FEEDING THE PRETERM INFANT

STANLEY H. ZLOTKIN, M.D., Ph.D., F.R.C.P.(C)
MAX PERLMAN, M.B., F.R.C.P.(Lond), F.R.C.P.(C)

Premature birth is formally defined as birth prior to 37 weeks' gestation. In the 1980s, the lower end of the spectrum of gestational age compatible with life is about 23 weeks. Survival rates of infants of 24 to 25 weeks' gestation (equivalent to birth weights of 600 to 900 g) are presently 50 percent or greater. The nutrient needs of premature infants differ qualitatively as well as quantitatively from those of full-term infants, owing to their relatively rapid growth rates (Table 1), their low nutrient reserves at birth (Table 2), and their functional immaturity (Table 3). Examples of the latter include low bile acid concentration, decreased pancreatic lipase activity, and reduced intestinal brush-border lactase activity together resulting in malabsorption of fats and lactose. In addition to a tendency toward nutrient deficiencies, the premature infant may be vulnerable to specific nutrient toxicities, owing to poor metabolic homeostasis, especially in liver and kidneys. Finally, the premature infant's nutrient needs are influenced by disease states that are specific to that age group. These include disorders initiated before birth, for example placental insufficiency, resulting in fetal undernutrition and poor fetal growth (so-called SGA or small-for-gestational-age infants).

The goals of feeding the premature infant are to promote growth, prevent specific nutrient deficiencies, and maintain metabolic equilibrium. Although the goal of promoting growth is well accepted, there is controversy as to the most appropriate rate of growth. We feel that duplication of the rates of intrauterine growth and nutrient deposition while

TABLE 1 Growth Rates During the First Year of Life

Age (days)	Growth Rate (g/kg/day)
−60 to −30 (premature)	15–20
8 to 24	10
42 to 56	6.5
84 to 112	3.5
365	1

maintaining metabolic stability is an appropriate goal. Since the fetus gains weight at about 15 to 20 g per kilogram per 24 hours during the early part of the last trimester of gestation, extrauterine feeding should result in a similar rate of weight gain. As the infant's "corrected age" approaches full term, the rate of weight gain decreases to around 10 g per kilogram per 24 hours.

TABLE 2 Nutrient Reserves

Tissues	Body Weight (kg)		
	70	3.5	1.0
Fat (adipose triglyceride)			
kg	15 (21%)[*]	0.53 (15%)	0.023 (2.3%)
kcal	141,000	4,800	200
Protein (mainly muscle)			
kg	6	0.45	0.085
kcal	24,000	1,800	340
Glycogen (muscle)			
kg	0.15	0.026	0.004
kcal	600	104	24
Glycogen (liver)			
kg	0.75	0.013	0.002
kcal	300	52	8

* Percentage of body weight.

TABLE 3   Relating Gastrointestinal Physiology to Feeding

Physiology	*Response*
Suck weak or absent	Tube feeding
Small stomach (tendency to reflux)	Small or continuous feeds
Decreased lactase activity	Formulas with low lactose or alternate carbohydrate
Low bile acid concentration	Use medium-chain triglycerides ·
Low lipase activity	Use medium-chain triglycerides
Immature water and electrolyte absorption by large bowel	Isotonic formulas
Decreased nutrient stores	Increased nutrient density of formulas
Enzyme immaturity	Formulas contain taurine, cystine, etc.
Poor intestinal motility	TPN
Immature renal function (increased losses of Na)	Augmented Na intake

SPECIFIC NUTRIENT REQUIREMENTS

Based on the intrauterine growth model and many studies examining the effect of varying combinations of nutrients on growth, the estimated protein needs of the premature infant are 3 g per kilogram per 24 hours; energy needs are 120 kcal per kilogram per 24 hours. It is important to note, however, that individual infants whose growth is unsatisfactory at 120 kcal per kilograms per day may need higher energy intakes.

The caloric density of the formulas specially designed for the premature infant is either 68 or 81 kcal per 100 milliliters. The energy content of the formula is supplied as a combination of fat and carbohydrate calories. Fat provides the major source of energy for growing premature infants. In human milk, about 50 percent of the energy is from fat, and in commercial formulas fat provides 40 to 50 percent of the energy. The saturated triglycerides of cow's milk are poorly absorbed and digested by the premature infant. Unsaturated long-chain triglycerides from vegetable oils, on the other hand, are much better absorbed. However, medium-chain triglycerides are even better absorbed, presumably because their digestion and absorption are not dependent on duodenal intraluminal bile salt levels, which are low in the premature infant. Thus the recently developed special formulas for premature infants contain a mixture of medium-chain triglycerides and predominantly unsaturated long-chain triglycerides. The essential fatty acid requirement of at least 3 percent of total calories in the form of linoleic acid is amply met by this fat mixture. Because of limited gastric capacity, the more calorically concentrated formula (81 kcal per 100 milliliters) allows the use of smaller feeding volumes. In order to achieve the recommended 120 kcal per kilogram per day energy intake, 150 ml per kilogram per day of the concentrated formula would have to be provided. At this intake, the formula provides sufficient water for the excretion of the renal solute load (urea and electrolytes). However, if lower volumes are given, there may be insufficient water provided for renal excretion due to the relatively constant extrarenal losses.

The type of protein most suitable for premature infants is currently under study. The choices include casein-predominant formulas (18:82 ratio of whey:casein cow's milk protein) versus whey-predominant formulas (60:40 ratio of whey:casein protein). When formula is given at a volume that provides the recommended protein intake, the significance of the type of protein (whey versus casein) is not readily apparent.

In the first few days of life, intestinal lactase activity may be low. Lactose that remains undigested will act as a substrate for bacterial proliferation in the lower intestine. In addition, the lactose may cause intestinal distention by its osmotic effect. Enzymes for the metabolism of glucose polymers are active in the premature infant early in gestation; thus glucose polymers in formula are well tolerated even at birth. On the basis of these physiologic considerations, the carbohydrate portions of the various special formulas for premature infants contain approximately 40 to 50 percent lactose and 50 to 60 percent glucose polymers.

MINERALS

Premature infants are not born with well-developed renal sodium conservation mechanisms. The use of mature human milk or commercial formulas designed for the feeding of term infants, both having low sodium content, has led to hyponatremia in preterm infants. Special formulas for premature infants, although higher in sodium than formulas for the full-term infant, provide less than 3 mmol per kilogram per day of sodium at full feeding levels. Formula alone, therefore, is unlikely to meet the needs of infants whose body weight is less than 1,500 g since this group may require from 4 to 8 mmol per kilogram per day of sodium to prevent hyponatremia. The potassium and magnesium needs of the premature infant are similar to those of the term infant at 2 to 3 mmol per kilogram per day and are met by breast milk or formula.

Human milk and formulas designed for term infants are deficient in calcium and phosphorus relative to the needs of the preterm infant. In order to duplicate the fetal retention rate for calcium and phosphorus in the very-low-birth-weight premature infant (less than 1,500 g), recommended intakes of these minerals are 185 to 210 mg per kilogram per day for calcium and 120 to 140 mg per kilogram per day for phosphorus. At the time of writing, the only "preterm" formula that has sufficient calcium and phosphorus when ingested at tolerable volumes is Similac Special Care (Ross Laboratories, Columbus, Ohio, Table 4).

There is no clear indication for iron supplementation before 1 to 2 months of age. The early physiologic anemia of prematurity is not affected by iron therapy. If an infant receives regular blood transfusions to maintain hemoglobin concentration, the introduction of oral iron supplements should be delayed until transfusions have ceased. When the infant reaches a weight of 2,000 g or is discharged home, the daily intake of elemental iron should be 2 to 3 mg per kilogram to a maximum of 15 mg per day (as ferrous sulfate drops) for the infant receiving breast

TABLE 4 Volume of Ingested Formula Needed to Meet Advisable Intakes of Specific Nutrients

| | | Volume (ml) to be Ingested to Meet Advisable Intake | | |
	Advisable Intake*	Enfamil Premature	SMA "Preemie"	Similac Special Care
Energy (kcal)†	120	148	148	148
Protein (g)	3.5	146	175	159
Sodium (mEq)	3.0	214	214	200
Chloride (mEq)	2.5	132	153	139
Potassium (mEq)	2.3	100	121	88
Calcium (mg)	185	195	247	128
Phosphorus (mg)	123	256	308	171
Magnesium (mg)	8.5	106	121	85
Zinc (mg)	0.6	75	120	50
Copper (μg)	108	148	154	54
Manganese (μg)	6	29	30	30

* For an infant between 29 and 31 weeks of gestational age (1,200 to 1,800 g).
† All data are expressed as kg/24 hours.

milk or unsupplemented formula. Supplements are not necessary for infants receiving iron-fortified formula. Iron supplements should be continued until the infant is on an adequate full-mixed diet (usually 12 to 15 months).

There are still no firm conclusions regarding the optimal concentration of trace metals to be included in a premature infant's diet. In order to prevent deficiencies, yet avoid toxicity, it is recommended that infant formulas contain 0.5 mg zinc, 90 μg copper, and 5 μg manganese per 100 kilocalories. Iodine uptake by the thyroid gland of the premature infant is similar to that of older children, thus the recommended dose of iodine for the full-term infant (5 μg per 100 kilocalories) is also the recommended dose for the premature infant. These recommended intakes can be achieved with any of the special "preterm" formulas (see Table 4). Although other minerals (such as cobalt, molybdenum, selenium, and chromium) are probably nutritionally essential in trace amounts, there is no information on which to base recommendations for intake dosages. Fluoride at 0.25 mg per day should be provided at age 6 months if the local water supply is not fluoridated, whether the infant is receiving breast milk or formula.

VITAMINS

The recommended oral intakes of vitamins A, K, B$_6$ (pyridoxine), thiamine, B$_{12}$, riboflavin, niacin, pantothenic acid, biotin, and folic acid for premature infants are the same as those for full-term infants. It is essential that all premature as well as term infants receive at least 1 mg of vitamin K at birth. Folic acid deficiency is unusual, although premature infants are prone to biochemical folate deficiency as demonstrated by hypersegmentation of their neutrophils. Premature infants weighing less than 2,000 g should receive 50 μg per day of folic acid (compared to 40 μg per day in the full-term). The prevention of severe bone disease in premature infants appears to rely on both high oral intakes of calcium and phosphorus and an intake of vitamin D between 500 to 1,000 IU per day. Because premature infants normally malabsorb fat, including the fat-soluble vitamins, the requirement for vitamin E, α-tocopherol, in the premature infant is higher than that of the term infant. In addition, vitamin E deficiency is exacerbated by a high intake of iron or polyunsaturated fatty acids, each of which increases the vitamin E requirement. The minimum recommended intake of vitamin E is 0.7 IU (0.5 mg of d-α-tocopherol) per 100 kilocalories and at least 1.0 IU of vitamin E per gram of linoleic acid. Dosages as high as 5 to 25 IU of supplemental vitamin E are considered acceptable because of the potential for intestinal malabsorption. Doubt has been cast on the use of large doses of vitamin E to prevent either retrolental fibroplasia or bronchopulmonary dysplasia.

All of the premature infant formulas provide the recommended dosages of vitamins as described above (except for vitamin D and folic acid), when more than 150 ml per kilogram per day is ingested. As a general rule, all premature infants, whether receiving breast milk or formula, should receive a daily multivitamin supplement. Folic acid is unstable in liquid form and therefore not included in multivitamin preparations. An intake of Similac Special Care 24 at 170 ml per kilogram per day will provide more than 50 μg per day of folic acid, or folic acid may be added to a multivitamin preparation in the hospital pharmacy.

THE USE OF HUMAN MILK

Premature infants who are fed banked human milk grow more slowly than infants fed formula. The reason for the slower growth is that the low concentration of energy, protein, and minerals in banked human milk is inadequate to sustain growth at intrauterine rates. Thus banked human milk is currently considered inadequate for the premature infant.

The milk produced by mothers who prematurely give birth ("preterm milk") is nutritionally different in composition from mature human milk. For the first 2 to 4 weeks of lactation, preterm milk has a higher concentration of energy (calories), protein, sodium, and chloride and a lower concentration of lactose. The concentration of other minerals, including calcium and phosphorus, is similar or even decreased in preterm compared to mature milk. The secretory immunoglobulin A (lgA) is also present in a higher concentration in preterm compared to mature milk. After 4 weeks, the nutritional composition of preterm and mature milk is similar.

Premature infants who are fed their own mother's milk at appropriate rates during the first month of life (180 to 200 ml per kilogram per day) exhibit growth rates comparable to intrauterine rates. However, the concentration of calcium, phosphorus, and possibly sodium, iron, copper, and zinc in preterm milk is still considered insufficient for the preterm infant. Mixtures of protein, carbohydrate, calcium, phosphate, trace minerals, and vitamins for addition to preterm milk have been developed by commercial formula manufacturers. When the fortifiers are added to preterm milk, the resultant nutrient, mineral, and vitamin concentrations approach those of the formulas developed for feeding premature infants. The clinical significance of this supplementation is presently under investigation and has yet to be adequately demonstrated. At the Hospital For Sick Children (Toronto), when the intake of "preterm" mother's milk is greater than 50 percent of an infant's daily fluid volume requirement, all infants receive a daily supplement of 700 IU of vitamin D_3 and increasing amounts of calcium (as calcium lactate) from 60 mg per day for infants weighing less than 1,000 g to 125 mg per day for infants between 1,500 and 2,000 g.

FORMULAS FOR THE PREMATURE INFANT

Many of the nutritional features of the specially formulated preterm formulas have been discussed above and are shown in Table 4. The common features of the formulas are that they include the whey-predominant proteins, carbohydrate mixtures of lactose and glucose polymers, and fat mixtures containing combinations of medium-chain and relatively unsaturated long-chain triglycerides. Because the use of soy-protein–based formulas for premature infants has resulted in hypophosphatemic rickets, they are not recommended for routine use.

METHODS OF FEEDING

Due to lower morbidity and cost, whenever possible feeding via the gastrointestinal tract should be used in preference to parenteral feeding. Coordination of sucking, swallowing and respiration appears at approximately 34 to 36 weeks of gestation: thus, before this time, unless a strong suck reflex is present, enteral feeding is contraindicated. Where enteral feeding is not possible, tube feeding (either nasogastric or nasojejunal) may be used. The contraindications to enteral feeding are listed in Table 5.

If gastric emptying is not a problem, the optimal feeding regimen for the premature infant of less than 34 weeks gestation is bolus feeds into the stomach every 2 to 3 hours. Continuous gastric feeds may be better tolerated than bolus feeds by some small infants when gastric emptying is unsatisfactory. Nasogastric feeding of boluses of milk is associated with disturbances of blood gas tensions in infants with respiratory problems; thus, in some circumstances, continuous transpyloric feeds (nasojejunal feeds) may be better tolerated. Although clinical results with transpyloric feeds are often acceptable, bypassing the stomach and duode-

TABLE 5 Feeding Contraindications

Contraindications to Nipple Feeding	Contraindications to Enteral Feeding
Extreme prematurity	Acidosis
Dyspnea/tachypnea	Hypotension/shock
Ventilatory support (IPPB or CPAP)	Sepsis or suspected sepsis
Altered level of consciousness	Abdominal distention
Neuromuscular disease	Repeated prefeed gastric aspirates of
Congestive heart failure	>1 ml/kg
	Bile-stained gastric aspirate
	Seizures
	During and following an exchange
	transfusion

num by a jejunal tube may cause inefficient utilization of the nutrients in the formula. Moreover, nasojejunal tube feeding with polyvinyl chloride tubes has been associated with jejunal perforation.

The first feed after birth is usually at 4 to 24 hours of age, depending on the infant's gestational age, severity of illness, and perinatal history. The first feed should be water. If the daily fluid intake requirement cannot be established or maintained with tube feeding, supplements with parenteral dextrose, saline, and, later, parenteral nutrition may be necessary. Guidelines for initial feed volumes, the interval between feeds, and the volume and timing of increments for tube feeding are shown in Table 6.

Generally, the volume of intake should be increased slowly, so that full feeding volumes are not established in infants weighing less than 1,000 g before 10 to 14 days, and in infants weighing more than 1,500 g

TABLE 6 Starting Volumes, Feeding Intervals, and the Volume and Timing of Increments for Tube Feeding

Weight (g)	Initial Volume of Feed (ml)	Interval Between Feeds (hr)	Volume of Increment (ml)	Frequency of Change (hr)
<1,000	0.5–1.0	1–2	0.5–1.0	>24
1,000–1,500	1.0–2.0	2	1.0–2.0	≥12
1,500–2,000	2.0–3.0	2–3	2.0–4.0	≥12
2,000–2,500*	4.0–5.0	3	4.0–7.0	≥8
>2,500*	10.0	3–4	10–15	≥3

* For infants >34 weeks gestation with good suck and swallowing-breathing coordination, consider ad-libidum on-demand feeding.

in 6 to 8 days. This gradual introduction of enteral nutrients theoretically allows for the adaptation of the intestinal tract without the complications of vomiting, distention, or diarrhea. The tolerance to increases in the volume of feeds depends on the volume of gastric aspirate and degree of abdominal distention. Gastric aspirates (drawn prior to the feed) of more than 1 to 2 ml may be regarded as excessive, in which case feeding volumes should be decreased or feeds temporarily discontinued. Although no causative relationship has been established, overzealous feeding may be associated with aspiration pneumonia and necrotizing enterocolitis. Feed volumes larger than those shown in Table 6 may be indicated (as tolerated) in infants with hypoglycemia (or a predeliction for hypoglycemia), small-for-gestational-age (SGA) infants and infants of diabetic mothers. For the SGA infant, the feed volumes should be adjusted based on the expected twenty-fifth to fiftieth percentile birth weight for gestational age.

There are a number of clinical situations that increase the risk of morbidity associated with enteral feeding. For example, a feed should be omitted prior to extubation. If the infant has moderate chest retractions with a respiratory rate above 60 breaths per minute or is in severe respiratory distress as manifested by an FiO_2 greater than 0.5, and a Pco_2 greater than 50 Torr, enteral feeds should be discontinued. Table 5 lists the relative contraindications for the start of enteral feeding (or indications for discontinuing feeds that have already started). When enteral feeding is contraindicated, the decision to initiate total parenteral nutrition (TPN) depends on predictions of the duration of the contraindications.

The chapter on *Total Parenteral Nutrition in Pediatrics* gives a detailed review of the indications for the initiation of total or supplemental parenteral nutrition. Briefly, all patients with obstructive lesions of the GI tract who are unable to tolerate oral or enteral nutrients prior to or following surgery should receive TPN. Patients with necrotizing enterocolitis who are on total gut rest (usually for 7 to 10 days) should receive TPN. Infants whose birth weight is below 1,000 g who cannot be expected to tolerate full enteral feeds within 3 days should be started on supplemental parenteral nutrition (start on day 2). Infants whose birth weight is 1,000 to 1,500 g who cannot be expected to tolerate full enteral feeds within 5 days should be started on supplemental parenteral nutrition within 2 to 3 days. Infants whose birth weight is above 1,500 g who cannot be expected to tolerate oral or enteral feeds within 7 days should receive supplemental parenteral nutrition by day 3. As detailed in the chapter on *Total Parenteral Nutrition in Pediatrics*, the adequacy of TPN is determined through a combination of clinical, anthropometric, and biochemical monitoring.

Although many therapeutic interventions, including nutritional care, have influenced the decreasing mortality and morbidity rates associated with premature birth, the role of providing optimal nutrition to improve the quality of life in the increasing number of survivors should not be understated.

SUGGESTED READING

American Academy of Pediatrics, Committee on Nutrition. Nutritional needs of low-birth-weight infants. Pediatrics 1985; 75:976-986.

Committee on Nutrition of the Preterm Infant, European Society of Pediatric Gastroenterology and Nutrition. Nutrition and feeding of preterm infants. Acta Paediatr Scand; Supplement 336, 1987 in press.

Pereira GR, Barbosa NMM. Controversies in neonatal nutrition. Pediatr Clin North Am 1986; 33:65-89.

THE PEDIATRIC SURGICAL PATIENT

ROBERT M. FILLER, M.D., F.A.C.S., F.R.C.S.(C)

Nutritional support in pediatric surgical patients can take several forms. When gastrointestinal (GI) function is absent or inadequate, total parenteral nutrition (TPN) is indicated. The choice of a central or peripheral vein for the infusion of nutrients is usually based on individual patient considerations. The major advantage of the peripheral venous route is the lower incidence of catheter-related sepsis. Central venous TPN is better suited to the child with unusually high energy requirements or one needing large amounts of concentrated hyperosmolar solutions. Central TPN is required when peripheral veins are not apparent or when experienced IV teams are not present to maintain peripheral infusions on a 24-hour basis. We prefer central venous feedings in older children and adolescents since multiple venipunctures over a prolonged period are not well tolerated. When some degree of GI function is present, supplemental enteral feedings are used.

INDICATIONS FOR TPN

TPN is reserved for infants and children whose health is threatened because feeding by means of the GI tract is impossible, inadequate, or hazardous. The common conditions for which nutritional support is needed in surgical patients are listed in Table 1. The decision to start TPN is sometimes obvious, as for the infant with complicated omphalocele or one in whom a large portion of the midgut has been resected because of volvulus. However, the need for TPN may not be so clear in others. For example, in a child with chronic diarrhea and malnutrition, one must be certain that enteral therapy has failed before beginning TPN. Similarly, TPN is not always necessary in a child with cancer who develops anorexia, vomiting, and diarrhea from radiation and chemotherapy. The need for improved nutrition to save life and reduce morbidity always must be weighed against the possibility of serious metabolic or septic complications. TPN is not indicated when adequate nutrients can be safely de-

TABLE 1   Indications for Nutritional Support in Pediatric Surgical Patients

Congenital or acquired anomalies of the GI tract
  Gastroschisis/omphalocele
  Necrotizing enterocolitis
  Short gut syndrome
  Meconium ileus
  Intestinal atresia
  Inflammatory bowel disease
  Chronic intestinal obstruction due to
    peritonitis or adhesions
  Fistulas
  Intractable diarrhea
Malignant disease
Multiple trauma/burns
Renal failure
Prematurity

livered and absorbed from the GI tract by oral feedings, gavage, or gastrostomy with or without the use of special diets.

COMPOSITION OF SOLUTIONS

The components of the basic diets used in our TPN program are listed in Table 2. We have chosen Vamin-N*, a mixture of crystalline amino acids, to supply the protein requirements. Glucose is the sole source of carbohydrate in our formula and is the major source of energy when fat emulsions are not administered. Solutions containing more than 10 percent glucose cannot be used when TPN is given by peripheral vein because its hyperosmolality causes venous thrombosis in veins with relatively slow blood flow. Intralipid, 10 or 20 percent emulsion, is our standard source of fat.

Standard IV formulations are used in most cases, which makes the ordering and maintenance of TPN simpler, safer, and more economical. The P solutions in Table 2 (P-5, P-10) are intended for premature babies, while the I solutions (I-10, I-20) are meant for older children. Our standard solutions are further subdivided according to their glucose concentrations. P5, for example is the 5 percent dextrose solution used in the

---

* Pharmacia, Montreal, Quebec, Canada.

TABLE 2 Composition of Vamin-N* Based Standard Solutions (per Liter)

Nutrient	Premature Babies and Infants				Children and Adolescents	
	P-5	P-7.5	P-10	PI-10	I-10	I-20†
Protein (g)	15	15	20	20	30	30
Glucose (g)	50	75	100	100	100	200
Energy (kcal)‡	248	340	455	455	495	870
Na (mmol)	20	20	14.3	30	30	30
K (mmol)	20	20	18.9	30	30	30
Cl (mmol)	21.1	21.1	15.7	31.3	32.1	32.1
Ca (mmol)	9	9	9	9	9	9
P (mmol)	9	9	9	9	9	9
Mg (mmol)	3	3	4	4	4	4
Zn (μmol)	46	46	46	46	46	46
Cu (μmol)	6.3	6.3	6.3	6.3	6.3	6.3
Mn (μmol)	1.8	1.8	1.8	1.8	5.0	5.0
I (μmol)	0.47	0.47	0.47	0.47	0.47	0.47
Cr (μmol)	0.076	0.076	0.076	0.076	0.076	0.076
Se (μmol)	0.25	0.25	0.25	0.25	0.25	0.25
Fe (μmol)§	—	—	—	—	18	18

Fat emulsion 10%–1,100 kcal/liter
Fat emulsion 20%–2,000 kcal/liter
* Pharmacia, Montreal, Quebec, Canada.
† I-20 is intended for central venous line therapy only.
‡ Energy unit 1 kcal = 4.2 kJ. The energy content includes the potential energy from the protein as well as that from the glucose.
§ Iron can be included in the "P" solutions in neonates who have been receiving TPN for 1 month or more and should therefore be ordered.

premature infant, whereas I-20 contains 20 percent dextrose and is used in the older child or adolescent on central venous feedings.

A complete mixture of vitamins and trace minerals designed to meet the needs of each patient is added to the total daily volume in the hospital pharmacy.

TECHNIQUES OF INFUSION

Infusion rates for children of different ages are given in Table 3. The superior vena cava is the safest site for delivery when the central venous route is used, although some centers have successfully used the inferior vena cava by way of the saphenous vein. In the infant and small child, access to the superior vena cava is achieved by passing a small silicone rubber catheter down the internal or external jugular vein, which has been exposed by cutdown technique. Venous intubation is best performed in an operating room or cardiac catheterization laboratory, where proper instruments, adequate exposure, and strict aseptic conditions can be provided. We have had very little experience with percutaneous catheter insertion in the small child.

The choice of catheter material is of considerable importance. The incidence of superior vena cava thrombosis and venous or right atrial perforation is much higher with stiff catheters made of polyurethane and polyvinyl than with soft silicone rubber tubing. Many types of silicone

TABLE 3 Regimens for Standard Solutions and Intralipid*

	Premature Infants	Infants and Young Children (0–7 years)	Children and Adolescents (7–18 years)
Total fluid (ml/kg)	120–200	100–140	80–120
Standard amino acid/glucose solution (ml/kg)	120–200	80–100*	80
Intralipid (ml/kg)	0–40	20–40	20–40

* I-10 and I-20 should not be used at rates exceeding 150 ml/kg/day or total intake of 3,000 ml/day.

rubber catheters are currently in use. Our catheter has a specially designed internal fixation device that avoids some of the problems seen with Broviac and Hickman type catheters.

The catheter is inserted under local or general anesthesia acccording to the age and status of the child. The external jugular vein is ordinarily the preferred site of insertion, but when the catheter cannot be passed centrally because of previous use or anatomical difficulties, the internal jugular vein is used. The internal jugular vein can almost always be cannulated even if it has been the site of previous cannulations.

The central venous line is left in place until completion of therapy, unless it is accidentally dislodged or septic complications develop. Many catheters have been in place for more than 1 year.

Routine catheter care includes weekly sterile dressing changes and application of povidone-iodine (Betadine) ointment to the venous exit site. The infusion tubing and administration set are changed every 2 days. Systemic antibiotics are not employed unless specifically indicated by the patient's primary illness. The IV feeding program must be supervised by specially trained personnel, alert to all potential hazards.

In the first days of TPN, daily measurement of body weight, urine volume, and extrarenal fluid losses is essential. Urine sugar content is monitored at each voiding. The most important blood tests and frequency of their study are given in Table 4. More frequent monitoring may be necessary in children with specific metabolic abnormalities.

Weight change during the period of IV feeding varies with overall clinical status and is an excellent guide to adequacy of treatment. Weight gains comparable to those of normal infants may be expected in children who are not malnourished at the time IV feeding is instituted or in whom sepsis is not a factor. In the patient with infection or other problems that increase metabolic requirements, a flatter growth curve is observed. Significant weight gain in the first 2 weeks is not usually seen in infants and children who are severely depleted at the start of treatment. Excessive weight gain usually means that the child is receiving too much fluid. Weight gains associated with peripheral venous infusions are comparable to those seen with central infusions as long as the planned volume of fluid to be infused can be maintained.

In most patients, the large quantities of IV glucose are usually well tolerated without the addition of exogenous insulin. Glycosuria sometimes indicates the onset of bloodstream infection, especially when it develops after many days of treatment.

**TABLE 4   Clinical Laboratory Blood Tests with
Minimum Frequency of Monitoring**

Weekly

Na, K, Cl
Urea
Glucose
Magnesium
Calcium, phosphorus
Total protein
Hemoglobin, hematocrit, white blood
   cell count
Blood culture

Every 2 weeks

SGOT, LDH, alkaline phosphatase
Bilirubin
Creatinine

As indicated

Copper
Zinc
Iron
Ammonia
Osmolarity
pH

HOME TPN

TPN at home should be considered for all patients requiring IV feeding for many months when the underlying cause no longer requires treatment in the hospital. Most of the candidates for home treatment have short bowel syndrome or chronic inflammatory bowel disease. A central venous catheter is necessary in these children.

Patients and their families must be instructed about catheter care, and a source for appropriate sterile nutrient solution must be provided. Back-up support from a TPN team and a pharmacy is necessary.

IV infusions are regulated at home by a constant infusion pump over a 10- to 14-hour period each day. Feedings are usually given at night, so that the patient can engage in normal activities during the day. After the daily ration is administered, the IV catheter is filled with a dilute heparin solution and capped to prevent clotting. Children with short-bowel syndrome usually tolerate additional feeding by mouth, whereas food is withheld completely in patients in whom the objective is to put the intestinal tract at complete rest. Catheter and metabolic complications are rare in these patients.

COMPLICATIONS

Metabolic Abnormalities

Potential complications are many, but most patients tolerate TPN well. Complications usually can be prevented by careful clinical and laboratory monitoring and appropriate adjustment of the infusate.

Persistent glucose intolerance and hyperglycemia, in the absence of sepsis, occur only in low birthweight premature infants and in children with severe renal and central nervous system abnormalities. Hypoglycemia has been reported when TPN is stopped abruptly, but we have not observed this complication despite many accidental interruptions of the infusion. Nevertheless, we recommend a slow weaning from the IV diet when TPN is no longer needed and oral feedings start.

Copper, magnesium, and zinc deficiencies have been observed in the past, especially in patients with chronic diarrhea and those on TPN diets containing insufficient trace metals. In the patient with depleted trace metal stores, overt clinical signs of deficiency are most likely to develop after nutritional therapy is begun, when weight gain and growth are being restored. Now that nutrient solutions contain copper, magnesium, and zinc, these clinical signs are no longer being seen.

Essential fatty acid deficiency does not develop in patients on Intralipid, and most of these patients have normal serum triglycerides and cholesterol during treatment. Serious elevations of serum lipid can be prevented by proper monitoring and adjusting the dose accordingly. The preterm infant is at greatest risk for hyperlipidemia.

Hypocalcemia, hypercalcemia, hypophosphatemia, and hyperphosphatemia have occurred in patients fed solely by vein, but these problems are not seen in the majority of patients receiving the quantities of calcium and phosphorus now administered.

Signs of abnormal liver function are frequently observed during TPN. Transient hepatic enlargement, with or without abnormal liver function tests, is noted during the first week of treatment in most small infants. Variable or transient elevations of SGOT, LDH, and serum bilirubin occur during treatment in many patients. Although cholestasis is a prominent feature histologically, the exact etiology is still unknown. Hepatic fibrosis with liver failure resulting in death occurs in the most severe cases and is the most serious hazard of TPN.

Children receiving TPN are at risk for the development of gallstones. This complication seems to be most common in children with abnormalities of the ileum. Periodic ultrasound examinations are indicated for children on long-term TPN to detect gallstones at a preclinical stage.

The fat overload syndrome is a rare complication of Intralipid administration, characterized by fever, irritability, respiratory distress, jaundice, and a bleeding diathesis. Although rare, the existence of this syndrome reinforces the need for monitoring of lipid levels in patients on TPN.

Metabolic acidosis and hyperammonemia are not problems with currently used IV diets.

Technical Problems

Many of the early technical problems associated with central venous catheter have now been corrected. The following problems have been experienced by us or noted in the literature:

1. Transient arrhythmias associated with insertion of the catheter, especially if the tip enters the heart.
2. Dislodgement of the IV catheter with subcutaneous accumulation of TPN solution.
3. Venous perforation with pleural or intrapericardial collection of TPN solution or blood. This has not been reported with silicone rubber catheters.
4. Thrombosis of the vein in which the catheter is placed, leading to venous distention and sometimes edema in the face and head. Pulmonary embolus is rare. We have had some success with the use of urokinase to lyse clots in thrombosed catheters.
5. Obstruction of the infusion system by kinking or clotting of the catheter.
6. Accidental uncoupling of joints in the infusion circuit, contaminating the system and allowing back-up of blood in the line with subsequent obstruction to flow.
7. Air embolus.

Infection

Sepsis remains the major complication of TPN in the pediatric patient. Long-term indwelling venous cannulae are a well-documented source of bloodstream infection. Organisms enter the bloodstream along the catheter tract or with contaminated IV solution. The catheter, as a foreign body in the bloodstream, acts as a focus for bacterial growth even when the organisms enter from a remote site.

The most common bacteria cultured from the blood of septic patients are *Staphylococcus epidermis* and coliform organisms. Candidial infections are now rare.

As a rule, catheter-related sepsis is treated by removing the line and administering appropriate IV antibiotics for 7 to 10 days. It is best to delay replacement of the central venous line during this period in order to prevent recolonization of the new catheter. In some cases, especially after repeated infections, catheter sepsis has been successfully treated by a 3-week course of appropriate IV antibiotics without removal of the catheter. This should be done only in selected cases and when there is a prompt clinical response to the antibiotics. Sepsis can be minimized by strict adherence to recommended catheter care techniques.

One should always remember that bloodstream infection can complicate peripheral TPN as well.

ENTERAL FEEDING

The indications for and techniques of delivery of chemically defined diets in pediatric surgical patients are similar to those in adults. We have found chemically defined diets to be most useful in infants and young children with short bowel syndrome, either as an alternative to TPN or during the weaning process, and in patients with inflammatory bowel disease. The most commonly used formulas are noted in Table 5.

TABLE 5 Chemically Defined Diets used for Enteral Feedings

Formula	Protein Source	Carbohydrate Source	Fat Source	Osmolality (mOsm/kg H₂O)	Calories/100 ml (Standard dilution)
SMA₂₀*	Cow's milk	Lactose	Vegetable oil	295	67
Pregestimil	Casein hydrolysate	Glucose polymer	Corn oil MCT† (40%)	338	69
Portagen	Sodium caseinate	Sucrose dextrose	Corn oil MCT (88%)	236	96
Vivonex	Crystalline amino acids	Glucose oligosaccharides	Safflower oil	550	100
Nutramigen	Casein hydrolysate	Sucrose Tapioca	Corn oil	443	66

* SMA₂₀ is a standard infant formula.
† MCT–Medium=chain triglyceride

SUGGESTED READING

Filler RM, Eraklif AJ, Rubin VG, et al. Long term parenteral nutrition in infants. N Engl J Med 1969; 281:589–594.

Heird WC, Greene HL. Panel report of nutritional support of pediatric patients. Am J Clin Nutr 1981; 34:1223–1234.

Roslyn JJ, Berquist WE, Pitt HA, et al. Increased risk of gallstones in children receiving total parenteral nutrition. Pediatrics 1983; 71:784–789.

Winthrop AL, Wesson DE. Urokinase in the treatment of occluded central venous catheters in children. J Pediatr Surg 1984; 19:536–538.

CYSTIC FIBROSIS

JOHN PATRICK, M.B., B.S., M.D.
MARGARET P. BOLAND, M.D., F.R.C.P.C.

The basic principles that guide our approach to the nutritional care of cystic fibrosis (CF) can be summarized as follows:

1. Document the functional failure of the pancreas by the demonstration of steatorrhea.
2. Treat insufficiency by replacement of pancreatic digestive enzymes with Cotazyme or Pancrease (enteric coated enzymes).
3. Give routine water-soluble forms of fat-soluble vitamins on the grounds that deficiencies have been documented. Mineral supplements and water-soluble vitamins are given on an empirical basis.
4. Provide an initial nutrition education package for parents.
5. Thereafter, monitor growth; if growth is normal, there is nothing further to do by way of nutritional support.
6. When wasting appears, check that the diet is of high energy density and that the prime importance of energy is understood by the parents and the child.
7. When wasting continues, despite maximal dietetic efforts, start long-term supplementary enterostomy feeding.
8. When carbon dioxide retention commences gradually, spread the daily energy intake over a longer period of time. This is greatly facilitated when enterostomy feeding is available.

It is not necessary to outline the features of cystic fibrosis here, but it is worth remembering that cystic fibrosis affects the cardiovascular, endocrine, neurologic, and reproductive systems as well as the lungs and the pancreas. The common link between these disparate features may be an abnormality in chloride transport. If that is the case, nutrition may modulate the effects of that transport defect by altering the structure of cell membranes; dietary lipids have already been shown to be capable of modifying membranes in this way.

422

GROWTH FAILURE

The more obvious effects of dietary inadequacies in CF are on growth, but one should emphasize that there are several patterns of growth failure. Some children have problems from the start, some never have problems, some are both stunted and wasted, some just stunted, and some just wasted. The final stages of the illness may be marked by a very slow, inexorable weight loss or by a series of episodic drops in weight associated with acute respiratory exacerbations. Occasionally, a child has a very rapid weight loss terminally that cannot be reversed even with enterostomy feeding. While growth failure is usually the response to a failure of energy supply, more specific nutrient deficiencies may also occur, secondary to the steatorrhea. The classification of growth failure will be described later.

STEATORRHEA

Assessing steatorrhea by signs and symptoms alone is not adequate; measurement of fecal fat excretion on a known fat intake is a necessary part of investigation. The focus should be on the correction of the nutritional consequences of steatorrhea. In the past, too much emphasis was placed on controlling the symptoms of malabsorption even if this required limitation of dietary fat. When children with cystic fibrosis begin to waste, dietary fat must be increased. This will lead to increased fecal excretion of fat, but if the child's energy balance is improved, this does not matter. Energy balance is more important than complete control of steatorrhea.

ENZYME REPLACEMENT—HOW MUCH AND HOW OFTEN?

Modern pancreatic replacement therapy has greatly improved the management of children with cystic fibrosis. However, even with these modern products, the amount of enzyme taken is greatly in excess of what should be biochemically necessary, implying that there are still problems with delivery of active enzyme to the small bowel. The critical enzyme is lipase, and we find that one capsule is required for approximately every 5 g of fat when added to enteral feed delivered to the jejunum. When the pancreatic replacement is taken with food, the requirement is much more variable from patient to patient because of the vagaries of gastric acid, gastric emptying, and small bowel pH. Some patients will consume enough replacements to raise their serum uric acid levels, but we have not seen any serious problems as a result. The role of bile salts in the absorptive problems of cystic fibrosis is still an area of active research, but as yet there are no definitive practical implications.

VITAMINS

What little data there are on water-soluble vitamins indicate that patients do not have serious deficiencies except for vitamin B_{12} in those patients with terminal ileum resection; these patients need appropriate parenteral supplementation. Supplementation with other B complex and C vitamins is probably unnecessary but is not dangerous. The fat-soluble vitamins are susceptible to loss with steatorrhea, and deficiencies of these have been documented despite pancreatic enzyme supplementation. Postmortem changes in the central nervous system compatible with vitamin E deficiency have been seen even in patients taking the currently recommended amounts of vitamin E. Measurement of vitamin E levels in relation to serum lipids may be necessary for optimization of dosage. The water-miscible forms are better absorbed than the fat-soluble forms, and it is recommended that patients be routinely supplemented with vitamins A, D, E, and K. Vitamin D and A are potentially toxic, but there are no reports of toxicity in patients with cystic fibrosis.

MINERALS

These can be conveniently divided into the macro minerals—Na, K, Ca, P, and Mg—and the trace minerals—Fe, Zn, Cu, Se, and Mn. The common practice is to supplement with NaCl in hot weather, and general dietary guidance for patients allows liberal use of table salt. Acquiring a taste for salty foods is not discouraged and at times is actively encouraged. This practice merits some serious review. The response of normal individuals who decrease Na intake from that of a normal North American diet (10 to 15 g NaCl per day) is to decrease urine and sweat loss of NaCl. This issue should be reexamined in cystic fibrosis. In the late stages of the disease, many patients develop cor pulmonale, and severe salt restriction in the diet is a necessary and rational treatment but one difficult to achieve in patients who, because of their habitual high salt intakes, crave salt. Some authors have warned of the potential for shock in patients who are severely restricted. We have restricted Na intake to 300 mg in teenage patients with no ill effects.

There are no data to support recommendations to supply anything but normal dietary amounts of Ca and P. Bone disease, when it occurs, relates to vitamin D deficiency, rather than mineral deficiency.

The trace minerals have been examined somewhat more closely. Iron deficiency anemia has been documented in cystic fibrosis patients, although iron absorption has been reported as normal. Gastroesophageal reflux with esophagitis, gastritis, and ulceration is not uncommon in sick patients, and this may be the site of blood loss causing iron deficiency. Treatment of the cause of blood loss should be combined with replenishment of body iron stores. Zn, Se, Cu, and Mn losses are stated to be increased with steatorrhea and high-fiber diets. Better control of the steatorrhea should result in better absorption of these nutrients. There are no descriptions of deficiency syndromes related to these nutrients in patients receiving appropriate dietary and enzyme treatment; however, some biochemical abnormalities are described, especially in patients with growth failure. The appropriate treatment for the biochemical abnormalities is not known. Some authors suggest routine supplementation of Zn and possibly Se. Children growing normally, with good hair, skin, and mucous membranes, are almost certainly not trace element deficient. Children receiving commercial enteral feeding products will be getting trace mineral supplements; therefore, the only group who may need mineral supplements are those attempting to correct weight loss by diet alone.

THE INITIAL EDUCATION PACKAGE

The diagnosis of cystic fibrosis carries with it so many implications and adjustments in living that the parents are often overwhelmed. Nutrition is only one small component. The development of educational materials that allow the parents to learn at their own rate and in an unstressed environment is the ideal. Not enough materials have been produced as far as we are aware, and dietitians should play a major role here. We feel that for efficient utilization of the dietitian's time, clear educational objectives should be set and the effectiveness of the educational process should be evaluated. The parents need to understand the effects of the disease on nutrient absorption, how enzyme replacement works, the importance of monitoring growth, and the energy density of foods. Once these objectives are met, further dietetic or nutritional treatment and counseling will not be necessary unless there is evidence of growth failure or the parents have specific questions.

MONITORING OF GROWTH

The first requirement for monitoring is to have a clear concept of which growth problems are nutritionally modifiable and which are not. A functional rather than an etiologic classification is therefore appropriate. Traditionally, protein-energy malnutrition (PEM) is classified into two main etiological categories.

1. Primary PEM: Kwashiorkor, marasmus, and undernutrition caused by starvation in the absence of any other disease process.
2. Secondary PEM: Loss or inadequate development of body cell mass or energy stores secondary to other disease processes that are associated with either increased nutritional requirements or a diminished capacity to feed.

However, it is more important to define malnutrition in terms that indicate the potential for worthwhile responses to treatment. The simplest and most convenient classification was described by J. C. Waterlow, who divided growth failure into two major categories, which he termed wasting and stunting. Stunting is the failure of statural growth. It does not carry a serious prognosis and is not responsive to acute nutritional intervention. Where stunting is a response to nutritional deprivation, it can be looked upon as an effective adaptation to limited energy supplies. Most cases of stunting in developed countries are of endocrine or metabolic origin. Attempts to correct stunting by intensive feeding can aggravate metabolic disorders.

Wasting, on the other hand, is a serious problem. In principle, it should be nutritionally remediable, unless there is also some ongoing metabolic or endocrine disease that precludes anabolism, as for example, chronic renal failure. It is defined as an inadequate body mass for length, and is detected by plotting weight against height on the appropriate standard charts. Intervention is necessary when a child falls off a previous track by more than 10 percentile lines or falls below 85 percent (not percentile) of the mean value. After the first year of life, weight for length is quite independent of age and sex until puberty. Severe wasting in primary malnutrition is associated with multiple functional abnormalities including those of cardiac, renal, endocrine, and fuel homeostasis. Description of these is beyond the scope of this chapter, but the practical consequences are that homeostatic mechanisms are impaired and maximal responses to all stresses are reduced. Hence, since these defects are corrected with refeeding, there are good a priori reasons for vigorous treatment of malnutrition in cystic fibrosis.

Our practice is to have all the children in the clinic measured at each visit by the same person, thus eliminating person-to-person error, and in an absolutely standardized fashion, thus reducing methodologic errors. A private area and wall-mounted stadiometer are essential for this purpose. When this is done, growth records are much more interpretable. Trends are picked up early and accuracy should be ±100 g for weight and ±0.5 cm for height. The need for nutritional counseling is eliminated in children who are growing normally, while conversely in children who are faltering, intense dietetic intervention is mandatory. Furthermore, growth data can then be used to determine for how long attempts should be made to achieve catch-up growth with oral supplements. Using these data to diagnose malnutrition has meant that we have not failed to increase body weight in any patient diagnosed as wasted who consented to follow our protocol for the treatment of malnutrition in cystic fibrosis.

DIETETIC MANAGEMENT OF WASTING

The first stage in the treatment of wasting requires enthusiastic and dedicated support from the dietitians. Their role is to carefully determine what and how frequently the child eats and then to help in the substitution of high-energy foods for low-energy foods and to encourage increased and appropriate snacking. Reference to recommended intakes is not useful—wasting is prima facie evidence of the inadequacy of the current energy intake, no matter what it is. Reference to particular goals like 150 percent of the RNI or RDA is likewise not helpful. Growth is the object of the exercise and that should determine the intake.

There is still too much emphasis on the quality of food in most clinics; quantity is far more important. For this purpose, it is apparent that fat at 9 kcal per gram is more valuable than protein or carbohydrate at 4 kcal per gram. Because protein requirements are met with 7 or 8 percent energy from protein, if enough food is eaten, enough protein will necessarily be eaten. It is very difficult to design a palatable diet that is energy sufficient and protein deficient.

The dietary prescription that results from these concepts needs to be carefully explained because it flouts the usual sound and correct public health advice such as is found in Canada's Food Guide. Vegetables, for example, have low energy densities (less than 50 kcal per 100 g for leaf vegetables); only legumes, pulses, and corn exceed 100 kcals. Fresh fruits also have a density of less than 100 kcal per 100 g, whereas dried and canned fruits are higher and preserved foods and confectionary items are in the 250 to 300 range because of their high fat content. Of course, there are important exceptions to these general rules, like avocadoes, with near 200 kcal per 100 g. Appropriate versions of food tables should be produced for parents as part of the educational package.

With the very best dietetic input, a child who falters in weight-for-height may regain weight for awhile, but it is probable that within 18 months dietary supplementation alone will be inadequate. It is important to be realistic about the likely outcome during this period. Family concerns over eating are not rare and it should be our objective to make everyone feel they have achieved all that could be achieved when supplementary enterostomy feeding becomes necessary.

It is important to put a definite time limit on how long oral supplementation can be accepted as adequate treatment without achieving preset weight-for-height goals. However, the psychological acceptance of the necessity for enterostomy feeds is a major barrier to the use of this form of treatment, and at present 12 to 18 months generally elapses from the first discussion of the possibility until the placement of a permanent tube.

INVASIVE METHODS OF SUPPORT

Indications

In this section we will outline the management of the child with wasting in whom attempts to correct the deficit in body weight by oral supplementation with high–energy density foods have failed. It is important to be aware that these approaches are still in the process of development and evaluation. If one carefully examines the weight charts of children with cystic fibrosis, several patterns emerge. Perhaps the most important pattern to recognize is that of the patients who lose a lot of weight (1.0 kg) with respiratory exacerbations. These patients then face the battle of achieving large "catch-up" weight gains between illnesses. These patients are very likely to benefit from enteral feeding, whether short-term nasogastric for rapid catch-up or long-term enterostomy for chronic support. For the first few episodes, nasogastric feeding may be the preferred route if the patient or family is reluctant to accept a permanent system. The other pattern is one of a slow inexorable downhill path. This group responds well to chronic enteral feeding but will achieve only transient benefit from short-term nasogastric feeding.

In our group of 13 patients started on jejunostomy feeding prior to the development of carbon dioxide retention and without any other disease except cystic fibrosis, we now have an approximate total of 30 patient years' experience ranging individually from 3 months to 4 years. Ten to 90 percent of daily intake is provided via the enterostomy tube. All patients use enterostomy feeding more intensively after a respiratory infection with weight loss and thereby minimize convalescence time. For example, we have recently had one patient gain 5 kg in 10 days after he had lost weight from a combination of traveling without using his enterostomy feeding system and an exacerbation of his chronic pulmonary infection. Patients use all of the commercially available standard enteral feeds, usually starting with an isotonic product such as Isocal but thereafter often moving to more energy-dense formulas.

The Quantitative Logic of Enteral Feeding

The logic of the treatment is clear once a quantitative approach to energy requirements is adopted. Measurements of energy expenditure in cystic fibrosis indicate that in the later stages of the disease, energy requirements are in the range of 130 to 150 percent of normal. In addition, even with optimal enzyme replacement, some malabsorption of dietary energy will occur, and the oral intake will therefore need to be in excess of 150 percent of normal. The easiest way to demonstrate this is to feed via an enteral tube with increments in energy intake every 3 to 5 days; the point at which weight gain just commences is a reasonable estimate of the daily maintenance requirements. Thereafter, weight gain requires the absorption of a further 25 to 50 kJ (5 to 10 kcals)* for every gram of tissue laid down. Thus a child with a 2 kg weight loss during an acute exacerbation of respiratory infection must consume 10 to 20,000 kcal in addition to the ongoing increased maintenance requirements in order to regain lost weight. This is an unreasonable burden to place on a sick, anorexic child and a concerned family.

As long as we avoid putting a number on the required intake, we avoid the realities of the situation. Once those realities are faced, supplements given via feeding tubes become inevitable. The short-term studies with parenteral feeding and nasogastric feeding have demonstrated that weight can be gained. Our unpublished experience with nasogastric feeding for a short period of catch-up growth was disappointing; weight was gained and subjective improvement occurred, but within 3 to 12 weeks most patients had lost the gains made. This seems to be a general experience. However, largely at the parents' request, we proceeded to investigate the effects of chronic enteral feeding.

Gastrostomy, Jejunostomy, or Nasogastric Feeding?

There are two papers demonstrating that either jejunal or gastric enterostomy feeding can be used effectively to maintain body weight over long periods; up to 4 years so far. Other studies document the use of nasogastric feeding for 6 to 12 months. Strength-related respiratory function appears to be stabilized, but the small airway disease process continues. One major benefit has been psychological in that all patients and families report an increased sense of well-being and increased involvement in social activities. For about one-third of our patients, insertion of an enterostomy and the establishment of adequate energy intake are associated with a degree of euphoria in the first month or so. Thereafter, there is a return to reality but the quality of life measured by an increase in discretional activities, such as attending parties, riding a bicycle, skating, and playing ball, is related to the level of energy intake. The body weight at which life and energy levels are acceptable and the weight at which lethargy and depression take over are not very different. Presumably, this is because there is an approximate range of + 30 percent of

---

* The large range for the cost of growth is due to the different cost for synthesis of muscle (5 kcal per gram) and adipose tissue (10 kcal per gram). These differences relate better to the energy stored in protein and fat, respectively, and to the much lower water content of adipose tissue.

energy intake at which weight is stable but metabolic adaptation is occurring.

The system we use is a Witzel jejunostomy. The tube is not sutured or otherwise permanently held in place and can be replaced when necessary. The only dressing is a transparent adhesive covering that is changed as necessary. Initial supplementation is night-time, pump-assisted feeding for 6 to 8 hours. We use a standard enteral feeding pump to control the rate of delivery into the jejunum (Biosearch Dobbhoff). We also use standard enteral formulas such as Isocal or Ensure and their higher energy density forms and add enzymes directly to the feeds or have the patient take them by mouth, depending upon individual preference. Currently, jejunostomy tubes can be made less obtrusive than gastrostomy tubes, and this is important, especially in teenagers.

The same gains can be made using a gastrostomy tube. Theoretical advantages to this are that it can be installed nonsurgically under local anesthesia, and it allows for larger or bolus feedings. There is no good reason to use elemental formulas in either case, although with gastrostomy feeding enzyme administration may be more problematic.

Problems

The problems encountered with the system have all been relatively minor. The tubes can become blocked or the material can break down, requiring tube replacement, which can easily be done as an outpatient procedure. In the more active patient, the tube can fall out, requiring reinsertion by the patient or parent as soon as possible. Intestinal secretions can leak around the tube, and several patients have developed a granuloma at the exit site. These problems are usually managed with local treatment. Tubes are changed every 6 months.

Carbon Dioxide Retention

When carbon dioxide retention develops, the total energy can be delivered over a longer period of time to maintain weight while spreading the carbon dioxide load, to avoid exceeding the limited capacity of the lungs. Thus a patient may feed for 16 to 20 hours per day at half the previous rate of intake. At present there is a trend toward the use of higher fat, lower carbohydrate products in chronic respiratory failure; the theoretical basis is simply that fat produces less carbon dioxide per unit of energy than carbohydrate and this will reduce the carbon dioxide load. However, within the acceptable range of diet composition the effect is only a few percentage points. Spreading the carbon dioxide load out with the use of a portable pump is more effective.

EVALUATION

The most difficult problem is the objective evaluation of long-term enterostomy feeding. Randomization within a clinic is not possible because the effects of enteral feeding are visible and activist parents will not join the control group and defeatist parents will not join the treatment group. Between-clinic studies would have too many confounding variables. We are currently examining the use of $n=1$ techniques for evaluating the benefits and risks for these patients.

FUTURE DEVELOPMENTS AND CONCLUSIONS

The rational nutritional treatment of cystic fibrosis patients is likely to mean patients will live longer and be more active, but it also means more of the complications of cystic fibrosis, such as diabetes, gastroesophageal reflux, and possibly liver disease, will develop. Management of these problems and nutritional therapy will have to be integrated into the cystic fibrosis clinic's team care, making coordination of services more complex. Once we are able to achieve normal growth via formula supplements or enterostomy feeding, the body's economy for the minor nutrients needs to be reexamined. Commercial formulas are rich in vitamins and minerals, and some of the present routine vitamin and mineral supplementation may be unnecessary. There are still some patients who are not asymptomatic with enteric coated enzymes. The development of an acid lipase should be of practical benefit in this group. Thus, there is abundant evidence that malnutrition can be corrected in cystic fibrosis and that a "better" nutritional state can be maintained with chronic enteral feeding; whether this treatment will affect the progress, longevity, or complications of the disease has not been established, but it will be a very dedicated therapeutic nihilist who will maintain that malnutrition is good for you.

SUGGESTED READING

Boland MP, MacDonald NE, Patrick J, Stoski D, Soucy P. Chronic jejunostomy feeding with a non-elemental formula in under nourished patients with cystic fibrosis. Lancet 1986; 1:232–234.

Golden, MHN, Jackson AA. Undernutrition: protein energy malnutrition. In: The Weatherall DJ, Ledingham JGG, Warrell DA, eds. The Oxford textbook of medicine. Oxford: Oxford University Press, 1983:8.12.

Levy L, Durie PR, Pencharz PB, Corey ML. Effects of long-term nutritional rehabilitation on body composition and clinical status in malnourished children and adolescents with cystic fibrosis. J Pediatr 1985; 107:225–230.

O'Loughlin E, Forbes D, Parsons H, Scott B, Cooper D, Gall G. Nutritional rehabilitation of malnourished patients with cystic fibrosis. Am J Clin Nutr 1986; 43:732–737.

Waterlow JC. Classification and definition of protein-calorie malnutrition. Br Med J 1972; 2:566–569.

Waterlow JC, Golden MHN, Patrick J. Protein energy malnutrition: treatment. In: Dickerson JWT, Lee HA, eds. Nutrition in the clinical management of disease. London: Edward Arnold, 1978:49.

TOTAL PARENTERAL NUTRITION IN PEDIATRICS

STANLEY H. ZLOTKIN, M.D., Ph.D., F.R.C.P.(C)

INDICATIONS AND TIMING FOR THE START OF TOTAL PARENTERAL NUTRITION

Nutrient reserves in infants and children are minimal; thus, the ability of this population to withstand an inadequate nutrient supply is markedly less than that of the older child, and certainly less than that of adults. Whenever possible nutrients should be provided via the gastrointestinal tract. If oral intake is precluded or inadequate, nasogastric (NG), nasojejunal (NJ), gastrostomy, or jejunostomy feeds should be considered before starting total parenteral nutrition (TPN). TPN is indicated only if it is not possible to provide an adequate nutrient intake via the gastrointestinal tract.

For those needing TPN for short periods of time, the goal is to provide the minimal amount of nutrients necessary to prevent acute nutrient deficiencies. For those needing long-term TPN, the goal is not only to prevent nutrient deficiencies, but also to provide an adequate amount of nutrients for growth.

For the small premature infant, who has limited nutrient reserves, TPN should be started as soon as the infant is made NPO. For the premature infant who is tolerating partial enteral feeds, supplemental parenteral nutrition should be started if the enteral (NG or NJ) intake is not meeting nutrient intake requirements within 2 to 4 days of the start of feeding. For the older infant or young child with good nutrient reserves, TPN should be started if the child is left NPO for 3 days or longer. For the older child or adolescent who is well nourished, TPN should be started if the patient is left NPO for 5 days or longer. For the malnourished infant, child, or adolescent, TPN should be used whenever oral (NG or NJ) intake is not meeting total nutrient intake recommendations for age and size.

TPN SOLUTIONS

If TPN is routinely used, then a manufacturing system that produces standard solutions is recommended. A standard solution contains amino acids, dextrose, minerals, and trace minerals at a concentration appropriate for a specific age group. The use of standard solutions makes the ordering and maintenance of TPN much simpler, safer, and more economical. Standard solutions can be manufactured by the pharmacy in large batches in anticipation of patient needs. Depending on the age range of the patient population, one or more sets of standard solutions may be prepared.

At the Hospital for Sick Children in Toronto, six standard solutions are routinely manufactured (Table 1). These solutions differ in their amino acid content, dextrose content, or mineral content. For example, solutions

TABLE 1 Composition of Standard Solutions (per Liter)

Nutrient	Premature Infants and Young Children			Children and Adolescents		
	P-5	P-7.5	P-10	PI-10	I-10	I-20*
Amino acids (g)	15	15	20	20	30	30
Glucose (g)	50	75	100	100	100	100
Energy (kcal)†	248	340	455	455	495	870
Na (mmol)	20	20	14.3	30	30	30
K (mmol)	20	20	18.9	30	30	30
Cl (mmol)	21.1	21.1	15.7	31.3	32.1	32.1
Ca (mmol)	9	9	9	9	9	9
P (mmol)	9	9	9	9	9	9
Mg (mmol)	3	3	4	4	4	4
Zn (μmol)	46	46	46	46	46	46
Cu (μmol)	6.3	6.3	6.3	6.3	6.3	6.3
Mn (μmol)	1.8	1.8	1.8	1.8	5.0	5.0
I (μmol)	0.47	0.47	0.47	0.47	0.47	0.47
Cr (μmol)	0.076	0.076	0.076	0.076	0.076	0.076
Se (μmol)	0.25	0.25	0.25	0.25	0.25	0.25
Fe (μmol)‡	—	—	—	—	18	18

* I-20 is intended for central venous line use only.

† The energy content is expressed as total energy and thus includes the potential energy from the protein as well as that from the dextrose.

‡ Iron can be included in the P solutions and is generally ordered if an infant has been receiving TPN for 1 month or longer.

intended for use in premature infants (the P solutions) generally contain less amino acids, dextrose, and electrolytes than solutions intended for use in older infants and children (the I solutions). The nutrient concentration of the standard solutions should meet the needs of most patients within the particular age group when infused at an appropriate rate. The nutrient solutions are placed in clear plastic intravenous bags, similar to those used in commercially prepared intravenous solutions. The standard bag sizes are 250 ml, 500 ml, and 1,000 ml. The size used will depend on the volume ordered.

When the nutrient content of the standard solution is inappropriate for a particular patient (e.g., a child whose diarrhea results in excessive electrolyte losses), a special solution can be prepared by the pharmacy that contains nutrients specific to the needs of an individual patient. Because of the increased cost and burden to the pharmacy, if the nutrient content of the special solution is not significantly different from the standard solution, then the standard solution should be used.

A complete mixture of vitamins is added to the TPN solution by the pharmacy each morning. The daily vitamin dose is added to one amino acid/dextrose bag per patient per day. For patients who receive more than one bag daily, the pharmacy should send one bag with the vitamins and the rest of the ordered volume without. When more than one bag is ordered, the vitamin bag should always be given to the patient first to ensure that the daily vitamin requirement is infused. The amounts of each vitamin added per day are listed in Table 2.

Ordinarily, each patient on TPN will receive two types of infusate: a standard amino acid/dextrose/mineral solution and an intravenous fat emulsion. The fat emulsion is available as a 10 or 20 percent solution, and comes in 100 ml or 500 ml bottles. Most patients will tolerate 2 to 4 g lipid per kilogram per 24 hours, although some, with careful monitoring, can tolerate more. Both strengths can be given by either peripheral or central vein infusion.

ROUTE OF INFUSION

The use of peripheral veins for TPN is preferred because of lower rates of infection, easier nursing care, and lower cost. Due to the small size and relative fragility of peripheral veins, the infusion volume will be limited as will the concentration of the nutrient mixture. In general,

TABLE 2 Daily Vitamin Additions to TPN*

Vitamin	All Age Groups
A (IU)	2300.0
D (IU)	400.0
E (IU)	7.0
C (mg)	80.0
Thiamin (B_1) (mg)	1.2
Riboflavin (B_2) (mg)	1.4
Pyridoxine (B_6) (mg)	1.0
Niacinamide (mg)	17.0
Pantothenic acid (mg)	5.0
Folic acid (μg)	140.0
Biotin (μg)	20.0
K_1 (mg)	0.2
B_{12} (μg)	1.0

* If more than one bag is used per 24 hours, the vitamins are added only to the first bag given to the patient.

for infants the maximum infusion volume by peripheral vein is 150 to 170 ml per kilogram per day. For older children and adolescents, the maximum infusion volume is 2.0 to 2.5 L per day. When the concentration of dextrose is greater than 10 percent combined with an amino acid concentration greater than 3 percent, the solution is hypertonic to the point where peripheral veins will be intolerant of even short-term use. In addition, older children will complain of pain and burning. Thus, the peripheral nutrient solutions must contain no more than 10 percent dextrose and 3 percent amino acids.

Failure to deliver an adequate nutrient intake (particularly energy) is an indication for switching from peripheral to central line TPN. If the patient is volume restricted, necessitating the use of very hypertonic solutions, then a central line must be used. Finally, if it is anticipated that a patient will need TPN for a prolonged period of time, central line TPN should be used.

PERIPHERAL TPN

For appropriate solutions to be used with peripheral TPN, refer to the preceding section on solutions. Metal butterfly needles are preferred over plastic cannulae for peripheral TPN. Since metal needles seldom remain in position for longer than 1 to 2 days, the risks of infection are minimized. With butterfly needles, especially, the nursing staff must frequently monitor the infusion site for early signs of extravasation of parenteral fluids and/or thrombophlebitis. Early detection of extravasated fluid can minimize the serious complications of skin and tissue necrosis that can occur after extravasation of large amounts of TPN solution. Thrombophlebitis may be prevented if the infusion site is changed every 72 hours and hyperosmolar solutions are avoided.

Plastic cannulae should be used only when it is not possible to maintain TPN with the repeated replacement of butterfly needles. If a plastic cannula is used, the following guidelines for skin preparation should be followed: (1) the operator should perform a basic hand wash before starting; (2) the skin at the entrance site should be prepared with povidone-iodine 10 percent solution and allowed to air dry for 60 seconds; and (3) the operator should also prep the hand that will be palpating for the vessel. As with the butterfly needle, the plastic cannula should normally not be left in place for longer than 72 hours. Color-coded dates on the cannulas can be used to note the day of insertion. If the only way of maintaining a peripheral line is by the continued use of plastic cannulae, then a central line should be inserted.

CENTRAL VENOUS LINE TPN

Since hyperosmolar solutions are most often used with central line TPN, the infusate should be delivered through a central, large-bore vein with high volume blood flow to minimize the risk of venous thrombosis and phlebitis. Placement of the catheter should be performed under full aseptic conditions, preferably in an operating room by a surgeon. The use of polyethylene or polyvinyl catheters has been associated with "sterile" inflammation due to tissue reactions with the plastic and, more importantly, venous perforations resulting in potentially life-threatening intrapleural or intracardiac collections of TPN solution or blood. Silicone rubber catheters (Silastic) which have a higher degree of flexibility and a soft nonwetting surface that works to resist clotting and is extremely durable, should be used whenever possible.

The choice of sites for insertion include the scalp, common facial, internal jugular, external jugular, cephalic, and subclavian veins. After the catheter is inserted and advanced into the superior vena cava to the junction of the right atrium (it should remain in the superior vena cava rather than in the right atrium), a separate incision is made on the chest or abdomen so that the distal end of the catheter can be directed through a subcutaneous tunnel between the two incisions. To decrease the risk of infection, the skin exit site for the catheter should be located in an easily accessible area away from any natural or acquired orifices, such as gastric or intestinal stomas, tracheotomies, and suprapubic catheters, and from any skin lesions, burns, etc. Care of the TPN system and catheters should be performed only by nurses and doctors who have specific training in this area. A procedures manual for the maintenance of central lines should be prepared and made available on the ward.

ADDITIONS TO TPN SOLUTIONS

Additions to TPN bags or bottles should not be made outside the pharmacy because of the risk of contamination. Urgent electrolyte additions to the amino acid/dextrose solutions may be made on the nursing unit only through the volume control set using appropriate aseptic techniques. If a patient requires frequent changes in electrolytes in order to remain metabolically stable, then TPN should be temporarily discontinued. If a patient requires individualized electrolyte additions (or deletions) on an ongoing basis, a special solution should be ordered and prepared in the pharmacy.

When drugs need to be administered to a patient receiving TPN, they should be given through a separate IV site. If a separate site is not possible, the drug may be administered through a separate line that has a Y connection to the TPN system as close as possible to the patient's infusion site. The TPN solutions should not be running and the common tubing must be adequately flushed before and after the drug administration. Only if the patient's clinical status requires uninterrupted TPN administration can certain drugs be administered through a separate set and Y connection with the TPN solutions still running. TPN solutions are of varied composition, and drug compatibilities can never be guaranteed. Lists of compatible drugs are available.

COMPLICATIONS

The major complications associated with TPN are related either to the catheter or to infections or metabolic imbalances. The purpose of monitoring patients on TPN is to detect and treat potential or actual complications. An individual or group of individuals, with training in the administration of TPN should be directly responsible for TPN monitoring. Each monitoring procedure should be linked to a specific complication. For example, as indicated in Table 3, urine and blood glucose determinations are made to rule out both hyper- and hypoglycemia. (Other examples are shown in Table 3). When monitoring procedures are not readily available, or the likelihood of complications occuring in association with the inclusion of the nutrient in the TPN solution are extremely low, such as with the use of zinc, copper, iodine, chromium, and selenium, the nutrients are included at recommended dosages, and monitoring is carried out only if signs or symptoms of excess or deficiency are present.

Catheter-related complications such as perforation or venous thrombosis have been markedly reduced with the use of Silastic catheters.

TABLE 3 Monitoring Recommended for TPN-Associated Complications

Complication	Monitored By	Frequency
Inadequate or excessive intake	Body weight, fluid balance, urea	Daily Daily Weekly
Protein depletion	Serum albumin	Weekly
Hypo/hyperglycemia	Urine glucose Blood glucose	Daily Daily–2× week
Electrolyte imbalance	Serum Na, Cl, K Urine Na, Cl, K	Daily–2× week As necessary
Mineral imbalance	Serum Ca, P, Mg	Weekly
Iron depletion	Blood count with smear	Weekly
Acid-base imbalance	Blood gases	Weekly
Lipid overload	Exogenous lipids Triglycerides	2× week 2× week
Hepatic cholestasis	Liver function tests	2× month

Sepsis, however, remains the major complication of central venous line TPN. Organisms may enter the bloodstream along the catheter tract, from contaminated solutions and additives, during catheter insertion, or from the manipulation of the administration system and catheter. Prevention of infection is the key to a successful TPN program. The rate of infection can be kept under control only if strict and carefully monitored infection control measures are employed. For example, fever in a patient receiving TPN should always be assumed to be of bacterial origin until proven otherwise. Appropriate samples from the patient and the TPN system should be sent for bacterial and fungal culture. Blood samples should be taken from both the central line and peripheral vein. If purulent drainage is present at the catheter exit site, the pus should be cultured and gram stained. While removal of the central line with appropriate antibiotic therapy is almost always curative, the use of appropriate antibiotic therapy without removal of the central line is often curative as well; however, careful long-term monitoring is manditory to ensure that the infection has been totally eradicated. When antibiotic therapy must be started before culture results are available (as in infants and children less than 1 year of age), broad-spectrum coverage should be provided, since both gram-positive and gram-negative bacteria are frequent causes of TPN-associated infection. A semisynthetic penicillinase-resistant penicillin should be used in combination with an aminoglycoside.

Although fungal infections are associated with TPN, "blind" antifungal therapy is usually not started until positive cultures are obtained. It is important to remember that malnourished and immunosuppressed patients with indwelling catheters and patients on long-term TPN are at increased risk for opportunistic infections.

STARTING AND STOPPING TPN

Very small neonates (less than 1000 g) are intolerant of high and low glucose loads. When starting TPN, they should receive a nutrient solution with 7.5 percent dextrose at a maintenance fluid intake rate of 120 to 150 ml per kilogram per 24 hours, run in over 24 hours. If blood glucose levels remain normal, then a 10 percent dextrose solution (P-10 solution, Table 1) may be given. Lipids may be concurrently started if the bilirubin level is within normal limits. Lipids should be started at 0.5 to 1.0 g per kilogram per 24 hours (infused over 24 hours) and increased slowly at increments of 0.5 to 1.0 g per kilogram per day. Serum lipid levels should be monitored daily while the lipid intake is being increased.

Older infants and children receiving peripheral TPN may start with 10 percent dextrose-nutrient solutions (P-10 or I-10 solutions, see Table 1), at maintenance fluid intake rates. Lipids should be started at 1 g per kilogram per 24 hours and increased by 1 g per kilogram per day until optimal intake is achieved (3 to 4 g per kilogram per 24 hours). For those on central line TPN, a 10 percent dextrose-nutrient solution is initially used for 24 to 48 hours, and then increased to the higher dextrose content if glucosuria and hyperglycemia are not detected.

TPN should initially be infused over a 24-hour period. For patients on long-term TPN who need time away from their infusion pumps, the time on TPN may be gradually decreased. Each day, the time on TPN may be decreased by 2-hour intervals with commensurate increases in the infusion rates over the shorter time period. Young children may be ultimately weaned to an infusion time of 12 to 14 hours per day, while older children and adolescents may need only 10 to 12 hours hooked up to the infusion pumps. For those with central lines receiving 20 percent dextrose-nutrient solutions, the infusion rate should be halved over the last 2 hours to prevent rebound hypoglycemia.

TPN can be discontinued rapidly only in patients who are receiving an adequate concurrent oral intake. For the neonate, TPN should be tapered slowly in concert with an increase in enteral intake calculated to meet daily nutrient requirements.

SUGGESTED READING

Kerner JA Jr. Manual of pediatric parenteral nutrition. Toronto: John Wiley & Sons, 1983.

Riordan TP. Placement of central venous lines in the premature infant. JPEN 1979; 3:381.

Zlotkin SH, Stallings VA. Total parenteral nutrition in the newborn: an update. In: Draper HH, ed. Advances in nutritional research. Vol 7. New York: Plenum Publishing, 1985.

FAILURE TO THRIVE

ROBERT I. HILLIARD, M.D., F.R.C.P.(C)

One of the most exciting aspects of being a primary care physician or pediatrician is watching children grow and develop physically, psychologically, socially, and sexually. One of the most frustrating and challenging problems both to physicians and parents occurs when children fail to grow and develop as expected. Failure to thrive is a descriptive term, not a specific diagnosis, and refers to a child's failure to grow physically, usually in respect to weight, that superficially has no obvious cause or explanation. There are two interrelated problems: "failure to thrive" refers to infants 2 years of age and under who fail to gain weight as expected; "short stature" refers to children, usually over 2 years of age, who fail to gain height as expected. Many parents are concerned about their child's growth, particularly between 1 and 2 years of age when the rate of growth or growth velocity falls dramatically and when a child's appetite or intake of food also seems less than in early infancy. The key to helping families understand the expected growth of their child is through the careful and appropriate use of growth charts. A child's height (length) or weight compared with other children of the same age at only one point in time is of limited value. It is critically important that all primary care physicians who are responsible for the child's total well-being follow and plot a child's weight, height (length), and head circumference over time.

Although families frequently worry about a child's growth, a child should be considered as failing to thrive only when (1) weight (or height) is significantly below the third percentile or less than 80 percent of that expected for age and height; or (2) the progress of the weight or height falls across and below two major percentile lines. Generally the cause of failure to thrive primarily affects weight, but as malnutrition becomes more severe and chronic, height will also be affected and later even head circumference.

When using growth charts for infants, one must recognize that the older standard growth charts—the Tanner Study in England and the Harvard Study in the United States—primarily studied Caucasian children in the locality of the study. As our population becomes more and more cosmopolitan, these graphs may not hold true for children of a variety of races and backgrounds.

PATHOGENESIS

In attempting to diagnose the cause of failure to thrive and in attempting to manage a child's poor weight gain, it is helpful to look at the nutrition and caloric intake. A child may fail to thrive for the following reasons:

1. An inadequate intake of food. This is by far the most important cause of failure to thrive, but the inadequate intake of nutrients and calories may be due to a wide variety of reasons, including poverty and an inadequate supply of food, an inadequate understanding by the care giver of the nutritional needs of the child, feeding difficulties, anorexia related to chronic or recurrent disease (e.g., chronic renal failure), or feeding difficulties related to recurrent pulmonary disease or chronic congestive cardiac failure.
2. Recurrent vomiting, as in gastroesophageal reflux.
3. Inadequate absorption and assimilation of calories, as with chronic diarrhea, cystic fibrosis, or celiac disease.
4. Failure to utilize nutrients and calories.
5. Loss of nutrients and calories, as with chronic diarrhea or diabetic glycosuria.
6. Increased requirements for calories, as with hyperthyroidism or various malignancies.

NUTRITIONAL NEEDS

There are various guidelines for the caloric needs for proper growth and development. Newborns need 100 to 120 calories per kilogram per day. For older children there is a useful formula indicating the caloric needs of a child—100 calories per kilogram per day for the first 10 kg of a child's weight, plus 50 calories for each kilogram greater than 10 for the range 10 to 20 kg and an additional 20 calories per kilogram for each kilogram over 20. For example, an 18-month-old girl weighing 11 kg would normally require about 1050 calories, a 4-year-old boy weighing 17 kg about 1350 calories. These, however, are the requirements for a child with normal metabolism and activity. Of this intake, 10 to 15 calories per kilogram per day are used for body growth. It is easy to see that the caloric deficit need only be small to result in inadequate weight gain and failure to thrive.

DIFFERENTIAL DIAGNOSIS OF THE UNDERSIZED CHILD

1. Familial.
2. Primordial, including some small-for-gestational-age infants, chromosomal abnormalities, intrauterine infections, and many pediatric syndromes.
3. Constitutional short stature with associated delayed growth and delayed adolescence.
4. Inadequate nutritional intake.
5. Endocrine disturbances including hypothyroidism, hyperthyroidism, hypopituitarism, and adrenal insufficiency.
6. Specific organic diseases.
   a. Gastrointestinal disorders, feeding problems, recurrent vomiting, chronic diarrhea and malabsorption, and chronic liver disease.
   b. Recurrent or chronic pulmonary disease, including cystic fibrosis.
   c. Chronic cardiac disease.
   d. Central nervous system (CNS) disorders, including mental retardation and cerebral palsy.
   e. Chronic renal disease, including chronic renal failure, recurrent urinary tract infections, and renal tubular disorders.
   f. Chronic metabolic diseases, including diabetes insipidus, diabetes mellitus, idiopathic hypercalcemia, and inborn errors of metabolism.
   g. Specific bone disorders and syndromes.
   h. Recurrent infections and immunologic disorders, chronic inflammatory diseases.
   i. Chronic hematologic disorders and malignancies.
7. Nonorganic failure to thrive.

In order to manage a child who presents with failure to thrive, we must have a broad understanding of why a child may be small. From the preceding list of differential diagnoses, it would appear that almost any disease in pediatrics might cause failure to thrive. With many of these conditions the child will present with a specific complaint, such as recurrent or chronic cough, recurrent vomiting, or chronic diarrhea, and the physician will note on examination that the child is underweight. There are, however a number of conditions in which the presenting concern of the family may be simply the child's poor weight gain. From the preceding differential diagnosis of the undersized child, important conditions to consider include:

1. Familial. Some children are small simply because it is inherent in their family background. For such children it is important to document the height and weight of the parents and siblings.
2. Primordial. Some children are inherently small and this often starts right at birth, as when the child is noted to be small for gestational age. Causes include a number of chromosomal abnormalities, intrauterine infections such as congenital rubella, congenital cytomegalovirus infection, or congenital toxoplasmosis, and a wide variety of syndromes with recognizable dysmorphic features.
3. Constitutional short stature with delayed growth. These children often present as short children who, after 2 years of age show a normal growth velocity but delayed bone age. These children eventually have a longer growth period because of delayed adolescence and growth spurt and reach normal adult size.
6. There are a wide variety of organic diseases that may cause failure to thrive. In most cases there is a specific presenting symptom or sign. There are a number, however, where the cause may be obscure and detected only by a very thorough history, physical examination and appropriate laboratory tests. These include such gastrointestinal conditions as celiac disease, chronic renal conditions, and certain metabolic disorders. Many children with CNS disorders (developmental delay, cerebral palsy, neuromuscular disorders) fail to thrive because of difficulty in ingesting sufficient food.
7. Nonorganic failure to thrive. This the most frequent explanation in children who present with failure to thrive that superficially has no obvious cause. Over the past 50 years this condition has received a number of different names. Initially it was called environmental or emotional deprivation; later the term "maternal deprivation" was used. This particular term is misleading because it assumes that the blame rests entirely on the mother. Surprisingly, in our culture where the traditional nuclear family is disappearing and where there are many single-parent families, there has rarely been any discussion of the

role of the father. In fact this condition involves poor interaction between the child and the parent, so that the responsibility for failure to thrive is shared by the child and the parent or care giver. Frequently there is a vicious circle of maladaptive behavioral interaction between the care giver and the infant associated with high emotional tensions.

Finally there may be a combination of causes for the child's failure to thrive including both an organic and nonorganic cause. A child with a chronic disease is more demanding and needy, and the parent may not be able to give the needed care and attention so that a deprivation situation is superimposed on a specific chronic disease. For example, a child born prematurely and having a number of the associated complications, such as hyaline membrane disease and intraventricular hemorrhages, may go home after a prolonged stay in hospital with a parent who has not yet bonded well with him. The parent may not be able to respond with the care and attention needed by an infant at risk.

NONORGANIC FAILURE TO THRIVE

When there are no obvious symptoms of any specific disease, failure to gain weight or thrive may have a number of nonorganic causes. There may be factors in the child or in the parents, or there may be an abnormal child-parent interaction. The child may be a poor feeder who recurrently vomits, colicky, restless and a poor sleeper, or suffer from a chronic illness. A parent may lack good parenting skills and not give adequate love and affection or stimulation. If the problem is severe the child may be neglected or even abused. Many authorities feel that nonorganic failure to thrive is part of the spectrum of child abuse and neglect. Frequently the parent was abused or neglected as a young child. The child's temperament may simply not match the temperament of the parent.

The child's poor weight gain is primarily related to an inadequate intake of calories. A number of biochemical abnormalities are found in these children, in particular a functional hypopituitarism. The cause of these has been debated (neuroendocrine derangement secondary to lack of stimulation versus a primary lack of caloric and nutritional intake), but it is now apparent that such abnormalities are readily reversed with hospitalization and adequate nutrition. There may be other clinical features such as a mild developmental delay that seem to be related to a lack of affection and stimulation.

This diagnosis should never be made simply by excluding other causes but should be actively considered and investigated particularly with a careful psychosocial and family history. The child is usually the youngest in the family and often born within 18 months of the next older sibling. In the majority the growth failure presents before 1 year of age and commonly before 6 months of age. Frequently these children come from single-parent families and those with financial instability and low socioeconomic status. It should be recognized, however, that nonorganic failure to thrive may be seen in all types of families from all socioeconomic groups. Often the children have frequent upper respiratory infections and episodes of vomiting and diarrhea. Feeding problems are common, including crying, colic, spitting up after feeding, and vomiting. On examination the child seems thin, pale, and unhappy, often bearing an expression of misery. The child may appear apathetic, avoiding eye contact with other individuals and withdrawing when approached. There is often some delay in psychomotor development, particularly in social adaptive and language skills. The children are noted to be hypotonic despite good muscle strength and frequently adopt a posture with the arms abducted, elbows flexed, and the hands held near or behind the head. There are often a number of laboratory abnormalities such as delayed bone age, elevated serum glutamic-oxaloacetic transaminase (SGOT), mild iron deficiency anemia, transient abnormalities of glucose intolerance, decreased adrenocorticotropic hormone (ACTH) release, decreased growth hormone response, and decreased levels of somatomedin. If these children are hospitalized, one is likely to find that they sleep less and are listless. However, with satisfactory adaptation to the hospital routine they show a good appetite, a dramatic weight gain, and often a craving for affection, so that they may become one of the favorites of the hospital and nursing staff. The unfortunate aspect of nonorganic failure to thrive is that even after recognition and an attempt to change the family and social conditions, there are usually long-term problems. One-quarter to one-half of these children remain small with weight below the third to tenth percentile. Many show below normal cognitive functions, especially verbal and reading skills, and there may be an abundance of behavioral problems. The poor family and social situation affects not only caloric intake and weight gain but also normal psychosocial development. Long-term studies have shown that only 20 to 30 percent of these children will have fully normal growth, behavior, and cognitive function.

DIAGNOSIS

The key to the diagnosis of failure to thrive is a complete history and thorough physical examination. The family history should include the height and weight and percentiles of the parents and siblings. A child's height and weight is usually between the percentiles of the two parents. A good pregnancy and birth history is required, including birth weight and gestational age of the infant. Previous heights and weights should be obtained, and the physician should obtain a history of the diet and feeding techniques. The physician may not be able to calculate the caloric intake but should be able to ascertain if the child is getting an adequate intake and balance of foods. A careful history of past illnesses and a full review of symptoms are needed, particularly appetite, intake of food and fluids, the presence of vomiting or diarrhea, and bowel and urinary patterns. There must be a careful family and social history and during the interview, the physician should watch the family and child to see how they relate to each other. Important social factors include: whether the parents are married; whether the pregnancy was planned; and whether family support from friends or relatives, financial difficulties or symptoms of family dysfunction such as irritability, sleep disturbances, excessive crying, tantrums, or feeding difficulties are present. The family medical history should include psychiatric and drug or alcohol problems. The physical examination should be thorough, remembering the large number of differential diagnoses possible in children who have poor weight gain. The height, weight, and head circumference should all be plotted on a growth chart. If a child is failing to thrive from lack of caloric intake it is usually weight that is affected, but profound malnutrition can also affect length and head circumference.

Laboratory investigations should only be ordered to make a specific diagnosis that is suspected from the history and physical examination. Ordering a large battery of laboratory tests as a protocol for failure to thrive is expensive and inappropriate. Simple useful tests might include:

hemoglobin, WBC, smear, ESR;
urinalysis, urine culture, and urine for specific gravity;
urine metabolic screen;
electrolyte and venous blood gases;
glucose, BUN, creatinine;
calcium;
thyroxine (T4) and TSH;
chest films and sweat chlorides;

Other investigations should depend on the presenting signs and symptoms and how strongly one suspects an organic cause for failure to thrive. If, for example, there is a chronic diarrhea or poor weight gain in spite of a history of adequate caloric intake, appropriate investigations should be done to diagnose the cause of the chronic diarrhea and possible malabsorption syndrome. If the child is also short, a bone age roentgenogram is indicated. If the child is developmentally delayed, sucks poorly, or is particularly hypo- or hypertonic, a neurologic work-up is indicated.

MANAGEMENT

Failure to thrive is usually a chronic and complex problem requiring a team approach. No physician should think or expect that he can deal with these children and their families alone. The team should include:

1. The family physician or pediatrician.
2. The hospital or ambulatory clinic nurse who can be helpful in observing the child/parent interaction and can often give advice about normal nutritional needs and how to deal with parenting problems.
3. The public health nurse, who can visit in the home, again to observe the family's interactions, but also to give counseling regarding diet, behavior, and development.
4. The dietitian, who can help to calculate a child's intake of calories and the various nutritional groups and who can advise families on how to improve their child's diet and give any nutritional supplements.
5. The social worker, who can meet with the family and discuss their feelings about the child's illness and help them to develop a healthier family atmosphere with love, affection and stimulation.

Most textbooks and articles that discuss failure to thrive present the problems as one of a hospitalized child but many children can be managed in an ambulatory setting. Most of the investigations today (including stool collections and caloric counts) can be done on an ambulatory basis either from a doctor's private office or through a hospital clinic. The indications for hospitalization of a child who is failing to thrive include:

1. When there may be a concern for the child's health or safety and when an improvement in family dynamics is not readily anticipated.

2. When the diagnosis is not obvious, and extensive investigations including a therapeutic trial in hospital may be required.
3. When abuse is suspected or when the family/social situation is so poor that the child should be separated from the parents.
4. When a trial of ambulatory care has failed.
5. When the child is referred to a secondary or tertiary pediatric center far from the family's home.

Hospital management of the child should include:

1. A thorough history and complete physical examination and only the simple basic laboratory investigations should be performed. A period of observation in the hospital is then needed before embarking on extensive or invasive laboratory investigations.
2. There should be a careful nutritional record with a calculation, usually by a dietitian, of the daily caloric and protein intake. The child needs to be weighed daily and intake and daily weight should be graphed to make a visible record of progress. "Catch-up" weight gain will not occur with the provision of only the normal caloric requirements; an intake of more than 150 calories per kilogram, based on the expected weight for age and height is required. If there is poor weight gain in spite of an adequate caloric intake, a malabsorption syndrome should be suspected and appropriate investigations initiated.
3. A child should have a program of activities and stimulation making use of the nursing staff, occupational therapists, child care workers, and recreational therapists and volunteers. Ward nurses are often too busy to achieve any appreciable degree of physical contact with the children in their care, but a well-intentioned volunteer can be very helpful in holding, cuddling, talking to, and playing with children.
4. The family needs to be involved in the child's care. The family should be encouraged to spend as much time with the child as possible, helping with meals and playing with, talking to, and holding him/her. This can help improve their parenting skills, their self esteem, and their confidence in caring for their child.
5. A child should be on a high-caloric diet with liberal amounts of high-calorie fats such as homogenized milk, butter, peanut butter, cheese, sauces, puddings, and gravies. Foods high in refined sugars and lacking other essential nutrients should be avoided. Also low-calorie fluids should be avoided as they are filling and do not provide a lot of calories.

If a child's food intake is poor, vitamin and iron supplements may be necessary, but in most cases these can be provided by a complete and balanced diet. Medications such as cyproheptadine (Vimicon) are not indicated.

6. Caloric supplements that provide a large number of calories and low volume can be helpful if the child does not get an adequate caloric intake from the regular diet alone. These include balanced liquid supplements such as Ensure or Isocal, glucose polymers such as Caloreen and Polycose, and MCT (medium-chain triglycerides) oil. These last two may be added to the child's regular diet in sandwiches, puddings, and cooked or prepared foods to increase the caloric density of the diet with minimal change in the volume of food intake. As long as the child has adequate digestion and absorption, enteral feeding or total parenteral nutrition is rarely indicated.

7. If the child is severely malnourished or neglected, he/she may be listless, apathetic, and feed poorly and may, in spite of admission to the hospital, continue to feed poorly. If there is an inadequate intake of regular foods, nasogastric (NG) tube feedings may be initiated using a soft indwelling silastic NG tube to supplement oral intake, especially during sleep. Nasogastric tube supplements should be given if the oral intake does not reach the daily caloric requirements (150 calories per kilogram based on expected weight).

8. If the child is severely neglected or abused, the child and family should be reported to the appropriate legal protective authority or social service agency. Occasionally the family may voluntarily accept help from such sources, but in general legal protection is much more difficult to obtain for children failing to thrive than for children physically abused.

After discharge or if the child does not need hospitalization, the same approach can be used outside the hospital with regular visits to a clinic or office and with regular home visits by a public health nurse and a social worker. If there is also concern about the child's psychomotor development, referrals should be made to an infant stimulation program or special developmental nursery school. *A child being treated on an outpatient basis should receive the same intensive team approach as a hospitalized child.*

SUMMARY

Failure to thrive is noted when a child's weight is significantly below the third percentile or when the weight falls across two major percentile lines on a height and weight growth chart.

1. The major cause for failure to thrive is inadequate caloric intake.
2. Most causes of failure to thrive can be diagnosed through a thorough history and complete physical examination.
3. In those cases where no specific organic diagnosis can be made through these measures, the majority are due to nonorganic causes. Nonorganic failure to thrive should be a positive diagnosis made from an appropriate family and social history and not just by exclusion of organic causes.
4. Laboratory investigations should be ordered for specific diagnoses suspected from the history and physical examination and not as part of a battery of screening tests.
5. The management of children failing to thrive involves a medical and paramedical team approach to provide a better nutritional intake and also counseling and family support to improve the child-family interaction.

SUGGESTED READING

Berwick DM. Non-organic failure to thrive. Pediatrics Rev 1980; 1:265–270.

Cupoli JM, Hallock JA, Barness LA. Failure to thrive. Curr Probl Pediatr 1980; 10:1–43.

Goldbloom RB. Failure to thrive. Pediatr Clin North Am 1982; 29:151–166.

Oates RK, Peacock A, Forrest D. Long-term effects of non-organic failure to thrive. Pediatrics 1985; 75:36–40.

Sills RH. Failure to thrive. The role of clinical and laboratory evaluation. Am J Dis Child 1978; 132:967–969.

NUTRITIONAL ASSESSMENT OF THE CHILD

NOEL W. SOLOMONS, M.D.
SUSANA MOLINA, M.D.

It is important for the reader to note that this chapter is written from the perspective of physicians in a developing country (Guatemala), a region with a substantial prevalence of childhood malnutrition where assessment of nutriture consequently plays a more central role in pediatric health evaluation. The causes of nutritional impairment differ in a Third World nation as compared to an industrialized country, but the final common pathways are similar.

The nutritional assessment of a child (Table 1) differs little, if at all, from any other type of focused health evaluation. Orientation to the major problem(s) is the initial and important first step. One should consider three orienting questions.

TABLE 1   Component Steps in the Nutritional Evaluation of a Child

Orientation to the clinical problem:

Clinical history:
  Specific disorders and diagnoses
  Social and environmental conditions
  Dietary intake and feeding patterns
  Review of systems

Anthropometry:
  Growth status
  Body composition
  Hydration

Physical examination:
  Clinical signs of nutritional abnormalities

Laboratory assays

Other diagnostic maneuvers and tests

1. Is there a clinical (or environmental or socioeconomic) situation in which abnormal nutrition is likely to exist? *Comment:* An appropriate suspicion of an underlying nutritional abnormality facilitates its recognition. Familiarity with specific disorders of nutrition common to specific health situations leads to even more precise identification, or ruling out, of malnutrition states.
2. Is the aberration in nutritional status in the direction of undernutrition or overnutrition? *Comment: Mal*nutrition means bad nutrition, and *too few nutrients is not the only cause*; there is an "up-side" scenario of faulty nutriture produced by too much of a nutrient or too much dietary intake.
3. Is the clinical problem an acute life-threatening condition or a chronic, stable one? There are true nutritional *emergencies* that require immediate skilled intervention. Hypomagnesia or hypophosphatemia in improperly managed parenteral or enteral alimentation are examples. Drastic changes in hydration states and electrolyte balance also require immediate therapeutic attention. Even apparently "uncomplicated" malnutrition, such as edematous protein-energy malnutrition (kwashiorkor) is fraught with potential instabilities during the dietary management and recuperation.

CLINICAL HISTORY

Here, as throughout medical practice, the *history* is the key to accurate diagnosis. The clinical history should be oriented to underlying disease processes or the impinging social, familial or environmental circumstances. Primary deficiencies or excesses are due to decreased or increased intake of a nutrient. The *dietary intake* history is an important element, but it need not be too formal or sophisticated. Knowledge of overall feeding behavior and patterns of food consumption and appetite is more valuable in the evaluation than the formal textbook approaches such as food-frequency questionnaires or 24-hour recalls. In the infant patient, the amount of breast milk taken, as well as maternal health and complementary feeding are important aspects to be noted.

As shown in Tables 2 and 3, however, the major promoters of nutritional imbalance are related not to the abundance of food in the diet but rather to other *conditioning* factors, such as impaired (hypo- or hyper-) absorption, impaired (over or under) excretion, changes in utilization or

TABLE 2   Causes of Manifestations of Nutrient Deficiency

Decreased intake
Diminished absorption
Increased excretion
Impaired utilization
Increased destruction
Increased requirement

accelerated destruction of nutrients, or altered requirements. Stated another way, *secondary* malnutrition is far more common in pediatric practice than primary malnutrition. In cystic fibrosis, celiac or Crohn's disease, parasitoses, or gastroenteritis, the malabsorptive component can reduce nutrient uptake while the inflammatory and tissue-necrosis components can produce nutrient catabolism and metabolic wastage. Different diseases have different recognized patterns of nutritional derangement, (e.g., extensive ileal disease will produce vitamin B_{12} deficiency; cholestatic liver disease predisposes to vitamin E depletion; hemorrhagic diseases lead to iron deficiency). Focusing on the diagnosis allows one to anticipate the likely nutritional disorders known to accompany specific disorders.

Child abuse (or rejection)—physical or psychological—can be reflected in a child's nutritional status. The history-taken should probe for evidence of abuse when obvious organic illness has been ruled out as a cause for malnutrition. If a child is overweight, the history of his activity pattern, sports participation, and television viewing is important, as is a familial tendency to obesity. As outlined below, the recent and remote patterns of growth in both height and weight (and sexual development in the adolescent patient) are crucial elements of the clinical history.

The review of systems portion of the history will reflect the physical examination and should focus on nutritional manifestations by anatomical system. Certain manifestations of nutritional disorders,

TABLE 3   Causes of Manifestations of Nutrient Excess

Excessive intake
Increased absorption
Decreased excretion
Decreased requirement

such as the nightblindness seen in vitamin A or zinc deficiency, are better elicited by history than by routine examination. The specific physical signs of nutrient depletion or excess are listed in Table 4. Questioning done before or during the physical examination, should systematically survey the symptom correlates of the specific clinical signs.

ANTHROPOMETRY

In children, perhaps the most sensitive index of nutritional health is growth. Virtually all nutrients, when severely limited, can retard growth, but especially protein, energy, zinc, chloride, certain vitamins, and most probably iron. Excessive accumulation of energy (obesity) is also detected as an alteration in growth. For these reasons, anthropometry

TABLE 4 Physical Diagnostic Elements of an Evaluation For Clinical Manifestations of Nutritional Deficiency in The Child

General appearance: (malnourished) _____

Skin: hyperkeratosis _____ dyspigmentation _____ pallor _____
pellagroid dermatosis _____ scrotal or vulvar scaling _____
petechiae _____ ecchymoses _____ seborrheic lesions _____
acrodermatitis lesions _____ flaky-paint dermatitis _____

Subcutaneous: adequate fat pads _____ edema _____

Hair: sparse _____ lusterless _____ thinning _____
easy pluckability _____

Nails: spooning _____ koilonchia _____

Eyes: conjunctival pallor _____ conjunctival xerosis _____
Bitot spot _____ corneal xerosis _____
blepheritis _____

Lips: cheilosis _____ angular stomatitis _____

Gums: gingivitis _____ bleeding _____

Teeth: caries _____ enamel hypoplasia _____

Tongue: atrophic papillae _____ magenta color _____

Throid gland: goiter _____

Cardiovascular: tachycardia _____ cardiomegaly _____

Thorax: rachitic rosary _____ Abdomen: organomegaly _____

Extremities: edema _____ bowing _____

Neurological: photophobia _____ apathy _____
gait _____ muscular weakness _____
vibration sense _____

emerges as the single most important indicator of nutritional status in pediatric practice.

The dimensions of anthropometric assessment are threefold: (1) growth attainment; (2) growth velocity; and (3) body composition. The most widely used concept is that of the "adequacy" of growth attainment, measured in terms of weight, height, or both combined. It is a static measure that refers to a point in time in a child's life or development. It requires an accurate and standard measurement of weight (body mass without clothing) and stature (supine, recumbent length in children below 24 months and standing height without shoes in older children). A suitably calibrated balance is required for weight determinations. A babymeter table is preferred for length measurements. A fixed, true vertical tape measure on a wall suffices for assessment of height.

Once the basic measurements are made, anthropometric adequacy is assessed by comparison to standard growth charts from a "healthy" reference population. The norms published by the U.S. National Center for Health Statistics (NCHS) for the North American child population are the standard currently in worldwide use. When the patient's datum is plotted on the graph, one can determine the relation of the body mass for chronological age (weight-for-age) or the stature for chronological age (height-for-age) to the 50th percentile (median) value for the NCHS standard. For instance, the generic formula is:

$$\frac{\text{actual weight/height of the patient}}{\text{expected (50th percentile) weight/height from NCHS}} \times 100$$

Thus, if a 12 month-old male weighs 8.16 kg, and the reference weight for that age is 10.2 kg, our subject would have an adequacy of weight-for-age of 80 percent. A similar calculation of adequacy is made for stature. The nutritional interpretation of these two indices bears mention, however. Presumably, since height changes slowly, a faltering of stature is a reflection of chronic undernutrition. The deficit in height-for-age is termed stunting. Interpretation of weight-for-age can be made legitimately only in a child of an acceptable height for age. Obviously, if a child is already stunted, it would be inappropriate to expect him to have the normative chronological weight. This has led us to place a more specific reliance on the weight-for-height as the index of acute malnutrition, the so-called measure of nutritional wasting (or conversely of true overweight) in a child.

The calculation of weight-for-height is a bit more tedious and complex, and it requires both growth charts (or a specialized graph specific for the weight-for-height approach). With the two chart method, one first determines on the height-for-age chart the age at which the measured height would be the 50th percentile height for a child. Let us say that our subject is a male child, 71 cm long. His height corresponds to that of a reference child of 8 months. Looking at the weight chart's growth curve, we find the 50th percentile weight for this age, in this instance, 9.24 kg; this becomes the expected weight for a child of our subject's height; i.e., the appropriate amount of mass on a given frame. Thus, our child who weighs 9.7 kg has 105 percent of his weight-for-height. The generic calculation of adequacy of weight-for-height is:

$$\frac{\text{actual weight of the patient}}{\substack{\text{expected weight (50th percentile) for a child} \\ \text{of one's patient's height}}} \times 100$$

Thus, even in a stunted child, some assessment of true weight loss, or weight excess, for actual stature can be made using the weight-for-height approach. The accepted interpretive norms for all three anthropometric indices are given in Table 5.

Height and weight cannot be measured with equal precision in a child, however. Thus, the anthropometrist must take into consideration certain intrinsic pitfalls in interpretation of adequacy of growth attainment derived from the relative precision of the measurement of height versus weight. Specifically, true length or height (stature) can be measured

TABLE 5   Classification of the Adequacy of Growth Attainment by Standard Anthropometric Indices of Height and Weight

Classification	Weight-For-Height (%)	Weight-For-Age (%)	Height-For-Age (%)
Above normal	120	110	—
Normal	90–119	91–109	95
Mildly deficient	80–89	75–90	90–94
Moderately deficient	70–79	60–74	85–89
Severely deficient	70	60[*]	85

[*] Or with clinical evidence of nutritional edema.

exactly. Moreover, there are only rare causes of loss of stature in a child, i.e., amputation, scoliosis, or kyphosis. Thus, repeated measures of height in the short term will be in close agreement and over time will increase progressively. On the other hand, several common factors influence the weight of a child, including food recently ingested, urine in the bladder, and stool in the ampulla of the lower colon. The sum of these elements can easily amount to 300 to 500 g. Since office visits rarely occur in the morning, in the fasting state, after first-morning micturition and a recent defecation, any two successive measurements will depend on the fullness of the various aforementioned body compartments. Thus, body weight, as measured routinely, can move up or down by half a kilogram depending on the relative influence of these factors. This has obvious consequences for the reliability of any given assessment of a static anthropometric index, such as weight-for-age or weight-for-height.

Another perspective on growth is growth velocity. We consider this to be more valuable for nutritional assessment than growth attainment. It is a dynamic index and can only be assessed with serial, longitudinal measurements. Its interpretation, however, is more reliable, we feel, than that of the simple, static anthropometric indices discussed previously.

Simply connecting with a line the serial measurements of height and weight made with the standard NCHS growth charts will establish a "growth channel" for a given patient. Normal growth is a curve that more or less parallels the curve for the weight or height percentile in which the child happens to fall. Abnormal growth would be a severely non-parallel course of change in weight or height relative to the expected trajectory. Most commonly this will manifest as a flattening of the rate of increase for weight or height over time when undernourishment is present. Alternatively, when a child is pathologically obese, the weight curve will have a nonparallel deviation in the upward direction. In frank growth arrest in stature, over periods of 6 to 12 months the height will change by less than 1 or 2 cm.

The advantage of this approach over the static indices is its greater sensitivity and specificity. For instance, a child who begins in the 95th percentile of height-for-age adequacy (Fig. 1) and suffers complete growth arrest, would still be assessed as having "normal" stature for many, many months. The pathology would be suspected only by looking at the pattern of growth velocity. Alternatively, if a child is in the 5th percentile of height-for-age, but grows along the expected growth channel, constitutional short stature, rather than true growth failure, is more probable (see Fig. 1).

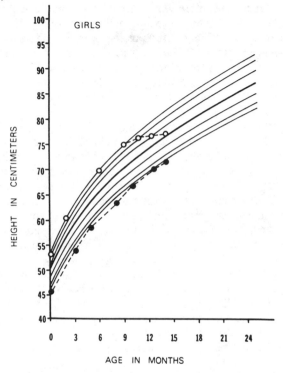

Figure 1 Illustrated is the NCHS growth curve standard for height for female children from 0 to 36 months. Serial measurement of height in two subjects has been plotted to emphasize the advantage of sensitivity and specificity of nutritional diagnosis with dynamic (growth velocity) data. For subject #1 (○), we have a situation of initial stature in the 95th percentile and adequate growth up to 9 months. At this point, although complete growth arrest has occurred, height remains well within the "normal" range of height-for-age. For subject #2 (●), we have a child who is in the 5th percentile of height-for-age from birth. Over time, the child remains more or less in this growth channel. It should be remembered that of every 100 healthy, well-nourished children in a normally distributed population, five will be at or below the 5th percentile purely by definition.

The issues of differential precision of measurement of height and weight also have implications for growth velocity. Since height generally does not recede, detecting a true change (or a true flattening) of growth in stature can be done more sensitively than a similar detection in weight gain or weight loss. The consequences of the several 100 g fluctuation due to extraneous influences such as food, urine, and stool, means that true changes in weight require up to 6 months to detect with serial weighing in the initially normally nourished child. Obviously, in the severely underweight or overweight child placed on a therapeutic regimen, changes of 500 g occur much more rapidly and thus can be detected in a shorter interval.

In anthropometry we think in terms other than weight and height, namely head circumference, skinfold thickness, and arm circumference. These are included because of another basic reality: in the final analysis, crude body mass (weight) provides only a poor approximation of the composition of the tissues that comprise the body. One would like to know more about the relation fat (energy reserves stored in adipose tissue) and lean (functional tissues including muscle, viscera, and bone) tissue in an individual. For instance, two children at the low end of the weight-for-height continuum could differ in the amount of fat-free (lean) body mass. The child with a greater percentage of body weight as lean tissue could just be "lean"; the child with a lesser fat-free mass would be at a high risk of malnutrition. At the upper extreme of the weight distribution, in excess of 120 percent of the expected weight for height, a similar issue obtains. The heavy child with a low percentage of body fat would be considered unusually muscular (but not obese). A child of equivalent weight with a high percentage of adipose tissue would be considered pathologically fat (obese).

For various technical reasons, the assessment of body composition—the distribution of weight between adipose tissue and muscle, viscera, and bone—is difficult in the child. In our experience, head circumference is not a useful index of body composition or nutritional status. Skinfold thickness merits discussion. It is performed with specialized spring calipers over a number of sites (triceps, subscapular, abdominal) and requires standardization and practice for reliability as the subcutaneous fat and skin (but not underlying muscle) are the tissues to be included in the fold. Norms have been developed to relate this to total body fat. Unfortunately, precisely at the extremes of thinness and fatness—the situations of greatest nutritional interest—the response becomes nonlinear and sensitivity and specificity become poorer. To look at body composition from the other component—lean body mass—a combination of an anthropometric index (height/length) and a biochemical, laboratory assay (24-hour creatinine excretion) has been proposed: the so-called creatinine-height index (CHI). It has several pitfalls in its application and interpretation, as well. Creatinine is a derivative of muscle, and tells us nothing about visceral proteins or bone. Also, the norms are based on underweight or normal weight situations. For overweight children, both the truly obese and the nonobese would have a greater muscle mass than a standard weight child of the same height. Thus, use of the CHI in the overweight child has severe limitations. Two electronic techniques, bioelectrical impedance analysis (BIA) and total-body electrical conductivity (TOBEC), offer promise as tools for pediatric body composition assessment. Both are noninvasive, nonradioactive and noninjurious even to premature children, involving the application of small currents of harmless electromagnetic current. Their validation and standardization for children, however, is not yet complete, and intrinsically, since electrical conductivity is proportional to the water and electrolyte pool, they will be more directly a measure of the fat-free mass. Fat mass will have to be calculated as the difference from lean mass and total body weight, propagating the error in the lean estimation into the estimation of adipose tissue mass.

The hydration state of children is certainly important in nutritional assessment. Water, it should be remembered, is a nutrient. A combination of anthropometry and physical examination techniques are used to detect and estimate degrees of dehydration (often a consequence of severe diarrhea) and overhydration (as nutritional edema in severe protein-energy malnutrition). If recent prior body weight is accurately known, the percent excess or loss attributable to fluid balance can be estimated. This can be a guide to rehydration therapy in the dehydrated child and to targeting of dietary refeeding in the edematous protein-energy malnourished patient.

PHYSICAL EXAMINATION

Given the foregoing arguments, malnutrition in children is usually a secondary phenomenon, especially in developed countries. Thus, the principal focus of a physical examination is the identification (or characterization) of the primary disorder. It is important, nevertheless, to examine the child physically for the classical nutritional signs. One must remember, however, that manifestations of nutrient deficit or excess occur late in the course of depletion or accumulation. It should also be borne in mind that physical signs are nonspecific in two ways: first, problems with several different nutrients can produce the same lesion; and second, the identical physical finding can be caused by both nutritional and nonnutritional factors. However, when a single, or better yet, a cluster of classical signs of nutrient imbalance are found on the physical examination, a strong argument for advanced malnutrition can be made. Unfortunately, the absence of physical findings is no guarantee of nutritional health or adequacy.

Bearing all of these caveats in mind, we present in Table 4 a regional review of manifestations associated with impaired nutrition. In fact, we use this system as a checklist in routine clinical work and in investigative survey work. In our experience, dental and gingival findings, pallor, and hair changes are the most commonly encountered physical signs related to nutrition. Less common are changes of the tongue or the skin. Occasionally, however, one will find a classical, almost diagnostic picture of a nutritional deficiency state such as a rachitic rosary, pathognomic for rickets, or the edema, apathy, flaky-paint dermatitis and hepatomegaly of kwashiorkor.

LABORATORY ASSAYS

Laboratory assays should be used prudently, both in routine and in directed nutritional assessment. Several pitfalls are present. An intrinsic limitation in blood analyses is the volume of blood that can be extracted, especially from small babies or sequentially in children of any age. Many assays have not been miniaturized in hospital laboratories to accomodate a smaller total specimen. Moreover, blood extraction is a painful and frightening experience for the young child. However, the most precise differential assays in the nutritional assessment, are based on the cellular elements or serum of human blood.

There exists a temptation to substitute more abundant and accessible, and less invasively procured, samples, such as urine (which can be of value) and hair and nails (of dubious clinical application) and even saliva, tears, and cerumen. Except for urine, we see little potential, in other than survey situations, for the examination of these secondary tissues and fluids for nutrients or metabolites. With respect to urine, the analysis of 24-hour creatinine excretion and the calculation of the creatinine/height index represent a formidable tool for the monitoring of the gain in lean body mass by a malnourished child. Moreover, in patients on total parenteral nutrition, urinary zinc examinations can provide useful information on the status of total body zinc nutriture.

Iron deficiency is common in children. Iron stores disappear and physiologic deficits ensue well before the failure of red cell production is reflected in a frank anemia. Anemia can be diagnosed (provisionally) by the measurement of hematocrit or hemoglobin concentration. There is, however, a wide overlap of deficient (for one child) and adequate (for another child) levels of these two indices. Serum ferritin has proven to be a useful and responsive index of the total-body stores of iron in adults, but in children, especially infants, its interpretation is complicated by several confounding factors. The response—a rise of 1 g per deciliter in the concentration of hemoglobin—to an adequate therapeutic trial with oral iron is the most definitive diagnostic test for iron deficiency anemia in the child. Inflammatory conditions produce a hypoplastic anemia that is not related to body iron deficiency. Copper deficiency produces an anemia morphologically indistinguishable from that produced by iron. Lead poisoning is another, not uncommon, cause of anemia in children. Infants, dependent as they are on milk or milk-based foods, are susceptible to iron deficiency anemia as are adolescent males in their growth spurt, when expansion of body mass often outstrips the ability to absorb and store dietary iron.

Albumin levels are a classic index of nutritional status. Circulating proteins are reduced in protein-energy malnutrition. However, in mild or moderate states, the albumin is unaffected, and even in severe deficiency it takes weeks before the levels fall below the 3.0 g per deciliter cut-off signifying a deficient level. Transferrin, retinol-binding protein, or pre-albumin, visceral protein products with a more rapid turnover, may be more sensitive "early alert" indices of protein deficiency. An abnormally low albumin is a significant diagnostic finding, but a normal level cannot provide assurance that the protein status of a child is not compromised. Here, body composition considerations and the creatinine height index can often provide better monitoring of protein status.

Fecal examinations for ova and parasites although not directly related to nutritional status, can often provide diagnostic clues to the causes of a compromised nutritional state and should not be overlooked. Casual, but valuable, information on nutritional status can often be culled from the complete blood count. Eosinophilia is compatible with a helminthic infection. Leukopenia is a laboratory sign of copper deficiency. Signs of hemolysis can be related to vitamin E deficiency.

If the nutritional problem is one of altered hydration, measurement of the serum electrolytes, sodium, potassium, chloride and bicarbonate, is indispensible. Knowledge of magnesium levels can also help in management if diarrhea has been prolonged and severe.

The specific assays to determine vitamin and mineral status should be reserved for situations when nutritional depletion has been chronic or when the underlying condition has clearly been associated with a high frequency of deficiencies. Vitamin A deficiency is a state that occurs commonly in association with protein-energy malnutrition. It is also not infrequent in liver disease and inflammatory bowel disease. Vitamin E levels (along with total lipoprotein concentrations) merit evaluation in malabsorption states and cholestatic liver disease. The diagnostic test of vitamin D status is the circulating level of 25-OH-vitamin D. Clinical rickets is obvious on physical examination, but milder forms of vitamin D defiency should be considered in a child with little sun exposure and a diet free of fish oils and fortified milk. A new radioimmune assay for abnormally carboxylated prothrombin is a sensitive index of vitamin K deficiency, but causes of that state in children are rare and there is little experience in pediatric populations with this index.

The status of water-soluble vitamins is assessed variously by circulating levels, activity quotients of the cofactor function in hemolysates of red cells, and by detection in the urine of abnormal metabolites, spontaneously or after a load test. With the possible exception of folate and vitamin B_{12} levels in cases of macrocytic anemias, specific diagnostic tests for vitamins are of little prospective clinical relevance. Empirically, therapy with the range of the water-soluble vitamins (vitamin C and B complex) in the severely malnourished child or the individual with malabsorption is indicated.

After iron, the most common mineral deficiencies in children are those of zinc and copper. The casual finding of a low ceruloplasmin or leukopenia merits consideration of copper depletion. Selenium deficiency has been described in children on total parenteral nutrition (TPN) without supplementation. Low red cell or plasma glutathione peroxidase activity confirms selenium deficiency. Deficiencies of chromium or molybdenum are too rare to merit consideration.

Recently, interest in two vitamin-like substances—carnitine and taurine—in child nutrition has surged. Both can be measured in the peripheral blood plasma but assays are not widely available. Again, in TPN a potential concern for carnitine and/or taurine deficiency is warranted.

Recently, the concept of *functional* assessment of nutritional status, as distinct from biochemical assessment, has been promoted to provide a more relevant, and individualistically specific, diagnosis, given the pitfalls in conventional tests and the overlap between levels in deficient and nondeficient individuals. Moreover, the functional tests are often rapid and noninvasive, whereas the conventional test is tedious or painful. Examples include rapid dark adaptation tests (for vitamin A or zinc deficiency) and taste acuity tests (for zinc deficiency). Red cell fragility is a suitable test for vitamin E or selenium status. At the present time, physicians should be aware of these alternatives, but in routine screening they are rarely of utility.

To conclude this discussion, primary nutritional problems (such as iron or copper deficiency) occur in children due to reliance on specific foods, i.e., milk. More common, however, are protein and energy deficits secondary to associated congenital or acquired illness. Plotting of growth and indices of body composition are perhaps the most revealing of the diagnostic tests for such states. They are more sensitive for early detection than physical signs, clinical symptoms, or most laboratory tests. Because blood is a precious and uncomfortably obtained commodity in the child, and because biochemical tests for specific vitamins and minerals are directed by specific health or environmental conditions, usual laboratory tests are of limited value in the pediatric nutritional evaluation. The best way to select the appropriate tests for a given child is through a thorough clinical history and a keen insight into the common consequences of the specific clinical, social, or environmental factors.

SUGGESTED READING

Dietz WH Jr. Body composition and nutritional assessment of the undernourished child.

In: Cohen SA, ed. The underweight infant, child and adolescent. Norwalk, CT: Appleton-Century-Crofts, 1986:1.

Maloch LD. Assessing and feeding the underweight infant. In: Cohen SA, ed. The underweight infant, child and adolescent. Norwalk, CT: Appleton-Century-Crofts, 1986:233.

Pencharz PB, ed. Symposium on nutrition. Pediatr Clin North Am 1985; 32(2).

ALLERGY AND INTOLERANCE

ARTHUR LEZNOFF, M.D., C.M., B.Sc., M.Sc., F.R.C.P.(C)
SUSAN M. TARLO, M.B., B.S., M.R.C.P.(UK), F.R.C.P.(C)

"I am sorry you're not feeling well, dear, it must be something you ate." This grandmother's empirical analysis exemplifies the fact and the fancy of the problem of food sensitivity. Reactions to food or additives may be due to allergic, metabolic, pharmacologic, or toxic mechanisms and are the cause of disease in from 5 to 10 percent of patients. Symptoms can be acute or chronic and vary from mildly annoying to life threatening. These true food sensitivities must be distinguished from an annual crop of trendy Designer Disease pseudosensitivity reactions, which engender much media sensationalism but lack scientific verification.

The heart of management of patients with food sensitivity is the identification of the offending product and its subsequent avoidance. Therefore, specific diagnosis and treatment are inseparable, and this chapter will discuss both aspects. A logical approach to the management is summarized in the accompanying flow chart (Fig. 1).

Allergic symptoms are most commonly due to IgE-mediated mast cell degranulation. Thus the patient commonly complains of itching of the mouth and palate, abdominal cramps with watery diarrhea, urticaria, eczema, and less frequently, rhinitis and asthma. Psychological symptoms, such as insomnia, hyperactivity, and anxiety fatigue syndrome, may well be due to pharmacologic properties of certain foods such as tea, coffee, chocolate, aged cheese, and alcohol, but claims that such symptoms are due to nonpharmacologically active foods, food dyes or preservatives or especially to "yeasts" or sugar, have never withstood objective scientific scrutiny. Several recent well-controlled studies have suggested an association between childhood migraine and food sensitivity. Additional investigations will be needed to confirm this association.

PRINCIPLES OF MANAGEMENT

Management of food sensitivity is based on the following principles:

469

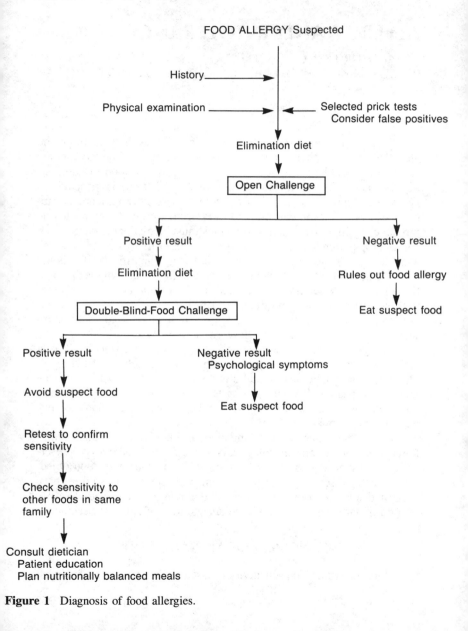

Figure 1 Diagnosis of food allergies.

1. When physical illness is caused by food sensitivity, the best treatment is avoidance of the causative food(s) or additives.

2. When food sensitivity is erroneously implicated, it is important to convince the patient that the food can be eaten safely. Many patients extrapolate from one food to another and avoid an increasing number of foods and additives. Their food phobias can come to dominate their personal and social lives and they may become nutritionally deprived.

3. A medical history associating symptoms with food sensitivity often yields false conclusions. Bock and May demonstrate that 50 to 75 percent of such associations are wrong, in that after negative double-blind challenges, the patient could ingest unlimited quantities of the suspect food.

4. Open challenges have limited reliability because of emotional overlay. However, these should always be done prior to double-blind challenges, since a negative open challenge rules out the sensitivity.

5. Double-blind challenge is the only definitive proof of food sensitivity. However, where the reaction is anaphylactic in nature or very severe, one should exercise great caution in these challenges and perform them, if at all, in a hospital setting. If capsules are used, the placebo or filler should be D-xylose rather than lactose.

6. Allergy prick testing is at least as sensitive as RAST testing but is cheaper and the results are immediately available. In patients with severe anaphylaxis, such tests should be done in a hospital setting.

7. Food skin testing or RAST testing often yields "false positive" results. About 50 percent of patients with clearly positive skin tests can eat the specific foods with impunity. False negative skin tests or RAST tests are less frequent in protein foods but commonly occur with commercial antigens of fruit, vegetables, and grains.

8. When "true" food allergies are present in a child under 3 years of age, there is a good chance (50 percent in one study) that it will disappear in 5 years. Therefore, judicious challenges may be repeated at 6-month intervals. When such an allergy is present in older children or adults, there is more chance (80 percent in one study) that it will persist.

9. A patient who is allergic to one member of a botanical or animal family, is sometimes allergic to other members of the same family. Continued ingestion of these other foods may perpetuate allergic symptoms. Consequently, it behooves the physician to be aware of food family associations and to eliminate all food family members

when a specific food has been identified, at least for a trial period.
10. Some food families lose their allerginicity when cooked. These include most nonprotein fruit and vegetables. In contrast, milk, eggs, nuts, legumes, and most other protein foods remain allergenic after cooking, although this may be diminished.
11. When the patient has multiple food sensitivities or allergy to important foods such as milk or wheat, the physician should utilize the services of a trained dietician to help educate the patient and plan nutritionally balanced meals.

ILLUSTRATIVE MANAGEMENT OF SUSPECTED TRUE FOOD ALLERGY

The following is a report of an extremely allergic child. Our discussion of management of this case illustrates the application of the preceeding principles. These will be italized for emphasis: A 2½ year old boy presented to our clinic with the major complaint of severe excoriated generalized atopic dermatitis, about five loose bowel movements per day, failure to gain weight in the previous year, a wheezy cough, and rhinorrhea. He had a history of an anaphylactic reaction to peanuts and repeated flares of eczema and diarrhea whenever cow's milk was reintroduced into his diet. His mother had noted other less dramatic associations between food and symptoms, but these were inconsistent. Prick tests showed a strongly positive reaction to cow's milk, chocolate, eggs, lamb, pork, oranges, garlic, peanuts, wheat, and tomatoes. There were negative reactions to other cereals, fish, bananas, and chicken. His diet had been restricted to soybean milk substitute, various cereals other than wheat, all meats, cheese, rice, peas, beans, and a few other items.

Our approach was based on the knowledge that, *although many food skin tests are false positives, this child was likely to be truly allergic because of the classic nature of his symptoms, because he had experienced an anaphylactic reaction after ingesting a small quantity of peanuts, and because milk elimination and (open) challenge had consistently indicated this specific allergy.* We were well aware that the only scientific proof was double-blind challenge, but so many foods were involved that such an investigation would have been very time consuming and would require hospitalization. Consequently, we used an approach that was easier and inexpensive. He was placed on a restricted basic diet of a few selected foods, which would meet his nutritional requirements and would be less likely to cause allergies. His history dictated that we *eliminate not only peanuts but all other legumes. This required the elimination of peas, beans, and soybean formula, as well as many other foods containing soybean meal, such as sausages and donuts. We avoided all milk-derived products and we interdicted wheat because of the strongly positive skin tests.*

Which foods to include? Soothill has described an "oligoantigenic diet," based on foods that are statistically less likely to cause allergies. He uses chicken or lamb as the only meat, but we selected well-done beef, since skin tests to the other meats were positive. The rest of the diet was as recommended. The cereal was rice, the fruit was cooked pears, and the vegetable was mustard family (cauliflower, broccoli, cabbage, and Brussels sprouts). Water was the only liquid and sugar, salt, and oil were allowed. He was given supplemental A, C, and D vitamins. We planned to continue the diet for 3 weeks but hoped to see an improvement in 1 week.

After 1 week the child was not significantly better and therefore, we reanalyzed our thinking. We suspected rice because of the 4+ reaction to wheat, both wheat and rice being in the same botanical family as grains. Consequently, we modified the diet by removing rice and adding sweet potato because the child had never eaten it and it is not related to any foods to which he had been allergic.

Within 1 week the child had improved dramatically. Eczema was reduced, he had one normal bowel movement a day, cough and rhinorrhea had lessened. We were concerned that he would not thrive on such a restricted diet, but after the 3 weeks he had gained 5 lb. *He was then rechallenged with four glasses of milk daily.* After 24 hours eczema flared, and his diarrhea returned. The basic diet was reinstituted and other challenges attempted. After 6 weeks it was determined that he could eat potatoes, turnips, all cooked fruit plus raw bananas, as well as lamb and fish, in addition to the basic diet. He could not tolerate carrots, celery, chicken, or any grain. He drank water and apple juice. He received a calcium supplement. Eczema was now reduced to patches on his legs, bowel movements were normal, and he had no asthma or rhinitis.

After 6 months we challenged him with milk and cereal grains because of the importance of these foods and because of the knowledge that immunologic tolerance to previously allergenic foods often develop with age. Wheat and rice were now tolerated but milk continued to produce the same symptoms as before. We also plan to challenge him with milk under cromolyn prophylaxis (see later).

Since double-blind challenges were not performed, scientific proof of his food sensitivities is lacking, but we are satisfied with his progress and quite confident of our assessment. It should be noted that blind challenges can be done in young children by "hiding" the test food in a milk shake or in mashed potatoes or by administering the test food by stomach tube.

DOUBLE-BLIND CHALLENGE

In contradistinction to the above case, we often perform double-blind challenges on adults or older children, in an out-patient setting, since they can swallow the necessary capsules of dehydrated food or placebo (unless there is a history of anaphylactic sensitivity). Many patients who claim psychological symptoms (i.e., anxiety, tension) to sugar or yeast or other unlikely antigens are perfect candidates for double-blind challenge. This is the only way to convince the patient that the "allergy" is fictitious. The patient receives a full and honest explanation of the challenge procedures. On six successive Tuesdays, the patient swallows enough capsules (determined by the amount of the product the patient declares will cause symptoms) of challenge substance or placebo, (three doses each.) He is observed by the doctor for 2 hours and then writes a diary of symptoms for 48 hours. After six doses the notes are compared. The patient is asked to identify which of the coded bottles contain the "allergenic" food. At this point most patients admit they cannot tell the difference, in which case it is not necessary to break the code. A few suspect they had more symptoms after certain challenges and then the code must be broken. *If there is a consistent response to the challenge substance and not the placebo, this confirms the sensitivity.* However, we have yet to meet a patient whose psychological symptoms proved to be due to food intolerance (in contradistinction to those with physical symptoms suggestive of true allergy.) After such double-blind challenge, these patients are finally convinced that their previous convictions about food allergy were nonsense, although some rationalize, in order to save face, that they had formerly been allergic but have now lost the sensitivity.

ADVERSE REACTIONS TO CHEMICALS AND ADDITIVES IN FOOD

In most cases of acute anaphylactic reactions to food, the patients or parent can identify the offending food, which is usually the only "new" food eaten in the preceding time interval, and this food and its relatives must subsequently be avoided. Where no food can be identified, then food additives should be suspect. These may be food derived such as vegetable gums, cotton seed, or soya meal or chemical additives. Sodium or potassium metabisulfite, an antioxident present in prepared foods such as commercial salads, dips, (i.e., gaucamole), french fried potatoes, cole slaw, dried colored fruit (e.g., apricots), some wines, and some lemonades, is a cause of dramatic, potentially fatal asthmatic or anaphylactic reactions. After proving that this is indeed the offender, by carefully graded provocative challenges (increasing doses from 1 mg to 200 mg at 20-minute intervals, in a hospital environment), the patient must be thoroughly and carefully instructed about the use of this preservative, (which is often unlabeled in food products), in the dose range that induces symptoms, so that it may be avoided. Sulphite oxidase impregnated strips are now commercially available to help the patient detect the relatively large amounts of metabisulfite that may be present in restaurant meals. Other additives such as dyes like tartrazine and preservatives such as benzoate can also cause anaphylaxis, asthma, or urticaria, but more often they are falsely implicated as causes of disease. Monosodium glutamate may cause Chinese restaurant syndrome, but is rarely a cause of asthma or urticaria. Before recommending a difficult change in eating habits and lifestyle, such as avoiding all food dyes and preservatives, it is wise to confirm sensitivity by appropriate double-blind challenge if the previous open challenge was seemingly positive. If the sensitivity is confirmed, then a consultation with a qualified dietitian is very helpful. It is not possible to describe here all the multiple adverse reactions to foods and additives. The report "Adverse Reactions to Foods" includes a listing of over 120 plant toxins and chemicals that can induce adverse symptoms, many of which may present to the physician as an "allergic reaction" to the food.

FOOD EXERCISE ANAPHYLAXIS

A few patients suffer from food exercise anaphylaxis, in which anaphylactic reactions occur if exercise is performed within 2 to 3 hours of eating. There is a different threshold for each patient. Some patients react after any food, while others suffer only after eating specific foods or classes of foods. In the latter case, the patient must avoid only a specific family of foods before exercising but can eat those foods at any other time. In the former case, all exercise is interdicted within 2 to 3 hours of eating any food.

USE OF MEDICATIONS

Is there any treatment for food sensitivity, other than avoiding the food family when the allergy is "real" or proving that the supposed sensitivity is false when psychologic factors are involved? There are several reports that 200 mg of oral cromolyn (disodium cromoglycate) taken as a suspension in warm water 15 minutes before eating may block a food allergic reaction. We have had limited success with this expensive drug. It is not recommended if the allergenic food causes severe anaphylaxis, but since it is essentially free of side effects it may be tried in other food allergies.

Antihistamines used prophylactically or therapeutically may blunt the food allergic reaction and are most useful when specific sensitivity has not been discovered or when the patient is unwilling to avoid the specific food. In acute reactions a double dose of short-acting antihistamines should be used; in chronic disease (eczema or urticaria), use a longer acting drug such as hydroxyzine or astemizole.

When a patient suffers from violent anaphylactic reaction to food or additives, more vigorous therapy is indicated. Some patients carry injectable Adrenalin in various preloaded syringe preparations to be administered subcutaneously. A short-acting antihistamine, twice the normal dose, (i.e., two 4 mg tablets of chlorpheniramine) is also taken orally. An asthmatic reaction requires the usual bronchodilator treatment. Occasionally, emergency support therapy such as intravenous aminophylline or hydrocortisone, oxygen and/or the use of an airway may be required.

Prednisone or its derivatives can be administered in severe cases. It should be noted that this drug will not take effect for several hours.

Once the committment to use prednisone is made, a sufficient dose , about 60 mg per day, must be used.

PHARMACOLOGIC REACTIONS TO FOODS

Unusual sensitivity to the pharmacologic actions of some food products can cause disease. Coffee, tea, chocolate, and carbonated beverages with caffeine can cause insomnia, irritability, palpitations, diuresis, and gastrointestinal symptoms and trigger migraines. Wine and beer, aged cheese, and bananas contain vasoactive amines and can precipitate flushing, migraines, and diarrhea. If the patient is taking medication for other illness, these drugs may interact with the above foods. Megadoses of vitamins can produce acute or chronic disease. Peculiar eating habits can cause unusual symptoms such as yellow pigmentation from excess carrot juice. Consequently, the physician should inquire diligently into the patient's dietary history.

UNORTHODOX METHODS

Unorthodox methods for diagnosis and treatment of food sensitivities are strongly promoted in some centers. There is no acceptable evidence that valid diagnosis or management can be achieved by administering drops of dilute solutions of the suspect food or additive under the tongue. There is likewise no scientific justification for rotating diets or for hyposensitization in any type of food sensitivity.

PROPHYLAXIS OF FOOD ALLERGY

Prophylaxis against allergic disease in infancy is a subject of current interest. Physicians have demonstrated that restriction of antigenic foods such as milk, eggs, and peanuts, in the late phases of pregnancy may be of benefit, but further studies are needed to confirm this data. There is no question that infants of atopic parents have a much higher risk of atopy, (up to 100 percent when both parents are allergic), and that sensitization of food can occur in utero, although this is not common. Fetal synthesis of IgE is detected in 20 percent of venous cord blood samples by 38 weeks of gestation.

Postnatal sensitization of atopic children is greatest in the first 3 years of life. Intestinal permeability is increased in infancy, especially in preterm infants, although even in adults some absorption of undigested food antigens occurs. This may in part relate to low concentrations of secretory IgA antibodies. These findings have led to the suggestion that infants of atopic parents should be breast fed rather than bottle fed. Since 1936, many studies have attempted to test this hypothesis with conflicting results. Nevertheless, a common finding in these studies was that breast feeding for at least 4 months and preferably 6 months, with late introduction to solid foods after 6 months of age, did seem to reduce the prevalence of eczema in the first 3 years. Therefore, this appears to be reasonable advice to atopic parents. There have been few cases reported in which breast fed infants have developed allergic reactions to food antigens ingested by the nursing mother and secreted into breast milk. In most cases the diet of the nursing mother should not be restricted on a prophylactic basis. However, if the infant does develop atopic manifestations such as atopic dermatitis, rhinitis, or angioedema, then the role of a possible sensitizer in maternal breast milk should be considered, and if investigations support this the relevant food should be eliminated from the mother's diet.

In summary, whether food sensitivity reactions are due to the common allergic factors or to other less prevalent causes, identification of the ingestant and its avoidance are the key to management. Patient education is important but drugs have only a limited role.

SUGGESTED READING

Adverse reactions to foods, A.A.A.I. and N.I.A.I.D. report, U.S. Department of Health and Human Services, N.I.H. Publication No. 84-2442, 1984.

Bock SA, May CD. Adverse reactions to food caused by sensitivity. In: Middleton E, Reed CE, Ellis EF, eds. Allergy, principles and practice. St. Louis: CV Mosby, 1983; 1115.

Symposium proceedings on adverse reactions to foods and food additives. J Allergy Clin Immunol 1986; 78, No.1, Part 2.

INDEX